PSYCHEDELICS

A CLINICAL GUIDE

Samoon Ahmad, MD

Clinical Professor
Department of Psychiatry
NYU Grossman School of Medicine
New York, New York

Wolters Kluwer

Philadelphia • Baltimore • New York • London
Buenos Aires • Hong Kong • Sydney • Tokyo

Acquisitions Editor: James Sherman
Senior Development Editor: Ariel S. Winter
Editorial Coordinator: Vinodhini Varadharajalu
Marketing Manager: Kirsten Watrud
Production Project Manager: Frances Gunning
Manager, Graphic Arts & Design: Stephen Druding
Manufacturing Coordinator: Lisa Bowling
Prepress Vendor: S4Carlisle Publishing Services

Copyright © 2026 Wolters Kluwer.

All rights reserved. This book is protected by copyright. No part of this book may be reproduced or transmitted in any form or by any means, including as photocopies or scanned-in or other electronic copies, or utilized by any information storage and retrieval system without written permission from the copyright owner, except for brief quotations embodied in critical articles and reviews. Materials appearing in this book prepared by individuals as part of their official duties as U.S. government employees are not covered by the above-mentioned copyright. To request permission, please contact Wolters Kluwer at Two Commerce Square, 2001 Market Street, Philadelphia, PA 19103, via email at permissions@lww.com, or via our website at shop.lww.com (products and services).

9 8 7 6 5 4 3 2 1

Printed in the United States of America

Library of Congress Cataloging-in-Publication Data

ISBN-13: 978-1-975220-59-4

Library of Congress Control Number: 2025930522

This work is provided "as is," and the publisher disclaims any and all warranties, express or implied, including any warranties as to accuracy, comprehensiveness, or currency of the content of this work.

This work is no substitute for individual patient assessment based upon healthcare professionals' examination of each patient and consideration of, among other things, age, weight, gender, current or prior medical conditions, medication history, laboratory data and other factors unique to the patient. The publisher does not provide medical advice or guidance and this work is merely a reference tool. Healthcare professionals, and not the publisher, are solely responsible for the use of this work including all medical judgments and for any resulting diagnosis and treatments.

Given continuous, rapid advances in medical science and health information, independent professional verification of medical diagnoses, indications, appropriate pharmaceutical selections and dosages, and treatment options should be made and healthcare professionals should consult a variety of sources. When prescribing medication, healthcare professionals are advised to consult the product information sheet (the manufacturer's package insert) accompanying each drug to verify, among other things, conditions of use, warnings and side effects and identify any changes in dosage schedule or contraindications, particularly if the medication to be administered is new, infrequently used or has a narrow therapeutic range. To the maximum extent permitted under applicable law, no responsibility is assumed by the publisher for any injury and/or damage to persons or property, as a matter of products liability, negligence law or otherwise, or from any reference to or use by any person of this work.

shop.lww.com

Dedication

*To my wife Kim, my son Daniel,
and my parents Naseem and Riffat
S.A.*

Foreword

One day in 2006, a colleague and my supervisor at the time, Dr Jeffrey Guss, walked into my office and started asking me what I knew of the history of psychedelic research in psychiatry. I was taken aback by the question since I knew nothing of what he was talking about. Dr Guss opened my eyes to something astonishing that was hidden in plain sight and had been absent from all of my medical training spanning from medical school to general psychiatry residency to addiction psychiatry fellowship training. The first wave of psychedelic research, conducted from the 1950s to the early 1970s, included over 40,000 research participants, mostly utilized lysergic acid diethylamide (LSD), and included evidence suggesting safety and efficacy of psychedelic therapy for alcohol addiction as well as pain and existential distress associated with advanced cancer. The first wave came to an abrupt halt in 1970 when the drugs escaped the lab, caused harm to the general public related to unsupervised recreational use, and got caught up in the war on drugs declared by Richard Nixon. Fascinated by this history, I was further surprised to hear that psychedelic research had restarted in the early 1990s.

Inspired by psychedelic researchers from the first wave of psychedelic research and mentored by pioneers such as Charles Grob at the University of California Los Angeles and the late Roland Griffiths at Johns Hopkins University in the second wave, Jeffrey Guss, Anthony Bossis, and I formed a psychedelic research program at New York University in 2006. In 2015, we recruited Michael Bogenschutz to join our group and collectively we have had the privilege of being part of the psychedelic research renaissance that has occurred over the last 25 years. Our work has focused on psilocybin-assisted psychotherapy to treat psychiatric and existential distress in advanced cancer, alcohol use disorder, and major depressive disorder, as well as 3,4-methylenedioxymethamphetamine (MDMA)-assisted psychotherapy to treat posttraumatic stress disorder (PTSD). In 2021, we established the NYU Langone Center for Psychedelic Medicine with the goal of further exploring the therapeutic potential of psychedelic therapy to target some of the most difficult-to-treat disorders in all of medicine, with a substantial unmet need, including end-of-life emotional and spiritual distress, addiction, major depression, PTSD, and chronic pain.

Having spent my entire career at Bellevue Hospital, I have had the great privilege of working with Dr Ahmad, who is one of the most compassionate and gifted clinical psychiatrists I have ever worked with. In addition, though, Dr Ahmad has the rare skill of being able to go deep into new areas of psychiatry and medicine and communicate vital and in-depth information to the public through his books.

In his newest book on the therapeutic potential of psychedelics, Dr Ahmad has once again done a masterful job of reviewing a topic that will be accessible to a broad range of people from the lay public to clinicians. Dr Ahmad skillfully balances the therapeutic potential of psychedelics with the known harm they can cause, especially when used in uncontrolled settings. We appear to currently be in a hype phase of psychedelic therapy, similar to what happened in the first wave of psychedelic research. Dr Ahmad points this out as a cautionary reminder to stay away from the polarization that occurs with psychedelics (eg, hype vs demonization) and to simply focus on the science and data, and to see where that leads.

The book is breathtaking in its scope and takes the reader on a tour of history, clinical applications, regulatory considerations, subjective effects, optimal conditions for administration regarding safety and efficacy, and putative mechanisms of action. In addition, the book extensively focuses on the neurobiology and therapeutic potential of a variety of serotonergic psychedelics (including psilocybin, LSD, N,N-dimethyltryptamine [DMT], 5-MeO-DMT, and mescaline), dissociative anesthetics (eg, ketamine), empathogens (eg, MDMA), and atypical psychedelics (eg, ibogaine, salvinorin A).

Given the resurgence in the clinical use of these drugs, the complexity of their pharmacology, and the current difficulty in finding books that focus primarily on the science of psychedelics, this is a truly timely book that will allow readers to better understand why psychedelics have generated so much optimism within the field of psychiatry.

Stephen Ross, MD
Professor of Psychiatry and Child & Adolescent Psychiatry
NYU Grossman School of Medicine
New York, New York

Preface

I first heard Stephen Ross speak about psychedelics approximately a decade ago. He was giving grand rounds at NYU Langone Medical Center on his research into the use of psilocybin to treat end-of-life anxiety and depression for patients with terminal illnesses, and what impressed me most was not his confidence, his public speaking ability, or even the data he presented. Rather, it was his courage to follow the science of psychedelics and to buck what was at that time conventional wisdom—namely, that psychedelics had no therapeutic value and that they were solely a drug of abuse. Therefore, I was honored when he agreed to write the foreword for this book. It never would have been possible without his work, as well as the efforts of other colleagues at NYU Langone Health Center for Psychedelic Medicine like Michael Bogenschutz and the hundreds (if not thousands now) of medical professionals around the world doing the clinical work to demonstrate the efficacy of psychedelic-assisted psychotherapy.

Looking back at the years during my residency in the 1990s, I could have never imagined authoring a book on psychedelics. The very idea and a proposal for such a book would have been a nonstarter. However, the last three decades have been nothing but transformative, and we have witnessed a massive biologic, psychological, and cultural shift that has shaped our understanding about these drugs. Gratitude and respect must be given to the researchers and organizations whose commitment and perseverance have prevailed, as they brought us to the cusp of having the first psychedelic approved by the Food and Drug Administration (FDA) in summer 2024. Though unsuccessful, ongoing trials suggest approval is more of a *when* rather than an *if*.

You might ask why I am writing this book. The simple answer is to educate myself and my fellow clinicians. I learned from my first experience while writing *Medical Marijuana: A Clinical Handbook* that we as physicians need to have a basic understanding about the risks and benefits of drugs that were once considered outside of the medical pharmacopeia if we are to provide our patients with the best possible care. Given the changing legal status of cannabis, many of us have seen an increase in use among our patients. Consequently, having up-to-date knowledge about the benefits and dangers of cannabis has become necessary for us to do our jobs, and our personal biases and opinions have no place when it comes to helping and serving our patients. After all, the word "doctor" is derived from the Latin "doceo," meaning a teacher. We are duty-bound to teach our patients since we are the ones prescribing medicines and should know and inform our patients on risks, benefits, and drug interactions—all of which are necessary and medicolegally important. The scientific shift toward acceptance of treatments that were once considered taboo is the new normal and the sooner we accept this fact, the quicker we can make a meaningful difference in our patients' lives. This framework has helped me evolve and I hope I can take my fellow clinicians on this fascinating journey into the world of psychedelic science to explore its therapeutic utility as we examine their risks and benefits, the psychiatric conditions they may help treat, and appropriate patient selection for psychedelic-assisted psychotherapy.

During our medical school and residency years (especially for those of us in the psychiatric field), the idea of a Schedule I drug being used for therapeutic purposes was contradictory to what we had learned or practiced. Schedule I is defined as a "drug or other substance that has a high chance of being abused or causing addiction and has no FDA-approved medical use in the United States." This is particularly relevant in the mental health field where our education and training have formulated our opinion to encompass all Schedule I drugs under the same umbrella. In addition, we are exposed to patients struggling with severe persistent mental illness who abuse these drugs with worsening of their symptoms, relapses, and deterioration in their overall functioning. It is not surprising that our inclination and assessment have been tainted by these experiences. Needless to say, there are a host of medicines that are not Schedule I but yet have the potential to worsen psychiatric conditions or lead to addiction. So why have we as physicians been so reluctant and rigid in our thinking in not accepting the fact that these drugs may have therapeutic utility in medicine? The answer may lie along a spectrum that shapes our thinking and is based on our medical school didactics, lack of research and data (remember it is very hard to do research on Schedule I drugs), witnessing only recreational use and abuse, addiction with certain Schedule I drugs, and more importantly seeing cause and effect of drug use and worsening of psychiatric conditions.

Fortunately, most of us have transcended this form of thinking and are now open to the idea that many of these drugs have therapeutic utility. Among them, psychedelics seem to hold an extremely important place, especially in psychiatry, where many disorders do not seem to respond to currently available therapies, or a host of other conditions only exhibit partial or poor response. Clinicians are clamoring for treatments to help end patient suffering in the shortest time frame, which has been a major obstacle in currently available treatments. Furthermore, such treatments require long-term maintenance and monitoring with risk of nonadherence. Psychedelic medicines seem to uproot these conventional treatment paradigms, exhibiting quick response and benefits with no long-term requirements for ongoing treatments and in some cases sustained benefits have been observed for months, which is antithetical to usual mental health treatment modalities.

However, I would be remiss to focus solely on the benefits of psychedelic medicine and to disregard important facts. It is essential that we curb our enthusiasm and not overestimate their potential, since there are numerous issues and concerns with the use of psychedelics. As we begin to explore its role in clinical practice, we must recognize that this is a new frontier and that it comes with its own challenges. Clinicians will have to undergo special certification and training, establish appropriate clinical settings with monitoring of patients that may last hours, and last but not least develop new frameworks with insurers to resolve issues with payment and reimbursement since these treatments require hand-holding and close supervision lasting hours in some instances. While daunting, these challenges are not insurmountable, nor do they change the fact that these treatments may be lifesaving if not cost saving and may radically change the landscape of psychiatric treatment in the future.

I hope that you will find the information presented in the following pages relevant both in terms of psychedelics' potential use in clinical practice as well as their historical significance. As medical science moves at warp speed, it does not negate the fact that mankind has utilized basic and rudimentary elements available in nature to heal themselves. Hopefully the coming decade will offer ways to merge these natural elements with increasingly sophisticated treatment options and to serve our patients who struggle with lifelong debilitating disorders.

> "Nature doesn't hurry, yet everything is accomplished."
> —LAO TZU

This book was written entirely by a human with no assistance from generative AI tools.

Acknowledgments

It is an honor and a privilege to reach the wider psychiatric and medical communities with this manuscript. My gratitude to all of you, and readers beyond who share my interest in this important subject matter, is immeasurable.

I would like to recognize my esteemed mentor and colleague Benjamin J. Sadock, MD, Menas S. Gregory Professor of Psychiatry, NYU Grossman School of Medicine, and his wife Virginia Sadock, MD, for their endless encouragement, guidance, and friendship. Their grace and role modeling continue to be a driving force behind my undertakings of authorship, for which I am perpetually thankful.

Maryanne Badaracco, MD, Director and Chief of Psychiatry, Bellevue Hospital, has been deeply supportive of my pursuit of academic excellence during my 30-year career at Bellevue. I additionally extend my gratitude to Charles Marmar, MD, Lucius R. Littauer Professor and Chair of the Department of Psychiatry, NYU Grossman School of Medicine, for his leadership and encouragement.

I am indebted to my research and editorial assistant, and proverbial right hand, Jay Fox, for his continued commitment. None of this would have been possible and nearly as enjoyable without your collaboration, Jay, and I thank you deeply for the privilege to depend on you as a friend, teammate, and partner.

To my publisher and the team at Wolters Kluwer, thank you for your ongoing support. Cranking out a book a year would not be possible without the seamless process you provide.

Lastly, to my life partner, Kim, and my son, Daniel, thank you for your patience and love. I recognize that the hours I commit to the endeavor of producing tomes means less with you, and I appreciate having you both by my side for what I hope and trust will be a worthwhile legacy.

Samoon Ahmad, MD
Clinical Professor
Department of Psychiatry
NYU Grossman School of Medicine
New York, New York

Contents

Foreword by Stephen Ross, MD iv
Preface vi
Acknowledgments ix

1. Introduction 1
2. Global History of Psychedelics 13
3. Clinical History 26
4. Regulations 46
5. The Psychedelic Experience 60
6. Psychedelic-Assisted Psychotherapy 75
7. How Psychedelics Affect the Brain 84
8. Potential Clinical Indications 95
9. Psilocybin 119
10. Lysergic Acid Diethylamide 155
11. *N,N*-Dimethyltryptamine (DMT) and Ayahuasca 171
12. Mescaline 190
13. Ibogaine 209
14. Ketamine 229
15. 3,4-Methylenedioxymethamphetamine 267
16. Miscellaneous Psychedelics 289
17. Patient Stories 300
18. Conclusion 311

About the Author 315
Index 317

1

Introduction

"I truly thought that I had experienced great pleasure upon many previous occasions, but the experience of this night was one quite unique in this regard in the history of a lifetime," wrote a 27-year-old chemist in 1895.[1] The unique experience that occurred almost 130 years ago was also important in the history of medicine, as it represents the first scientific trial ever conducted on a human with a psychedelic: peyote. It would be another 2 years before the isolation of mescaline, the alkaloid responsible for the effects described by the bewildered chemist. How long it will take until we finally have a full understanding of the benefits, risks, and mechanisms of action for this class of drugs remains to be seen.

One thing that is for sure is that the conversation around psychedelics has dramatically shifted within the last 15 years. Once widely considered to have a high potential for abuse and no medicinal value, psychedelics have become a topic of intense interest and there is a palpable sense of optimism about the direction of research. One would be hard pressed to go to any major psychiatric conference within the last few years and not find numerous sessions on the promise of ketamine, psilocybin, lysergic acid diethylamide (LSD), or 3,4-methylenedioxymethamphetamine (MDMA). Throughout this time, stories about the potential benefits of psychedelic-assisted psychotherapy have also made regular appearances in mainstream television, newspapers, and magazines. Back in 2021, the *New York Times* even proclaimed, "The psychedelic revolution is coming."[2]

Opinions are clearly changing, and it's not only among researchers and the public. A growing number of people who work on the clinical side of health care are also recognizing that psychedelics may serve a practical and therapeutic role in psychiatry. A paper published in *Psychedelic Medicine* by Barnett and colleagues sent surveys about the use of psychedelics to 1,000 attending psychiatrists and resident fellows between 2022 and 2023. The same researchers had sent a similar survey in 2016. What they found was that large majorities in the more recent survey supported research into the potential applications of psychedelics in treating psychiatric conditions in general (93.9%) and specific conditions like substance use disorders (88.6%). The 131 who responded to the more recent survey also showed far more optimism about psychedelics, and the percentage of participants who said psychedelics were unsafe even under medical supervision dropped from 24.6% to 9.9%. Just over half expressed a moderate or strong interest in incorporating these drugs into their practice.[3]

There is no doubt that the revolution is underway, and the most vocal proponents of psychedelic medicines—whether they are researchers, activists, startup owners, investors, or journalists—earnestly believe that these drugs will change our approach to mental health, particularly within psychiatry, and may even transform our understanding of consciousness. Their optimism is certainly understandable, and even some of the most ordinarily skeptical members of the medical community share this attitude.

It is a tempered optimism, however. There are real-world obstacles to the widescale use of these drugs within a clinical setting. First and foremost, research into psychedelic medicines still faces significant headwinds because the regulatory environment in the United States makes it difficult to access samples of these drugs for research. Consequently, many of the clinical studies involving psychedelic medicines have been conducted in a relatively small number of people.

However, there is hope that the regulatory environment will experience a seismic change soon, which is both driving and being driven by the flood of investment and researchers into psychedelics. As Sara Reardon of *Nature* wrote in November 2023:

> With the regulatory landscape shifting, legal psychedelic research is becoming easier—and potentially more profitable. Neuroscientists, psychiatrists, pharmacologists, biochemists, and others are entering the field, bringing fresh ideas about what the drugs do at a cellular and molecular level and trying to unravel how these mechanisms might help to relieve symptoms of psychiatric conditions.[4]

There is good reason to believe that we are at an inflection point with respect to regulations and that therapies involving psychedelics are not part of a passing fad. Psychedelics have been used by various cultures throughout the world for millennia for spiritual, ritualistic, and medicinal purposes. Although the religious use of psychedelics is most commonly associated with cultures indigenous to the Americas, perhaps most familiarly in the United States by the Native American Church, there is strong evidence to suggest that psychedelics were also used by cultures in Asia, Africa, and Europe.[5]

Though it would be a stretch to assert that psychedelic medicines have been utilized by all cultures, there is no doubt that their use has been central to the evolution of religions and the spiritual lives of people across myriad cultures, as explored in Chapter 2. There is reason to believe that these substances can also help patients struggling with chronic psychiatric conditions, especially when they are administered responsibly and in controlled clinical settings under the supervision of trained professionals.

Why Are Psychedelics Controversial?

It may come as a surprise to many that this is not the first time that psychedelics have attracted such immense interest from the medical community. During the last quarter of the 20th century and for much of the 21st century, conventional medicine largely overlooked the potential value of these compounds, characterizing them primarily or solely as drugs of abuse. However, within the 27 years following the discovery of LSD's psychedelic properties in 1943 by Swiss chemist Albert Hoffman, more than 1,000 clinical papers were published discussing the use of psychedelics, and an estimated 40,000 individuals took part in experiments or treatments involving psychedelics.[6] As described in Chapter 3, researchers became intimately familiar with the effects of drugs like mescaline, LSD, and psilocybin, and protocols were created for the safe and effective administration of these drugs before, during, and following psychedelic sessions.[7]

Although the work from this fecund period created the foundation for today's research, its tail end was accompanied by a surge in recreational drug use that included not only psychedelics like LSD but also illicit drugs like cannabis and heroin, as well as pharmaceutical drugs like Milltown (meprobamate) and Benzedrine (amphetamine).[8] According to Hoffman, "The joy at having fathered LSD was tarnished after more than ten years of uninterrupted scientific research and medicinal use when LSD was swept up in the huge wave of an inebriant mania that began to spread over the Western world, above all the United States, at the end of the 1950s."[5]

Hoffman notes that the laissez-faire attitude toward casual drug use and sensationalized descriptions of LSD's effects and benefits in mainstream publications in the 1950s and early 1960s helped fuel this "inebriant mania." Demand for the drug was further exacerbated in the mid-1960s, driven by the growth of the hippie counterculture and controversial advocates of LSD, most notably Harvard psychiatrist Timothy Leary, who encouraged a generation of young people: *Turn on, tune in, drop out.* By the end of the decade, recreational LSD use had become extremely widespread, and its reputation in the scientific community had been irrevocably harmed.[5] Stigmas against LSD quickly calcified, and few would maintain publicly that it possessed therapeutic utility, as they would risk losing credibility.

This stigma extended to virtually all psychedelics and became part of a larger cultural backlash against the excesses of the 1960s, one that precipitated the legislation that undergirded the War on Drugs—the Controlled Substances Act (CSA) of 1970.[9] As Chapter 4 details, the CSA continues to place all regulated substances in one of five schedules that are stratified based on the substance's accepted medical use, potential for abuse, and ability to do harm. Schedule V drugs are the most benign, with established medical uses, low potential for abuse, and the lowest capacity to harm patients. Schedule I drugs are believed to have no accepted medical value, the highest potential for abuse, and the greatest ability to do harm.[10] The list of Schedule I drugs includes heroin, cannabis, and virtually every psychedelic discussed in this book.

It's worth remembering the words of historian John Barry, who in 2020 wrote, "When you mix science and politics, you get politics."[11] Though this was said in the context of a larger debate about public health directives and how to best contain the spread of SARS-CoV-2, it is a keen observation that one should keep in mind while reading the following chapters because psychedelics have been unfairly politicized. Consequently, this politicization has prevented researchers from studying the effect of these drugs, as well as denied clinicians and patients from accessing potentially helpful therapeutic tools.

Though the CSA remains in effect, its stranglehold on research is beginning to loosen and psychedelic research is once again blossoming. Consequently, it now seems appropriate for clinicians to learn about the history, risks, and potential uses of psychedelic medicines in general (Chapter 7), as well as the pharmacology of specific drugs like psilocybin (Chapter 9), LSD (Chapter 10), *N,N*-dimethyltryptamine

(DMT) (Chapter 11), mescaline (Chapter 12), ibogaine (Chapter 13), ketamine (Chapter 14), and MDMA (Chapter 15). This book hopes to provide that knowledge in a manner that is well organized, unbiased, and based on the latest available evidence. It is by no means a comprehensive work. Rather, it is meant to provide clinicians and other practitioners with an introductory text that also includes patient experiences (Chapter 17), data about the many trials that have been conducted with these drugs, and information about how these drugs have been administered in traditional and clinical settings.

Although some drugs may be adequately described by focusing solely on their pharmacologic properties, psychedelics demand a more multidisciplinary approach. To understand why, we must first answer the question: What makes a particular drug a psychedelic?

What Is a Psychedelic Drug?

The term "psychedelic" was first coined by the British psychiatrist Humphrey Osmond in the 1950s and is a combination of the Greek words *psyche* (meaning "mind") and *deloun* (meaning "show"), which translates into "mind-manifesting."[12] In most cases and throughout this book, the word "psychedelic" (or "psychedelics") will be used as an umbrella term to denote a drug or class of drugs capable of inducing powerful alterations in sensory perception, mood, and consciousness. Another key characteristic of psychedelics is that they can facilitate mystical-type experiences in patients, which has led some to use the word "entheogenic" when describing them. "Entheogenic" is a neologism meaning "spiritually inspiring." These experiences, especially in conjunction with psychotherapy, can lead to profound changes in perception, revelations, and psychological breakthroughs. More will be said about what is entailed by a mystical-type experience in later chapters, particularly Chapter 5.

Of course, mystical-type experiences are not necessary for one to have a dramatic change in perspective. In Aldous Huxley's book *The Doors of Perception*, which is probably one of the most important works on the psychedelic experience, he mentions that one also has a sense of wonderment. Following an experience with mescaline, Huxley wrote, "Visual impressions are greatly intensified and the eye recovers some of the perceptual innocence of childhood, when the sensum was not immediately and automatically subordinated to the concept." Huxley also described the experience as one in which the brain's ability to filter out excessive stimuli diminished. Instead, what one perceives is "something more than, and above all something different from, the carefully selected utilitarian material which our narrowed, individual minds regard as a complete, or at least sufficient, picture of reality."[13]

To glimpse this alternative picture of reality, one that is often free of the conceits of the Freudian ego, psychedelics offer many patients more than just a fresh perspective; it affords them the opportunity to recognize problematic patterns, to enter into nonordinary states of consciousness (NOSCs) and to even have mystical-type experiences. Individuals who experience NOSCs or mystical-type experiences often experience improved introspection and enhanced empathetic reasoning, which can in turn lead to psychological breakthroughs.[14] These psychological breakthroughs then allow them to begin healing, especially when they occur within a properly designed therapeutic container. In other words, their efficacy is not due to their pharmacology alone.

Of course, not everyone has a pleasant experience while under the influence of psychedelics. It can oftentimes be psychologically challenging, especially for patients with deeply traumatic backgrounds or patients who are reconciling the fact that they have a terminal illness. However, it should be noted that unpleasant or challenging experiences are not necessarily negative. They can be therapeutically useful and lead to positive changes in the long run if the patient has proper guidance.

The fact that the phenomenologic experience and subjective effects of psychedelic drugs can influence their efficacy in treating psychiatric disorders is part of what makes them so distinct. As researchers have long recognized, the tone of the psychedelic experience can be impacted by several other factors, most notably set, setting, and support, which are things over which therapists have control.

Set, Setting, and Support

One of the phrases that one frequently encounters when reading about psychedelics is "set and setting." Coined by Timothy Leary in the early 1960s while he was researching the effects of psilocybin, the phrase refers to two extrapharmacologic factors that can influence an individual's psychedelic experience. More recently, the concept of "support" has also become vital to ensuring a positive psychedelic experience.

Set refers to the mindset of the patient and the therapist. It has a relatively broad meaning that encompasses their personality, level of intelligence, current mood, expectations about psychedelics, and concern about past or upcoming events. It can also refer to their experience with psychedelics, which is of extreme importance for patients within a clinical setting. On the one hand, psychedelic naive patients may be easily influenced by expectancy or find the experience to be emotionally difficult. On the other hand, patients with significant psychedelic experience may be somewhat accustomed to NOSCs, which could diminish the impact of the experience.

Setting refers to the environment in which the psychedelic is administered. This can refer to the physical area the patient occupies, as well as the social space in which they find themselves. As earlier researchers found, leaving a person in a sterile examination room or strapped to a bed exacerbated their anxiety and fear. Conversely, when psychedelics are administered in more naturalistic and comfortable settings, patients tend to have a better experience.

Finally, *support* refers to the support systems before, during, and after the administration of the psychedelic. Friends and family will typically be involved in providing this support, but creating a therapeutic container that is conducive to generating a therapeutically beneficial experience is the purview of the therapist. This responsibility will be explored in greater detail in Chapter 6.

Classic Psychedelics and Atypical Psychedelics

Under the umbrella term "psychedelics" are *classic psychedelics* and *atypical psychedelics*. The former include psilocybin, LSD, mescaline, and DMT (the active ingredient in ayahuasca). Classic psychedelics share a similar mechanism of action (ie, demonstrating agonistic activity at serotonin receptors, especially $5\text{-}HT_{2A}$), though each compound appears to be capable of affecting several distinct targets outside of the serotonergic system. Moreover, each compound is capable of inducing a unique experience, and they all have unique pharmacokinetics and pharmacodynamics that will be explored in later chapters.

The term "atypical psychedelics" is a blanket description for any substance that induces altered NOSCs without primarily targeting serotonergic pathways. There are dozens of drugs that fall under this loose description, including dissociative psychedelics like phencyclidine (PCP), ibogaine (which is also referred to as an *oneirogen*, meaning "dream-inducing"), and ketamine; muscarinic receptor antagonists like atropine and scopolamine; some cannabis receptor agonists; and a unique class of drugs known as either empathogens ("generating a state of empathy") or entactogens. The latter term, coined by Dr David E. Nichols, refers to certain drugs' abilities to facilitate the process of internal retrieval of repressed or traumatic memories (the neologism "entactogen" combining Greek roots "en-" and "gen-" (meaning "within" and "to generate," respectively) with the Latin root *"tactus"* (meaning "touching").[15] The entactogen that has received the most attention is MDMA. Research has indicated that it may help individuals process trauma successfully, allowing for significant reductions or even the resolution of symptoms associated with posttraumatic stress disorder (PTSD). As explored in Chapter 15, recent phase 3 clinical trials have validated the notion that MDMA can help treat the symptoms of PTSD, though there are concerns with the data that will be discussed below and in Chapter 15.

The Potential of Psychedelics and Psychedelic-Assisted Psychotherapy

Beyond PTSD, research suggests that classic psychedelics, in conjunction with psychotherapy, can aid in the treatment of numerous psychiatric conditions, including anxiety, mood and affective disorders, as well as substance use disorders, particularly alcohol use disorder (AUD). They may also provide comfort to patients who have a terminal illness with a poor prognosis and are struggling with the existential distress of facing their own mortality.

Most of these benefits appear to be related to the mystical-like experience produced by these drugs, which is believed to be mediated by the activation of 5-HT_{2A} receptors.[16] However, there is also evidence to suggest that psychedelics promote neuroplasticity by binding to tropomyosin receptor kinase B (TrkB), the protein receptor for brain-derived neurotrophic factor (BDNF), or via other means to be explored in Chapter 7.[17] Meanwhile, research has found that the therapeutic efficacy of psychedelic-assisted psychotherapy may be mediated through critical period reopening for social reward learning.[18]

This is not only theoretical. Ketamine has shown efficacy in alleviating symptoms associated with treatment-resistant depression and major depressive disorder with acute suicidality. Esketamine (Spravato), a nasal spray consisting of only the (S)-ketamine enantiomer, even received approval from the Food and Drug Administration (FDA) in 2019 for treatment-resistant depression.

Clinical trials are indicating that psychedelic-assisted psychotherapy with classic psychedelics can produce results that are significantly better than placebo. As an example, a randomized clinical trial of 25-mg doses of psilocybin administered with psychological support was associated with a 19.1-point reduction in Montgomery-Åsberg Depression Rating Scale (MADRS) scores from baseline to day 43, whereas the control group (who received a 100-mg dose of niacin) experienced only a

6.8-point reduction in MADRS score.[19] Within a palliative care setting, Holze and colleagues administered LSD during two treatment sessions in a double-blind, placebo-controlled, randomized phase 2 trial. Of the 44 participants in the trial, 21 were assigned to the group who received LSD during the first session while 23 received placebo in the first session. Following the study, the authors reported that LSD "induced rapid and lasting reductions in anxiety, depression, and general psychiatric symptomology for up to 16 weeks."[20]

Meanwhile, a retrospective study involving the use of ibogaine in the treatment of 33 individuals with opioid use disorders found that 25 (76%) experienced complete resolution of opioid withdrawal and did not exhibit subsequent drug-seeking behaviors.[21]

Ongoing Limitations

Despite these promising results, there are still several limitations with many of the studies that will be described in the following chapters. In some cases, sample sizes of clinical trials, especially phase 1 trials, are no more than a dozen or two. Similarly, participants may only participate in studies that last for a few weeks or months, which makes it difficult to make claims about the long-term efficacy of these treatments. Psychiatric disorders can be afflictions that last a lifetime and cycle through periods of increased symptomology and periods of remission. Knowing that participants in a study experienced remission for 2 weeks or even 2 months following psychedelic-assisted therapy is excellent news, but it leaves open the possibility that patients may need intermittent boosters of psychedelic-assisted psychotherapy as opposed to a total of only one or two sessions to make the most of the treatment modality. As these sessions are labor- and time-intensive for mental health practitioners, oftentimes lasting upward of 8 to 10 hours during which time clinicians cannot see other patients, this could seriously impact the scalability of psychedelic-assisted therapy.

Another limitation is that there is often a lack of diversity in these studies. Retrospective studies and studies that involve surveys are particularly lacking in diversity, with the majority of respondents being affluent, White non-Hispanic males. Of note, males were overrepresented in early clinical trials, though more recent trials have made strides in remedying gender disparity. However, non-Hispanic White participants continue to be overrepresented in most trials, but acknowledgment of this issue within recent years is likely to change practice, and papers based on studies conducted after this recognition will have more diverse cohorts.

Finally, blinding continues to be a major challenge in psychedelic research. Psychedelics induce extremely unique alterations in perception, cognition, and emotion, and participants in blinded studies (as well as researchers) can typically discern who received the psychedelic drug and who did not. In phase 3 trials involving MDMA for the treatment of PTSD, participants in the treatment arm were able to correctly guess roughly 90% of the time that they received the drug, whereas those in the control arm were able to correctly guess that they received placebo 75% of the time.[22] This was one of the major determining factors why an advisory panel for the FDA encouraged the agency to not approve the use of MDMA in the treatment of PTSD. The June 2024 decision rejected the notion that MDMA is an effective treatment for PTSD by a vote of 9-2 and stated that the risks of MDMA outweigh the benefits by a vote of 10-1. In August 2024, the FDA formally sided with the panel's advice and withheld their approval of MDMA until more evidence is available to support its use. In addition to concerns about blinding, they noted flaws in the reporting of adverse events (particularly the potential for adverse cardiovascular effects), some possible bias among researchers and therapists involved in the study, and an alleged case of misconduct involving a patient and therapist.[23]

Despite these issues and safety concerns that are unique to each drug, clinical trials have reported that psychedelic therapies work in controlled settings and their efficacy is not based on mere anecdotal evidence. Even though there are some dissenting voices and critiques about the methodologies of these trials, some of the leading experts from the National Institute on Drug Abuse (NIDA) have begun to take notice, despite the fact that NIDA has historically considered psychedelics solely within the context of abuse. In an opinion piece coauthored by the head of NIDA, Dr Nora Volkow, that was published in the October 2023 volume of *JAMA Psychiatry*, the authors note, "Although existing pharmacologic treatments such as antidepressants and medications for opioid use disorder are valuable for many people with these conditions, a large proportion are not helped by those treatments. In this context, psychedelic drugs represent a promising psychotherapeutic frontier." They continue, "An important research question is whether the subjective experiences associated with psychedelic drugs are intrinsic to or separable from their therapeutic effects."[24]

Although this is far from a full endorsement for psychedelics, it is certainly a positive change that NIDA is considering the possibility of psychedelic medicines having potential therapeutic applications. In addition to calling into question psychedelic drugs' status as Schedule I drugs and being emblematic of the evolving perception of psychedelics within the medical community, the authors' concerns beg several questions that will be addressed throughout this book and concern the drugs' mechanisms of action, safety profiles, and ability to be used in controlled settings without fear of adverse reaction. This book will also explore the major question proposed by the authors, one that strikes at the heart of their therapeutic applications: *Must patients experience the subjective effects of psychedelics to realize the full benefits of psychedelic therapy?*

REFERENCES

1. Prentis DW, Morgan FP. Anhalonium lewinii (mescal buttons). A study of the drug, with especial reference to its physiological action upon man, with report to experiments. *Ther Gnz*. 1895;11(9). Accessed May 21, 2024. https://collections.nlm.nih.gov/bookviewer?PID=nlm:nlmuid-101751140-bk
2. Jacobs A. The psychedelic revolution is coming. Psychiatry may never be the same. *New York Times*. Updated November 11, 2021. Accessed November 1, 2023. https://www.nytimes.com/2021/05/09/health/psychedelics-mdma-psilocybin-molly-mental-health.html
3. Barnett BS, Arakelian M, Beebe D, et al. American psychiatrists' opinions about classic hallucinogens and their potential therapeutic applications: a 7-year follow-up survey. *Psychedelic Med*. 2023;2(1). doi:10.1089/psymed.2023.0036
4. Reardon S. The science behind psychedelic therapy. *Nature*. 2023;623:22-24.
5. Hofmann A. *LSD: My Problem Child*. Multidisciplinary Association for Psychedelic Studies (MAPS); 2009.
6. Richard WA. *Sacred Knowledge: Psychedelics and Religious Experiences*. Columbia University Press; 2016:3.
7. Freedman DX. Perspectives on the use and abuse of psychedelic drugs. In: Efron DH, ed. *Ethnopharmacologic Search for Psychoactive Drugs*. Vol I. Synergetic Press; 1967:77-102.
8. DeGrandpre R. *The Cult of Pharmacology: How American Became the World's Most Troubled Drug Culture*. Duke University Press; 2006.
9. Richert L, Dyck E, Turner A. Psychedelic wards: LSD as mental medicine in a battle for hearts and minds. In: Farber D, ed. *The War on Drugs: A History*. New York University Press; 2022:186-211.
10. Gabay M. The federal controlled substances act: schedules and pharmacy registration. *Hosp Pharm*. 2013;48(6):473-474. doi:10.1310/hpj4806-473
11. Barry JM. The pandemic could get much, much worse. We must act now. *New York Times*. Published July 14, 2020. Accessed November 1, 2023. https://www.nytimes.com/2020/07/14/opinion/coronavirus-shutdown.html
12. Tanne JH. Humphrey Osmond. *BMJ*. 2004;328(7441):713. PMCID: PMC381240.
13. Huxley A. *The Doors of Perception & Heaven and Hell*. HarperCollins Publishers; 2009:24-25.
14. Timmermann C, Bauer PR, Gosseries O, et al. A neurophenomenological approach to non-ordinary states of consciousness: hypnosis, meditation, and psychedelics. *Trends Cogn Sci*. 2023;27(2):139-159. doi:10.1016/j.tics.2022.11.006. PMID: 36566091.
15. Nichols DE. Entactogens: how the name for a novel class of psychoactive agents originated. *Front Psychiatry*. 2022;13:863088. doi:10.3389/fpsyt.2022.863088
16. Gattuso JJ, Perkins D, Ruffell S, et al. Default mode network modulation by psychedelics: a systematic review. *Int J Neuropsychopharmacol*. 2023;26(3):155-188. doi:10.1093/ijnp/pyac074. PMID: 36272145; PMCID: PMC10032309.
17. Moliner R, Girych M, Brunello CA, et al. Psychedelics promote plasticity by directly binding to BDNF receptor TrkB. *Nat Neurosci*. 2023;26:1032-1041. doi:10.1038/s41593-023-01316-5

18. Nardou R, Sawyer E, Song YJ, et al. Psychedelics reopen the social reward learning critical period. *Nature*. 2023;618(7966):790-798. doi:10.1038/s41586-023-06204-3
19. Raison CL, Sanacora G, Woolley J, et al. Single-dose psilocybin treatment for major depressive disorder: a randomized clinical trial. *JAMA*. 2023;330(9):843-853. doi:10.1001/jama.2023.14530
20. Holze F, Gasser P, Müller F, Dolder PC, Liechti ME. Lysergic acid diethylamide-assisted therapy in patients with anxiety with and without a life-threatening illness: a randomized, double-blind, placebo-controlled phase II study. *Biol Psychiatry*. 2023;93(3):215-223. doi:10.1016/j.biopsych.2022.08.025. PMID: 36266118.
21. Köck P, Froelich K, Walter M, Lang U, Dürsteler KM. A systematic literature review of clinical trials and therapeutic applications of ibogaine. *J Subst Abuse Treat*. 2022;138:108717. doi:10.1016/j.jsat.2021.108717. PMID: 35012793.
22. DePeau-Wilson M. FDA staff questions safety of MDMA treatment for PTSD. *MedPage Today*. Published May 31, 2024. Accessed June 4, 2024. https://www.medpagetoday.com/psychiatry/anxietystress/110423
23. Jacobs A. F.D.A. panel rejects MDMA-aided therapy for PTSD. *New York Times*. Updated June 5, 2024. Accessed June 5, 2024. https://www.nytimes.com/2024/06/04/health/fda-mdma-therapy-ptsd.html
24. Volkow ND, Gordon JA, Wargo EM. Psychedelics as therapeutics—potential and challenges. *JAMA Psychiatry*. 2023;80(10):979-980. doi:10.1001/jamapsychiatry.2023.1968

Global History of Psychedelics

Psychedelic compounds have been used by numerous cultures for thousands of years, though their consumption was particularly prevalent among shamanistic cultures in the Americas and Central Asia. However, there is circumstantial evidence that psychedelic concoctions were also used in Europe, particularly by the Greeks, and in parts of Asia. Although a discussion of each culture's use of psychedelics is beyond the scope of this book, this chapter is intended to provide historical and cultural context with respect to the use of psychedelic compounds. Moreover, it will include a review of the archaeological and historical evidence concerning early psychedelic use and how these drugs have been used by various cultures as a medicine and sacrament.

Of note, some of the drugs covered in this book will not be discussed in this chapter since their discovery took place in the lab during the 20th century. These drugs include 3,4-methylenedioxymethamphetamine (MDMA), which was first synthesized in 1912 by the German pharmaceutical company Merck[1]; lysergic acid diethylamide (LSD), which was first synthesized by Swiss pharmacist Albert Hoffman in 1938[2]; and ketamine, which was first synthesized in 1962 by Calvin Stevens.[3]

This leaves **psilocybin**, a tryptamine alkaloid found in psychedelic mushrooms primarily of the genus *Psilocybe*, which has nearly worldwide distribution; **ibogaine**, an alkaloid found in the iboga plant (*Tabernanthe iboga*), which grows in Central Africa, primarily in Gabon; **mescaline**, a phenethylamine alkaloid found primarily in the North American peyote cactus (*Lophophora williamsii*) and the South American San Pedro cactus (*Echinopsis pachanoi*); and ***N,N*-dimethyltryptamine (DMT)**, an indole alkaloid and derivative of tryptamine found in a wide variety of plants and animals, including humans. DMT is the active ingredient in ayahuasca (also known as yagé or hoasca), which is a psychedelic decoction that has been used in the Amazon basin of South America. There is no singular recipe for ayahuasca, but it typically consists of at least two ingredients: DMT-containing leaves of *Psychotria viridis* and *Banisteriopsis caapi* vines. The vines contain monoamine oxidase inhibitors (MAOIs), which are important since without them, the DMT would be inactive via oral administration.[4] Close relatives of DMT (eg, bufotenin, 5-methoxy-*N,N*-dimethyltryptamine [5-MeO-DMT]) have also been used by indigenous peoples of South America and the West Indies, primarily as snuffs.[5]

The Archaeological Record

There is evidence that humans began using psychotropic drugs thousands of years ago—the most common example being alcohol. The establishment of permanent settlements and more advanced forms of agriculture is believed to have begun close to 12,000 years ago,[6] but evidence of beermaking appears to predate even this era of history. Circumstantial evidence of beermaking by the Natufian culture—which was a semi-sedentary group of people based in the Levant from approximately 15,000 to 11,500 years ago—dates back even further.[7]

One benefit of searching for sites of ancient breweries is that they are relatively easy to find. On the one hand, it requires at least a semipermanent settlement where the brewing process can happen. Consequently, archaeologists can detect the detritus of the settlement and focus their search there. Second, the process of brewing beer leaves behind residual evidence on pottery that may then be discovered at the site.

However, discovering evidence of psychedelic use is far more difficult. If psychedelic plants or fungi were used by nomadic or semi-nomadic peoples, the search for remnants of a camp that would suggest temporary settlement is like looking for a needle in a haystack. A second challenge would be detecting the remnants of psychedelic alkaloids at such a camp. Although the process of making beer or wine leaves behind residual compounds that can be collected at archaeological sites, the preparation of most psychedelic alkaloids is far simpler.[i] Psychedelic mushrooms, peyote, San Pedro cacti, and ibogaine require minimal preparation (as they can be consumed orally fresh or dried), and physical evidence of their remains lasts only so long.

For example, mushrooms are soft-bodied organisms, and physical evidence of their culinary or medicinal use has been recovered rarely from archaeological sites (typically burial sites) even from a few 1,000 years ago. Ötzi, the Tyrolian "iceman" who lived over 5,300 years ago, represents one famous example. His body was discovered entombed in ice and in possession of a birch polypore mushroom (*Piptoporus betulinus*), which he may have used as a vermifuge.[8] Another example is the Red Lady of El Mirón, who is believed to have lived in Spain between 18,000 and 19,000 years ago. A close examination of the dental calculus of her remains revealed a diet that consisted of ibex, red deer, salmon, the seeds and underground storage organs of plants, and mushrooms.[9,10] It should be noted that some of the mushroom spores found in her fossilized teeth were of the order *Agaricales*, which does leave open the possibility that at least some of the mushrooms in her diet were capable of inducing psychedelic effects.

The oldest indisputable physical evidence of psychedelic use dates back to 3780 to 3660 BCE.[11] Dried buttons of peyote were discovered in the Shumla caves, which are located in Texas not far from the Rio Grande. The specimens still contained concentrations of 2% mescaline.[11] Specimens of peyote have also been recovered from northern Mexico, indicating pre–Columbian use.[12] Other archaeological finds in the Americas point to the use of snuffs to administer either tobacco or relatives of DMT (5-MeO-DMT) prior to European contact. The oldest to be discovered was found at a site along the central Peruvian coast and dates back to 1200 BCE.[13] Smoking pipes containing residual 5-MeO-DMT date back to 2130 BCE and were discovered in northern Argentina.[13] Carvings at the Peruvian site Chavlín de Huántar, which sits over 10,000 feet above sea level, suggest that the ceremonial use of San Pedro cacti dates back to at least 1200 BCE.[14(p15)] In Africa, archaeological evidence from approximately 2,000 years ago suggests that the iboga plant was being used medicinally by people within present-day Gabon.[15]

---

[i] One notable exception is ayahuasca, which requires an advanced knowledge of botany to create. This decoction does not have one formal recipe and may be composed of dozens of ingredients, but it would have required extensive research and experimentation to figure out that DMT from *P. viridis* or another plant needs to be administered in conjunction with an MAOI to slow the breakdown of DMT and make it orally bioactive. Knowledge of how to locate the plants capable of creating such a brew was not something that one simply picked up casually.

Though the fragility of physical specimens makes it very difficult to find direct evidence to support the theory that the widespread use of plants and fungi containing psychedelic alkaloids was common among prehistoric cultures, enough evidence has been uncovered to make a very strong case that these drugs are not recent discoveries.

Ancient Artworks

In most cases, truly ancient evidence of the use of psychedelics has been gleaned through their representation in artworks like mushroom statues, which are found throughout Central America (Figure 2.1), and cave art. The most well-known example of the latter is from Algeria (at the site Tassili n'Ajjer), which dates back to approximately 7,000 years ago.[16] As shown in Figures 2.2 and 2.3, there are clear figures in the petroglyphs that resemble mushrooms. Moreover, the abstract nature of the artwork has led many to suggest that the artist (or artists) had some first-hand knowledge of the effects of psychedelics.

Although the petroglyph should not be considered *proof* of psychedelic mushroom use, it is worth noting that similar drawings portraying mushrooms have been found in Spain (likely *Psilocybe hispanica*) and Siberia (likely *Amanita muscaria*, otherwise known as the fly-agaric mushroom).[16]

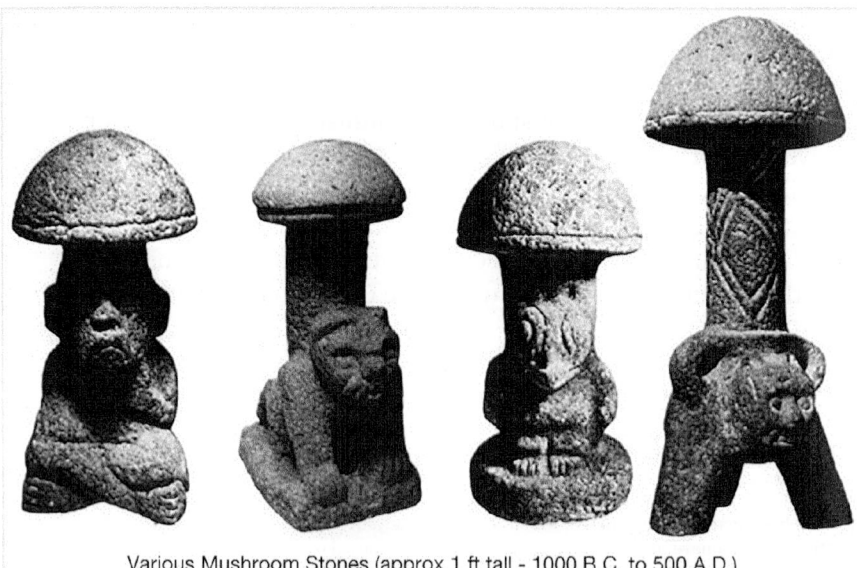

Various Mushroom Stones (approx 1 ft tall - 1000 B.C. to 500 A.D.)

Figure 2.1 Example of mushroom statues from Central America dating to between 1,500 and 3,000 years ago.

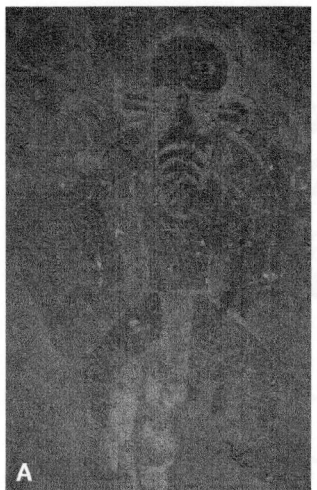
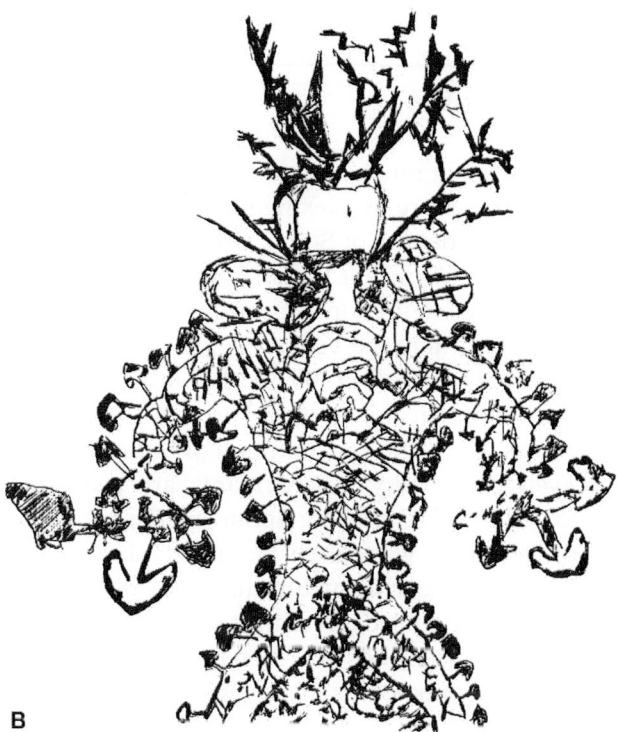

Figure 2.2 A. Photograph of the wall of a cave at Tassili n'Ajjer in Algeria. B. Drawing of the figure featured in the photograph.

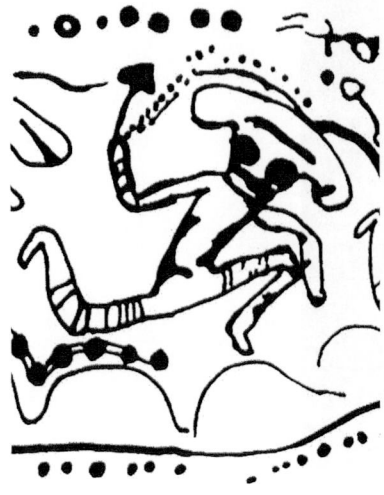

Figure 2.3 Closeup drawing of the mushroom figures from Figure 2.2B.

The Historical Record

The historical record is not much clearer with respect to many psychedelics. One of the more perplexing mysteries in the history of religion is the botanical identity of Soma, which is described as a god, a plant, and an entheogen in ancient Indian hymns known collectively as the Rigveda. The text was written in Sanskrit between 1500 and 1000 BCE. In addition to being central to the Vedic religion (which thrived among the Indo-Aryan peoples between ~1500 and 500 BCE), the Rigveda is still recognized as one of four sacred canonical texts in Hinduism.

Within the texts, the ritual consumption of Soma grants strength, brilliance, and even immortality to participants, and a significant portion of the Rigveda is dedicated to praising Soma and describing how to prepare the Soma potion. It was clearly not a metaphor. According to comparative religion scholar Huston Smith, "Dried plants were steeped in water and their juice pounded out with stones and wooden boards covered with bull hides. This juice was then forced through wooden filters and blended with milk, curds, barley water, ghee, and occasionally honey."[17]

Though R. Gordon Wasson made what was considered a compelling argument that identified the fly-agaric mushroom as Soma more than 50 years ago, the matter remains unresolved to this day. Other proposed candidates of Soma have included psilocybin mushrooms, hops, ephedra, and *Cannabis sativa*.[18]

Like Soma, *kykeon* was central to a sect of Ancient Greeks who engaged in the Eleusinian Mysteries. The Mysteries were based on Greek mythology and involved Demeter, goddess of agriculture and fertility, and Persephone, Demeter's daughter by Zeus. As the story goes, the god of the underworld, Hades, fell in love with Persephone and asked Zeus for her hand. Hoping to not offend, Zeus neither objected nor gave his consent to Hades, who then kidnapped Persephone at the site of Eleusis, and then took her home to the underworld. After 10 days of searching for her daughter, Demeter discovered the news, and in her distress caused a drought to befall the people of Greece. As the people starved, they could no longer provide sacrifice to the Olympian gods, which convinced Zeus to pressure Hades to release Persephone to Demeter (at Eleusis). As Persephone had consumed several pomegranate seeds while in the underworld and the Fates required anyone who ate or drank in Hades to remain there, a deal was struck where Persephone would return to Hades for several months of the year (one for each pomegranate seed) and spend the rest of the time with her mother. Mythologically speaking, the tale represents a fertility rite, the triumph of life over death, and a cosmologic story to explain the return of spring each year.[19]

Central to this tale is Eleusis. Located just outside of Athens, the ancient village became the site of a temple where Persephone's return from the underworld was celebrated starting in approximately 1500 BCE. The ceremony, known as the Eleusinian Mysteries, then continued uninterrupted for nearly 2,000 years until the Mysteries, like all pagan practices, became illegal under the Roman Emperor Theodosius I at the end of the 4th century CE. Those who participated in the Mysteries included great playwrights like Euripides and Sophocles, philosophers like Aristotle and Plato, and even the Roman emperor Marcus Aurelius. Evidently, he was the only layperson ever allowed within the *anaktoron*, the inner sanctum of the temple, after he rebuilt the site in 170 CE following its destruction at the hands of Kostovoks.[20]

Initiates to the Mysteries walked away evidently knowing that a life continues after death following the consumption of *kykeon*, which many have speculated was an entheogen. Like the rites of the Mysteries, the active ingredient in kykeon remains a mystery, though some have speculated that it was an as-yet unidentified ergot derivative similar to LSD, psilocybin mushrooms, or even a combination of a plant containing DMT and an MAOI like Syrian rue (thus making a potion similar to ayahuasca). For a detailed account of the mysteries surrounding *kykeon*, psychedelic beer, and spiked wines from the ancient Mediterranean, see Brian C. Muraresku's *The Immortality Key*.

Historical evidence of psychedelic use in South America, Central America, and Southwestern United States is far less mysterious, largely on account of three factors. First, the images showing the ritualistic use of psilocybin mushrooms and mescaline-containing cacti prior to European contact remain well preserved even to this day. Second, the Spanish and Portuguese individuals (predominately members of the clergy) who were tasked with chronicling the conquest and destruction of the many empires throughout South America and Mesoamerica were surprisingly thorough in their descriptions of the rites and ceremonies observed by indigenous Americans. Finally, the ceremonies involving the use of psilocybin, mescaline, ayahuasca, and snuffs containing DMT (or its relatives) did not vanish—they merely went underground. Although the practice of using plant-based entheogens has certainly evolved since the 1500s, the use of specific drugs and the conceptual frameworks through which healers operate appear to have remained intact. In the more remote parts of South America or Mexico, where Western influence remains limited even to this day, some of these practices have continued with minimal interruption."[14(pp33-49)]

Perhaps one of the most thorough ethnographic products to come from the era was *La Historia General de las Cosas de Nueva Espana* (*The General History of the Things of New Spain*). It is more commonly known as the *Florentine Codex* because the best-preserved version is held at the Laurentian Library in the Italian city of Florence. The 12-volume work was written in Spanish and Nahuatl by the Franciscan friar Bernardino de Sahagún with the help of indigenous elders between his arrival in Mexico in 1529 and his death in 1590. In his writings, Sahagún describes the ceremonial and religious use of psychedelic mushrooms and peyote cactus by the Nahuatl people (referred to as the Aztecs by the Spanish). On mushrooms, he wrote, "They ate these little mushrooms with honey, and when they began to be excited by them, they began to dance, some singing, others weeping."[21] He notes that not all of them participated in the revelry. "Some did not want to sing but sat down in their quarters and remained there as if in a meditative mood. Some saw themselves dying in a vision and wept; others saw themselves being eaten by wild beasts; and imagined that they were rich and possessed many slaves," he wrote.[21] Finally, he describes what could be thought of as an integration session: "When the intoxication from the little mushrooms had passed, they talked over among themselves the visions which they had seen."[21]

On account of the similarities between the Christian Eucharist and the indigenous use of cacti and mushrooms (psilocybin mushrooms were referred to as *teonanacatl*, "flesh of the gods"), the use of plant-based entheogens became prohibited in the European colonies in the Western hemisphere. At best, these plants were thought to merely produce a state of intoxication. At worst, they were considered to be an outright mockery of Christianity.[14(pp33-49)]

Despite the risk of persecution and severe punishment if they were discovered, shamanistic traditions persisted throughout the Americas.

Shamanism

Well into the 20th century, the terms "shaman" or "shamanism" were met with derision by Western physicians and the public at large. This should not come as a surprise, as the terms were largely pejorative and meant to define a person who was governed by superstition and irrationality.

However, some of the earliest traits of religion as practiced by hunter-gatherer societies were shamanistic, with a strong focus on the worship of ancestors and natural spirits.[22] Anthropologist Michael Winkelman defines shamanism as a "cross-cultural concept derived from recognition of a similar complex of spiritual healing practices in pre-modern cultures around the world."[23] The role of the shaman eventually developed to be one defined as a conduit between the material realm and spiritual/sacred realm. In order to access this realm, the shaman would enter into a nonordinary state of consciousness (NOSC) using ritualistic fasting or sleep abstention; sensory deprivation; yoga; meditation; breathwork; or exhausting physical and communal activity that may include chanting, singing, dancing, or drumming. Psychedelics were also a crucial part of shamanism, Winkelman notes, and that shamans were responsible for managing "the therapeutic and other adaptive effects that can be obtained by using psychedelics to integrate information in consciousness."[23] "Consciousness" here could refer to the individual consciousness of the shaman or a person from the community or the collective consciousness of the community.

Unlike allopathic medicine, where health concerns are viewed as physiologic problems that have physiologic solutions, the line between spirituality and medicine is considerably more blurred among many cultures that operate within a shamanistic framework. Even today, many indigenous individuals see illnesses not solely as physiologic or neurobiologic problems but potentially spiritual ones as well. Accordingly, patients may request that a shaman (also known as a folk healer) combat the spiritual effluvia afflicting them, friends, members of their family, or their community as a whole. They may also request the services of a folk healer to remove a curse or even find a lost object.[14(pp26,27)]

Specific practices of folk healers are anything but uniform. However, they tend to require entering into an NOSC with the use of psychedelics or one of the nonpsychedelic methods described previously. In some cases, both the patient and the healer will consume a psychedelic substance, and then work together to resolve the issue. This may involve a one-on-one ceremony or a group ceremony overseen by the healer/shaman. The latter seems to have been quite common in the past and continues to this day. One example is the communal chanting and drumming which has long been a vital part of the peyote ceremonies of the Native American Church.[14(pp41-55)] South American ceremonies involving the use of San Pedro cacti and northern Mexican ceremonies involving the use of peyote frequently include all-night dancing ceremonies.[14(pp24,41-43)] Like other psychedelics, mescaline encourages stereotypic and rhythmic movements while (unlike many other psychedelics) producing a stimulant effect.[14(p24)] Meanwhile, drumming, singing, and dancing are regular features of the iboga ceremonies of the Bwiti in Gabon.[24]

One-on-one sessions tend to be less outwardly joyous. In these scenarios, the healer may only administer a psychedelic to their patient and then guide them through the experience with the goal of allowing the patient to discover a solution or cure to their problem, have an epiphany or revelation, or gain insight into something with which they are struggling. In still other scenarios, the shaman may choose to be the sole individual entering the NOSC.[14(pp25,26)]

The Benefits of Nonordinary States of Consciousness

Though there is no formal definition of an NOSC, there are three distinct features. First, they are transient. Second, they are phenomenologically distinct from ordinary states of consciousness (ie, typical waking life). A person recognizes that the experience of an NOSC is distinct from the experience of their ordinary state of consciousness. Finally, they are neurobiologically distinct from ordinary states of consciousness, as well.

What appears to be common across all NOSCs—whether they are induced by a psychedelic, hypnosis, deep meditation, or some other practice—is that they decrease activity in key parts of the brain and allow for shifts in perspective or experiential structure.[25] In more extreme cases, the NOSC may temporarily disrupt the narrative sense of self, allowing for a dissolution between subject and object in a phenomenon known as "ego dissolution," which may be associated with oceanic boundlessness and a sense of unity with others, nature, the universe, or the divine. Studies involving the use of magnetoencephalography

(MEG), electroencephalography (EEG), and functional magnetic resonance imaging (fMRI) indicate that the sensation of ego dissolution is associated with disruptions in the functional connectivity of specific nodes within the central nervous system, most notably the default mode network (DMN), which includes the precuneus, medial prefrontal cortex (mPFC), posterior cingulate cortex (PCC), and angular gyrus.[26] Functional connectivity may be disrupted between the nodes of the DMN and other brain networks, as well.[25] (These mechanisms will be explored in greater detail in Chapter 7.)

During this window of opportunity where the "voice" of the extended narrative self is quieted or even silenced, individuals *can* experience deeper introspection and enhanced empathetic reasoning, while also reshaping self-related models and beliefs.[25] If properly integrated, this work *can* result in long-term trait changes and therapeutic benefits.

> *"Can" is the operative word in both sentences, and this is where the therapeutic benefits of psychedelics, as well as NOSCs in general, run into limitations. To truly seize the opportunity afforded by this temporary window of plasticity, individuals must receive proper preparation and guidance during the experience so that they are in the correct mindset (set); be situated in the right environment (setting); and have a supportive network before, during, and after the experience to help them process the experience (support). In other words, to optimize the therapeutic benefits of psychedelics, well-trained guides who can offer psychedelic-assisted psychotherapy will be necessary to ensure proper set, setting, and support.*

Conclusion: Shamanism and Psychiatry

To enhance the therapeutic benefits of psychedelic medicines and to help patients integrate the psychedelic experience, Gary Bravo and Charles Grob argued many years ago that psychiatrists must recast themselves as modern-day shamans.[27] Though many psychiatrists may find this recommendation to be strange, Bravo and Grob note that working within the psychedelic-assisted psychotherapy paradigm is very similar to the shamanistic conception of the spiritual world, especially since psychedelic experiences are often ineffable unless couched within religious terminology, metaphor, or the language of the unconscious. "Something can be learned from the shamanistic paradigm, where healing is inextricably set within a preternatural frame of reference," they write.[27]

Does this mean that psychiatrists must become shamans? No. However, it does mean that operating within a paradigm that utilizes psychedelics requires rethinking why drugs are administered and, perhaps more crucially, *how* these drugs are administered. As the following chapters will explore, Western medicine spent a good part of the 20th century learning what shamanistic healers already seem to have known: psychedelic drugs are only as useful as the guides administering them.

REFERENCES

1. Freudenmann RW, Oxler F, Bernschneider-Reif S. The origin of MDMA (ecstasy) revisited: the true story reconstructed from the original documents. *Addiction*. 2006;101(9):1241-1245. doi:10.1111/j.1360-0443.2006.01511.x
2. Hoffman A. *LSD: My Problem Child*. Multidisciplinary Association for Psychedelic Studies (MAPS); 2009:35-47.
3. Kolp E, Friedman HL, Krupitsky E, et al. Ketamine psychedelic psychotherapy: focus on its pharmacology, phenomenology, and clinical applications. In: Wolfson P, Hartelius G, eds. *The Ketamine Papers: Science, Therapy, and Transformation*. Multidisciplinary Association for Psychedelic Studies; 2016:97-197.
4. Nichols DE. Psychedelics. *Pharmacol Rev*. 2016;68(2):264-355. doi:10.1124/pr.115.011478. Erratum in: *Pharmacol Rev*. 2016;68(2):356. PMID: 26841800; PMCID: PMC4813425.
5. Wassen SH. Anthropological survey of the use of South American snuffs. In Efron DH, ed. *Ethnopharmacologic Search for Psychoactive Drugs: Proceedings of a Symposium held in San Francisco, California January 28-30, 1967*. Vol. I. Synergetic Press; 2018:233-289.
6. Arranz-Otaegui A, Carretero LG, Ramsey MN, Fuller DQ, Richter T. Archaeobotanical evidence reveals the origins of bread 14,400 years ago in northeastern Jordan. *Proc Natl Acad Sci U S A*. 2018;115(31):7925-7930. doi:10.1073/pnas.1801071115
7. Hayden B, Canuel N, Shanse J. What was brewing in the Natufian? An archaeological assessment of brewing technology in the Epipaleolithic. *J Archaeol Method Theory*. 2013;20(1):102-150.
8. O'Regan HJ, Lamb AL, Wilkinson DM. The missing mushrooms: searching for fungi in ancient human dietary analysis. *J Archaeol Sci*. 2016;75:139-143.
9. Strauss LG, González Morales MR, Carretero JM, Marín-Arroyo AB. "The Red Lady of El Mirón". Lower Magdalenian life and death in the oldest Dryas Cantabrian Spain: an overview. *J Archaeol Sci*. 2015;60:134-137.
10. Power RC, Salazar-Garcia DC, Strauss LG, González Morales MR, Henry AG. Microremains from El Mirón Cave human dental calculus suggest a mixed plant-animal subsistence economy during the Magdalenian in Northern Iberia. *J Archaeol Sci*. 2015;60:39-46.
11. El-Seedi HR, De Smet PA, Beck O, Possnert G, Bruhn JG. Prehistoric peyote use: alkaloid analysis and radiocarbon dating of archaeological specimens of Lophophora from Texas. *J Ethnopharmacol*. 2005;101(1-3):238-242. doi:10.1016/j.jep.2005.04.022. PMID: 15990261.
12. Terry M, Steelman KL, Guilderson T, Dering P, Rowe MW. Lower Pecos and Coahuila peyote: new radiocarbon dates. *J Archaeol Sci*. 2006;33(7):1017-1021. Accessed May 14, 2024. https://www.sciencedirect.com/science/article/abs/pii/S0305440305002451
13. Samorini G. The oldest archeological data evidencing the relationship of Homo sapiens with psychoactive plants: a worldwide overview. *J Psychedelic Stud*. 2019;3(2):63-80. doi:10.1556/2054.2019.008
14. Jay M. *Mescaline: A Global History of the First Psychedelic*. Yale University Press; 2021.
15. Nuwer R. This psychoactive plant could save lives—and everyone wants to cash in. *National Geographic*. Published March 8, 2023. Accessed February 27, 2024. https://www.nationalgeographic.com/animals/article/ibogaine-pschedelic-drug-root-fair-trade-gabon

16. Guzmán G. New taxonomical and ethnomycological observations on Psilocybe s.s. (Fungi, Basidiomycota, Agaricomycetidae, Agaricales, Strophariaceae) from Mexico, Africa, and Spain. *Acta Bot Mex*. 2012;100:79-106. Accessed May 14, 2024. https://www.redalyc.org/pdf/574/57424406004.pdf
17. Smith H. *Cleansing the Doors of Perception: The Religious Significance of Entheogenic Plants and Chemicals*. Jeremy P. Tarcher/Putnam; 2000:45-63.
18. Ingalls DHH. Not hashish, hops, datura, ephedra, sacrostemma or rhubarb. New York Times. Published September 5, 1971. Accessed May 15, 2024. https://timesmachine.nytimes.com/timesmachine/1971/09/05/79152637.html?pageNumber=83
19. Graves R. *The Greek Myths*. Vol 1. Penguin Books; 1974:89-96.
20. Muraresku BC. *The Immortality Key: The Secret History of the Religion with No Name*. St. Martin's Press; 2020:1-36.
21. de Sahagún FB. *Historia General de las Cosas de Nueva España*. Alfa. Quoted in Spiers N, Ciauby Labate B, Ermakova AO, Farrell P, González Romero OS, Gabriell I, Olvera N. Indigenous psilocybin mushroom practices: an annotated bibliography. *J Psychedelic Stud*. 2024;8(1):3-25. doi:10.1556/2054.2023.00297
22. Peoples HC, Duda P, Marlowe FW. Hunter-gatherers and the origins of religion. *Hum Nat*. 2016;27(3):261-282. doi:10.1007/s12110-016-9260-0
23. Winkelman MJ. The evolved psychology of psychedelic set and setting: inferences regarding the roles of shamanism and entheogenic ecopsychology. *Front Pharmacol*. 2021;12:619890. doi:10.3389/fphar.2021.619890. PMID: 33732156; PMCID: PMC7959790.
24. Goutarel R, Gollnhofer O, Sillans R. Pharmacodynamics and therapeutic applications of iboga and ibogaine (Gladstone WJ, trans). *Psychedelic Monogr Essays*. 1993;6:71-111.
25. Timmermann C, Bauer PR, Gosseries O, et al. A neurophenomenological approach to non-ordinary states of consciousness: hypnosis, meditation, and psychedelics. *Trends Cogn Sci*. 2023;27(2):139-159. doi:10.1016/j.tics.2022.11.006. PMID: 36566091.
26. Gattuso JJ, Perkins D, Ruffell S, et al. Default mode network modulation by psychedelics: a systematic review. *Int J Neuropsychopharmacol*. 2023;26(3):155-188. doi:10.1093/ijnp/pyac074. PMID: 36272145; PMCID: PMC10032309.
27. Bravo G, Grob C. Shamans, sacraments, and psychiatrists. *J Psychoactive Drugs*. 1989;21(1):123-128. doi:10.1080/02791072.1989.10472149

3

Clinical History

This chapter gives the reader insight into how clinical work involving psychedelics fits within the broader cultural and historical context of the first seven decades of the 20th century. It also highlights how these drugs were used by medical professionals prior to being subject to increasingly strict regulations that ultimately culminated in the Controlled Substances Act (CSA) of 1970. Consequently, the CSA made researching psychedelics prohibitively cumbersome. Many of the cultural figures typically associated with psychedelics during the 1960s (Ken Kesey, Tom Wolfe, the Grateful Dead, etc) will be omitted from this history, as this chapter's focus is less cultural and more clinical. This chapter should not be considered a chronicle of psychedelics in the 20th century but an abridged history of the clinical work of scientists and researchers.

Psychedelics From the 1800s to 1950

The majority of psychedelics described in this book are alkaloids, which are nitrogen-containing compounds that occur naturally in plants as secondary metabolites (sometimes also referred to as allelochemicals). Secondary metabolites primarily prevent predation or regulate growth, and alkaloids can be found in varying quantities in approximately 20% of plant species.[1] Many of these alkaloid-containing plants have been used as medicines (eg, quinine), drugs of misuse (eg, cocaine), poisons (eg, strychnine), or all three (eg, opioids).[2]

While traditional healers use the entire plant when providing care to patients, beginning in the 19th century, Western chemists began isolating the therapeutic alkaloids found in these plants. The first of these compounds to be isolated, by Friedrich Wilhelm Sertürner, is still in use today and is perhaps one of the most well-known drugs in the world: morphine.[3] Sertürner first published his findings in 1806 on what was originally referred to as "morphium"—in reference to Morpheus, the Greek god of dreams—leading researchers across Europe to begin hunting for other useful alkaloids. Strychnine was isolated in 1817, followed by caffeine in 1820, and then nicotine in 1828.[3] Additional alkaloids discovered in the 19th century include capsaicin, quinine, atropine, harmine, cocaine, and ephedrine.

Mescaline, ibogaine, *N,N*-dimethyltryptamine (DMT), and psilocybin are also alkaloids. The first of these compounds to be isolated was mescaline by Arthur Heffter just before the turn of the century—in 1897.[4(p70)] The compound was isolated from a sample of peyote cactus, while ibogaine was first isolated from the iboga plant in 1901 by Dybowski and Landrin.[5] DMT was synthesized in 1931 by Richard Helmuth and Frederick Manske and was then discovered in the root bark of *Mimosa hostilis* by Oswaldo Gonçalves de Lima in 1946.[6] Lysergic acid, "the nucleus common to all ergot alkaloids" was discovered by W. A. Jacobs and L. C. Craig of the Rockefeller Institute of New York in the early 1930s.[4(pp40,41)] Of note, lysergic acid diethylamide (LSD) was first synthesized by Albert Hofmann in 1938,[4(p44)] and, 20 years later, Hofmann isolated psilocybin from mushroom specimens (*Psilocybe mexicana*) taken from Mexico.[4(pp125-129)]

Early Studies With Mescaline

The use of psychedelics had been commonplace among many cultures throughout the Americas prior to European contact, but thereafter the practice became so suppressed that, by the 19th century, knowledge of these drugs' existence was rare outside of a few remote locations where authorities had little influence. In most cases, these areas were deep in the jungles of Central and South America or in the desert regions of northern Mexico.

However, this began to change in the 1850s when the use of peyote began to spread among Native American cultures who had no prior history of use. Reports of peyote use began to appear in American newspapers, where it was sometimes referred to as "whiskey root."[7(p65)]

The phenomenon was largely a result of many different tribes being forcefully relocated to Oklahoma, where they were introduced to cultures and healers who had traditionally used the cactus. Despite several bans on peyote trading and sales, as well as an effort to disrupt what became known as "the peyote cult," use continued to spread into the 20th century and eventually led to the founding of the Native American Church in 1918 (see Chapter 4).

Though some studies involving peyote had occurred during the 1880s and early 1890s, it was not until 1895 that the very first human trial was conducted by Daniel Webster Prentiss and Francis Morgan at what is today George Washington University in Washington, DC.[8] The team administered peyote to several individuals, the first being the 27-year-old chemist who was introduced at the beginning of Chapter 1 and had been given five buttons but developed nausea soon after consuming three, and only later continued taking the rest. According to the chemist's notes that were published in Prentiss and Morgan's paper, he began to notice brilliant designs and colors about 2 hours after the experiment began. "These visions were so pleasing that I at once decided to continue the experiment, and I placed the fourth and part of the fifth button in my mouth," he wrote. "Then followed a train of delightful visions such as no human being ever enjoyed under normal conditions."[8]

Other reports soon followed, eventually piquing the interest of Havelock Ellis, a British doctor, who was also a progressive, writer, and social reformer. On Good Friday in 1897, he performed a self-experiment with peyote (which he referred to as "mescal") and later described it in an article, "Mescal: A New Artificial Paradise," that first appeared in *The Lancet* in 1897.[7(pp91-93)] A more substantial version was published in early 1898 in the *Contemporary Review*, a progressive literary quarterly. The article was clearly written for a more literary audience and centered on the visual content of the experience, which Ellis described as "an orgy of vision" and "an optical fairyland, where all the senses now and again join the play."[9] "Mescal," he wrote, "does not wholly carry us away from the actual world, or plunge us into oblivion; a large part of its charm lies in the halo of beauty which it casts around the simplest and commonest things."[16] At one point, Ellis even insinuates that a mescaline experience is necessary if one wants to fully appreciate the works of the poet William Wordsworth. He concludes with the following: "It may at least be claimed that for a healthy person to be once or twice-admitted the rites of mescal is not only an unforgettable delight but an educational influence of no mean value."[9]

Ellis's glowing review of the mescaline experience and flagrant encouragement of use among aspiring poets looking for inspiration successfully created a demand for mescaline among artists, though use never became widespread. Some of the most well-known individuals within Ellis's circle of friends to experiment with mescaline were the poets W.B. Yeats and Arthur Symons.[7(pp79-100)] Mescaline use continued in certain circles well into the 20th century, particularly among artists and intellectuals like Walter Benjamin, Stanisław Ignacy Witkiewicz, Gheorghe Marinescu, Antonin Artaud, and Maurice Merleau-Ponty. It would also become popular among occultists, the most notorious of which being Aleister Crowley.[7(pp147-223)]

Mescaline was first synthesized in 1919 by Ernst Späth.[7(pp79-100)] The following year, the manufacture of synthetic mescaline began by Merck, and it stirred increased clinical interest.[4(p70)] Of particular note, are the studies conducted by Kurt Beringer at Heidelberg University. Beringer administered mescaline in doses ranging from 200 to 600 mg to 60 study participants during the 1920s. He published his results in the 1927 book *Der Meskalinrausch* (Mescaline Intoxication), where he concluded that there were no therapeutic applications for the drug.[7(pp131-146)]

Despite an apparent lack of therapeutic applications, studies involving mescaline continued into the 1930s.[7(pp171-198)] Many researchers (including Beringer) found that its administration led individuals to exhibit symptoms akin to psychosis, with Beringer suggesting that mescaline intoxication and psychosis might share a similar biologic basis.[7(pp131-146)] Consequently, mescaline began to be referred to as a psychotomimetic drug, meaning that it mimics psychosis.[10] While some psychiatrists, such as Walter Frederking, found that smaller doses of mescaline could facilitate the exploration of patients' memories and symbolic associations during talk therapy, by the end of the 1930s and the beginning of the 1940s, the growing consensus among psychiatrists was that mescaline might prove useful in the study of model psychosis—an experimentally produced psychotic state.[7(pp171-198)]

Ergot and the Precursors to Lysergic Acid Diethylamide

Claviceps purpurea is an ergot fungus that grows parasitically primarily on rye (*Secale cereale*), though it has been known to grow on other cereal grains and grasses. Ergot poisoning can lead to ergotism, which may come in two forms. Convulsive ergotism (*Ergotismus convulsivus*) is characterized by convulsions, paranoia, and hallucinations, while gangrenous ergotism (*Ergotismus gangraenosus*) is characterized by peripheral neuropathy, edema, and the death and loss of affecting areas (oftentimes fingers and toes).[11] The burning sensation associated with the latter affliction was once known as St. Anthony's fire.[11]

Ergot was identified as early as 1100 BCE in China and was referred to as a "noxious pustule in the ear of grain" on an Assyrian tablet dating back to approximately 600 BCE.[12(pp39-41)] As rye flour was a relatively common part of the European diet during the Middle Ages, epidemics of ergotism appear sporadically in the historic record, perhaps the most significant of which occurred in France during 944 and 945 CE, when an estimated 20,000 people died after consuming contaminated rye flour.[13] Even though rye contaminated with ergot was eventually recognized as the pathogen responsible for these afflictions, cases of ergotism were still being reported in Russia, England, Ethiopia, and India well into the 20th century.[11]

In addition to causing mass deaths, ergot poisoning may have also led to mass delusions, with some historians arguing that witch trials (including the ones that took place in Salem, Massachusetts, between 1692 and 1693) may have been caused by paranoia brought on by convulsive ergotism.[11] Some mystic religious movements during the Middle Ages may have also been influenced by ergotism.[14] As mentioned in the previous chapter, an ergot derivative similar to LSD may have been an ingredient in *kykeon*, which was consumed ritualistically by participants in the Eleusinian Mysteries.[15]

Recognition that grain contaminated with the fungus could lead to disease was made in Europe during the 1500s and 1600s, and in 1853, Louis René Tulasne formally identified ergot as being the pathogen responsible for ergotism.[11]

Medicinal Uses of Ergot

Though ergot is poisonous, as early as 1100 BCE, Chinese physicians recognized that it could be used in obstetrics as an ecbolic to induce uterine contractions, and similar claims were made by Hippocrates and Ayurvedic doctors in the 4th century BCE. Midwives in Europe were also using ergot to accelerate parturition or as an abortifacient at least as far back as the 1500s.[13]

Throughout the 1800s and early 1900s, ergot was only rarely used as an ecbolic in the United States and Europe due to difficulties in assessing proper dosage, though it was somewhat regularly employed to stop excessive bleeding during or after childbirth.[4(p40)] The alkaloid largely responsible for this effect, ergometrine, was isolated in 1932 by Harold Dudley and John Chassar Moir and is currently on the World Health Organization's List of Essential Medicines.

Just a few years earlier, the British scientists Henry Hallett Dale and George Barger had isolated ergotoxine (a combination of ergocristine, ergocornine, and ergocryptine—not a pure alkaloid) from ergot and subsequently found that the alkaloid mixture inhibited sympathetic nerve function, which helped lay the foundation for Dale's future work on chemical neurotransmission, as well as the development of β-adrenergic agonists.[16] Dale and Otto Loewi would eventually share the 1936 Nobel Prize for their work on neurotransmission and acetylcholine.[12(pp29-88)]

Albert Hofmann and Lysergic Acid Diethylamide

Like many research chemists before him, Albert Hofmann hoped to isolate the active principles of medicinal plants and to develop more effective and stable medicines that could be mass produced and easily distributed around the world. In 1929, not long after finishing his studies at the University of Zurich, he joined the Sandoz Company's pharmaceutical-chemical research laboratory in the Swiss city of Basel, where he worked under Professor Arthur Stoll, who had isolated ergotamine from ergot in 1918.[4(pp35-38)]

One of the first tasks Hofmann sets his mind to was devising a novel way to prepare ergometrine synthetically, which he did by combining lysergic acid with propanolamine, an amino acid. According to Hofmann, he was able to improve upon the therapeutic properties of ergometrine by combining lysergic acid with butanolamine, producing methylergometrine (Methergine).[4(p44)] This drug is also on the World Health Organization's List of Essential Medicines.

Hofmann continued his work with ergot alkaloids, combining lysergic acid with more than two dozen amines. In 1938, Hofmann produced the 25th substance within this series (lysergic acid diethylamide 25 or LSD-25), which produced no special interest during animal testing. The ostensibly boring drug was shelved and forgotten.

Bicycle Day

In the Spring of 1943, Hofmann decided to synthesize LSD-25 once again for further testing. This was not a common practice, since substances without clear pharmacologic purposes are typically abandoned following initial testing. However, on April 16, 1943, as Hofmann underwent the final step of purifying and crystalizing LSD-25 in the form of a tartrate, he began to feel strange and went home. As he later wrote to Professor Stoll:

> At home, I lay down and sank into a not unpleasant intoxicated-like condition, characterized by an extremely stimulated imagination. In a dreamlike state, with eyes closed (I found the daylight to be unpleasantly glaring), I perceived an uninterrupted stream of fantastic pictures,

extraordinary shapes with intense, kaleidoscopic play of colors. After some two hours this condition faded away.[4(p47)]

Hofmann immediately recognized that LSD-25 was behind these bizarre effects, but he was puzzled. He had always kept a meticulously clean workstation due to the toxicity of ergot, so Hofmann surmised that a very small amount of LSD had caused the effects, likely after being absorbed through his skin. To test this hypothesis, he decided to conduct a self-experiment with what he believed would be a very small dose: 0.25 mg.[4(pp47,48)]

The following is from Hofmann's laboratory journal:

> *4/19/43 16:20: 0.5 cc of ½ promil aqueous solution of diethylamide tartrate orally = 0.25 mg tartrate. Taken diluted with about 10 cc water. Tasteless. 17:00: Beginning dizziness, feeling of anxiety, visual distortions, symptoms of paralysis, desire to laugh. Supplement of 4/21: Home by bicycle [emphasis added]. From 18:00-ca.20:00 most severe crisis.*[4(p48)]

Recent studies have found that modest drug effects of LSD may be felt at dosages as low as 25 μg and that psychedelic experiences occur at dosages as low as 50 μg.[17] Hofmann had taken 5 times that amount. As he recounts in his memoir, the experience was not initially pleasant. Once home, objects that had once been familiar began to morph into grotesque, animated forms, and he felt that he was either going mad or dying; however, this was temporary. By the time a doctor arrived and observed that Hofmann was not in mortal danger, the subjective effects had become less horrifying. He eventually began to experience synesthesia (in this case experiencing sounds as optical perceptions), which he enjoyed. Once the effects wore off, he then slept and felt invigorated upon waking. "When I later walked out into the garden, in which the sun shone now after a spring rain, everything glistened and sparkled in a fresh light," he wrote. "The world was as if newly created. All my senses vibrated in a condition of highest sensitivity, which persisted for the entire day."[4(pp50,51)]

Incredulous that such a small dose of a substance could produce such profound effects, three colleagues from Sandoz took one-third of the dose Hofmann had taken. Any doubt about the potency of Hofmann's new discovery quickly vanished.[4(p52)] By 1947, Sandoz had begun marketing LSD under the name Delysid for use in analytic psychotherapy. In addition, experimental studies involving model psychosis began in which LSD was self-administered or administered to "normal subjects" at the psychiatrist's discretion.[4(pp63-78)] LSD became available in the United States in 1949. By today's standards, the notion that any researcher (which was quite liberally defined) could request and receive a freely distributed drug would clearly seem like a recipe for disaster, but this policy remained in effect until Sandoz halted production of Delysid in 1965.[18(p143)]

Psychedelics From 1950 to 1970

Psychiatry during the first half of the 20th century had been dominated by the practice of psychoanalysis. This began to change in the late 1940s and early 1950s, as greater emphasis began to be placed on neurobiology and psychopharmacology, especially given the promise of recently discovered drugs such as lithium and chlorpromazine. The former was a highly effective mood stabilizer, while the latter was the first antipsychotic, and this helped contribute to a larger sense of optimism within psychiatry.

LSD fit within this positivistic and optimistic zeitgeist in a way that mescaline did not. The latter was far less potent than LSD and was more likely to cause nausea and some other unpleasant side effects, and LSD very quickly overtook mescaline as the drug of choice among psychedelic research. The isolation of psilocybin in 1958 and its subsequent rise in popularity led to a further decline in interest in mescaline. To this day, the use of mescaline (either plant based or synthetic) in clinical settings is relatively rare.

Throughout the 1950s, researchers who regularly used psychedelics began to gain an appreciation of how "set and setting" affect the psychedelic experience, but while early researchers had no such appreciation. Moreover, regulations were extremely lax when it came to the testing of experimental pharmaceuticals, and the conditions in which early experiments were conducted are almost beyond comprehension. In fact, prior to the passing of the 1962 Kefauver-Harris Amendments to the 1938 Food, Drug, and Cosmetic Act, researchers did not even need to obtain informed consent before administering experimental drugs. However, these amendments were made primarily due to the scandal involving the unrestricted experimental use of thalidomide (which causes severe birth defects in children).[18(p146)] It is worth noting here that prior to the early 1960s, clinicians also regularly self-administered drugs—something that was extremely common with psychedelics.

Suffice to say that many studies from this time lack the standards of what would be considered credible research today. At best, they serve as anecdotal reports or observational studies, and many failed to record any objective data at all. Concerns about lost objectivity are also rampant throughout pre-prohibition studies, as researchers became psychedelic zealots or simply biased study participants via the subject-expectancy effect. Still, the volume of research is quite impressive, as there were an estimated 40,000 individuals who received doses of classic psychedelics (primarily LSD) from the 1950s through 1965.[19] Over 1,000 papers on these drugs were published throughout the mid-late 20th century.[20]

Model Psychosis and M-Substance

At the beginning of the 1950s, the prevailing opinion about mescaline and the newly discovered LSD was that the two drugs were psychotomimetic. Their clinical utility came from their ability to induce temporary psychosis.

To further understand the relationship between psychedelics, such as LSD and mescaline, and psychotic disorders, several research teams in the early 1950s administered these drugs to hospitalized patients with schizophrenia or bipolar disorder. They found that the drugs typically exacerbated symptoms of schizophrenia or mania. Of note, a distinguishing feature between psychosis and the psychedelic state emerged, as researchers found that auditory hallucinations were common among the former and that psychedelics primarily produced visual disturbances.[21]

It was also during the 1950s that Humphry Osmond and John Smythies introduced the notion that psychedelics did not merely induce a state akin to psychosis; they hypothesized that psychedelics were chemically similar to an undiscovered and endogenous hallucinogen that caused schizophrenia and other psychotic disorders. They argued that the administration of psychedelics produced short "trips" (psychotic episodes), while the endogenous hallucinogen ("M-substance") was part of a "chemical imbalance" that produced the long-term symptoms of psychosis.[10] Upon moving to Weyburn Mental Hospital in the Canadian province of Saskatchewan, Osmond paired up with Abram Hoffer where they continued to try and identify the mysterious M-substance. They also began conducting clinical tests to see if these drugs could treat alcoholism based on the notion and hypothesis that the psychedelic experience would induce a kind of conversion experience similar to delirium tremens.

Lysergic Acid Diethylamide and Alcohol Use Disorder

The theory that M-substance plays a role in schizophrenia or psychosis did not stand up to scrutiny and was largely dismissed by the end of the 1950s. Similarly, Osmond and Hoffer's belief that the psychedelic experience is akin to delirium tremens did not hold water. However, LSD did seem capable of treating alcohol use disorder by granting patients the power of increased introspection and clear self-reflection, as well as other mechanisms that are still unclear and being studied.

The team in Saskatchewan treated more than 700 individuals with alcohol use disorder over the course of approximately a decade, finding that about half of the patients became sober and remained sober for at least several months.[18(pp144-152)] Even Bill Wilson, the founder of Alcoholics Anonymous, believed in the therapy and participated in LSD-assisted psychotherapy sessions while in California during the 1950s.[18(pp152,153)] By the end of the decade, the Saskatchewan provincial government had begun writing a policy that would make LSD a standard treatment option for individuals with alcoholism, but some skepticism about LSD's seemingly miraculous results persisted.

This skepticism appeared justified when the Addiction Research Foundation in Toronto attempted to replicate the findings of Osmond and Hoffer by isolating the effects of the drug from other variables, including set and setting. More specifically, they strapped study participants to a bed, administered doses of LSD as high as 800 μg, and then watched what happened.[22] It should be noted that 800 μg represents a dose 3 times higher than Hofmann's first self-administered dose.

Set and Setting

As it turns out, clinicians play a vital role in optimizing the efficacy of psychedelics in treating alcohol use disorder or any other psychiatric condition. This is something that the team in Saskatchewan had understood implicitly. Even if one patient had a solely blissful, transcendent experience and one endured something that was ostensibly horrifying, both individuals could walk away from the experience with a new appreciation if they received appropriate clinical support from therapists. In other words, a challenging experience is not necessarily a bad experience from a therapeutic perspective.

That said, the team still wanted to avoid putting patients through terrifying experiences, and over a period spanning hundreds of sessions they learned that they could minimize "bad trips" by administering the drugs in a supportive environment with an attentive therapist. While they did not coin the phrase "set and setting" (that would be Timothy Leary in the early 1960s), they recognized that the variability of the psychedelic experience was not entirely random, and that proper preparation and the creation of a comfortable environment helped to minimize bad trips. Conversely, sterile environments often made patients feel alienated, white lab coats made patients fearful of being interrogated or judged, and locks and restraints made patients paranoid.[10]

Unfortunately, this was all lost on the team at the Addiction Research Foundation. In addition to restraining patients and giving them an exceptionally high dose, those who administered the LSD were instructed not to talk with volunteers.[18(pp144-152)] It should have come as no surprise that the study failed to replicate the results reported by Osmond and Hoffer.

Psycholytic and Psychedelic-Assisted Psychotherapy

During the 1950s, psychedelics became associated less with psychotic models and more as a means to enhance the therapeutic utility of psychotherapy. *"In LSD inebriation the accustomed worldview undergoes a deep-seating transformation and disintegration,"* Hofmann wrote in his autobiography, *LSD: My Problem Child*. *"Connected with this is a loosening or even suspension of the I-you barrier. Patients who are bogged down in an egocentric problem cycle can thereby be helped to release themselves from their fixation and isolation."* Hofmann continues, noting that, *"LSD does not act as a true medicament; rather, it plays the role of a drug aid in the context of psychoanalytic and psychotherapeutic treatment and serves to channel the treatment more effectively and to shorten its duration."*[4(p74)]

From this new conceptual understanding stemmed two distinct types of therapy involving LSD, mescaline, and (eventually) psilocybin. Though related, they are distinct. In both treatments, patients undergo extensive preparatory sessions, as well as subsequent integration sessions, and they are accompanied by at least one therapist (more commonly two) during their psychedelic sessions.[4(p75)]

The first, *psycholytic treatment*, relies on moderately strong doses of psychedelics administered across multiple therapy sessions. It is more popular in Europe and oftentimes involves group discussions and expression therapy following sessions when the psychedelic is administered. During the 1950s, it was also quite popular in the United States as a treatment for "neurotic disorders" that may have included anything from personality disorders to "sexual disorders" or even "residual schizophrenia."[21] In studies that took place in both Europe and the United States prior to 1970, patients often reported significant improvements, but there were no real objective measurements for said improvements and no controls.[21]

The second, psychedelic therapy or *psychedelic-assisted psychotherapy*, relies on a very large dose of a psychedelic meant to induce a mystical-type experience. It was and continues to be more popular in the United States. Once again, there had been a lack of objective measures and control groups in studies published prior to 1970.

A notable exception concerns the work at Spring Grove State Hospital and the Maryland Psychiatric Research Center, both located in Baltimore. A total of 243 patients with a variety of conditions participated in LSD and mescaline studies there during the 1960s and even into the 1970s. A formal framework was developed to include emotional support from two therapists (typically one man and one woman) but without interpretation of the psychedelic experience during the session. Follow-up occurred the following day and thereafter at 1, 2, 4, 8, and 12 weeks and once again at 6 months. Doses ranged between 200 and 300 μg for LSD, with 200 to 400 mg of mescaline to potentiate the effect in some patients. Of the first 113 patients to receive a questionnaire following their experience, 93 replied and 83% reported a lasting benefit, while 76% reported improvement in symptoms 3 months after dosing and 85% reported improvements both in the 3- to 6-month range and even after 1 year.[21]

It should be noted that though both psycholytic and psychedelic-assisted therapies have shown efficacy over the years, the vast majority of the clinical trials discussed in this book use the psychedelic-assisted psychotherapy model, which was pioneered by Osmond and Hoffer. In fact, Osmond coined the term *"psychedelic"* in the following couplet:

> *To fathom Hell or go angelic*
> *Just take a pinch of psychedelic.*

One Bright May Morning

In addition to introducing the term "psychedelic" to the world, in May 1953 Osmond introduced the famed British intellectual Aldous Huxley to 400 mg of mescaline.[7(pp171-202)] In fact, the above couplet appeared in a letter written to Huxley a few years later.

Following the experience, Huxley went on to produce one of the most well-known books within psychedelic literature, *The Doors of Perception*. Published in 1954, it laid much of the intellectual groundwork that would characterize the kind of psychedelic-associated mysticism that emerged in the 1950s and 1960s and persists even today.[18(pp159-164)] One of the most enduring tenets of Huxley's thought was perennialism, a philosophical position that regards all earnest spiritual and religious teachings as manifestations of a core metaphysical truth.

Mystical-type experiences that are achieved through non-ordinary states of consciousness, whether under the influence of psychedelics or not, oftentimes leave individual's feeling as though they have glimpsed this truth.

Psychedelics began to permeate some of the most notable works of fiction to emerge from the avant-garde movements of the 1950s, perhaps most clearly within the novels of William S. Burroughs and the poetry of Allen Ginsberg. Of course, by the end of the Psychedelic Sixties, this would expand into popular books, music, film, television, and virtually all other forms of art.

The Arrival of Psilocybin

Up until the 1950s, people in the West were not sure if the stories about psychedelic mushrooms originating from the jungles of Central America were real or exaggerations of early Spanish conquistadors. Some scholars contended that the early chroniclers had simply mistaken peyote for a mushroom.[4(p120)]

This changed with the publication of a *Life* magazine article in 1957 in which R. Gordon Wasson introduced the world to the Mexican town of Huautla de Jiménez; as well as a Mazatec woman named "Eva Méndez" (real name María Sabina); and the *velada*, a ceremony that involved the use of psilocybin mushrooms.[18(pp104-114)] Wasson—a retired banker and amateur mycologist who would later propose the identity of soma to be fly agaric (*Amanita muscaria*)—described the ceremony in vivid detail and his article, "Seeking the Magic Mushroom," caught the attention of the world. It would prove ruinous for Sabina and Huautla de Jiménez, as the previously quiet community became a destination for beatniks, then hippies and celebrities seeking their own magic mushroom experience. Sabina's home was even burned to the ground, and, unfortunately, she even spent time in jail.[18(p114)]

Samples of the magic mushroom (*Psilocybe mexicana*) ultimately made their way to Europe for analysis.[4] In 1958, Albert Hofmann isolated psilocybin from the specimens, and psilocybin was synthesized that same year. Starting in 1960, Sandoz briefly began marketing Indocybin, the trade name for synthetic psilocybin.[23] As was the case with Delysid, Sandoz made Indocybin freely available to researchers.

Timothy Leary and Extra-Scientific Uses of Psychedelics

Psychologist Timothy Leary was first introduced to psilocybin in Mexico in 1960.[18(pp185-203)] The experience changed him and his colleague at Harvard University, Richard Alpert (later known as Ram Dass), who are often credited or blamed (depending on one's perspective) for introducing a generation of young people to psychedelics and/or allowing psychedelics to "escape from the lab."

This is a gross oversimplification. Members of the general public were well aware of psychedelics such as mescaline, psilocybin, and LSD prior to Leary's first psychedelic experience. Throughout the 1950s, articles had been regularly published in popular magazines, journals, and newspapers about these drugs. Just a few examples include:

- Sidney Katz's "My Twelve Hours as a Madman," published in *MacLean's* ("Canada's National Magazine") on October 1, 1953
- Wilfried Zeller's "Ein kuhnes wissenschaftliches Experiment," [a daring scientific experiment] published in the German magazine *Quick* on March 21, 1954
- Robert M. Goldenson's "Step into the World of the Insane," published in *Look* magazine on September 21, 1954
- Aldous Huxley's "Drugs That Shape Men's Minds," published in *The Saturday Evening Post* on October 18, 1958
- Laura Bergquist's "The Curious Story Behind the New Cary Grant," published in *Look* magazine on September 1, 1959

Cary Grant, one of the most well-known stars from Hollywood's Golden Age, became especially vocal about his support for psycholytic therapy, which he credited with giving him peace of mind. However, Grant's endorsement, at least in the *Look* article noted earlier, was not for psychedelics—it was for psycholytic therapy. Conversely, Leary endorsed the unsupervised use of psychedelics while proselytizing about a cultural and spiritual revolution.

The beginnings of this revolution were rather modest when Leary and Alpert launched the Harvard Psilocybin Project in 1960 at five Divinity Avenue in Cambridge. The two were given a great deal of latitude with the project, but one of the lines they were told not to cross concerned the distribution of psychedelics to undergraduate students. Meanwhile, the graduate students who took part in the project's seminars were given the opportunity to participate in "consciousness-expanding" experiences with psilocybin, which they were meant to document almost as a form of fieldwork.[18(pp185-203)]

The sessions quickly began to look more like parties, which led to concerns, and then complaints. Eventually, a meeting was called in March 1962 in the hope of reigning in the project's "naturalistic" use of psychedelics and cavalier approach to research. A journalist for the *Crimson*, the university's newspaper, was in attendance, and the publication of their article about the Psilocybin Project's freewheeling use of psychedelics led to a national scandal. The project was ultimately shut down in 1963 amidst more controversy stemming from the allegation that Alpert had provided undergraduate students with psychedelics. Leary was dismissed that same year for failing to show up to class.[18(pp185-203)]

Ultimately, for all the sound and fury of the Harvard Psilocybin Project, it produced little of scientific merit. Leary can be credited with coining the phrase "set and setting," but the Concord Prison Experiment, which tested recidivism rates between individuals who received psilocybin versus those who did not and is the study for which Leary is most famous, was found to be deeply flawed by later analysis (conducted by Rick Doblin).[24] A major exception was the Good Friday Experiment, with which Leary was only tangentially involved.

The Good Friday Experiment

Walter Pahnke was a graduate student at Harvard Divinity School in the early 1960s. Though he was a medical doctor, he also had a strong interest in mysticism and had become intrigued by the use of psychedelics and their ability to occasion mystical experiences. Pahnke believed that psychedelic drugs could facilitate mystical experiences in individuals with religious inclinations if they were given the drug in a religious setting. This ultimately became the subject of his doctorate, and as part of his research, he designed a double-blind, placebo-controlled experiment where he would give 10 volunteers an active placebo (nicotinic acid or niacin) and 10 volunteers psilocybin.[25(pp99-105)] Additionally, 10 guides were recruited. One of the guides was Huston Smith, a highly esteemed scholar of philosophy and religious studies, who was a professor of philosophy at the Massachusetts Institute of Technology from 1958 until 1973 and authored what was for many years the standard textbook on world religions, aptly titled *The World's Religions*.

While designing his experiment, Pahnke worked with Leary and Alpert, but he also received the blessing of Rev. Howard Thurman, the Dean of Marsh Chapel at Boston University, to use the basement of the building to conduct the experiment.[25(pp99-105)] The basement was home to several conference rooms and a self-contained chapel with an altar, pews, stained glass windows, and religious symbols. On Good Friday, April 20, 1962, the 20 subjects and 10 volunteer guides entered the basement of the chapel. From the main chapel upstairs, Thurman's two-and-a-half-hour service was broadcast. Subjects were divided into five groups of four and each group had two guides. Half of the subjects and half of the guides in each group received niacin. Half of the subjects in each group received 30 mg of psilocybin, while half of the guides also received psilocybin, though at a smaller dose than subjects (15 mg).[26]

Smith was one of the guides who received psilocybin. He was already a well-known scholar of religion who had received his PhD in 1945 and had already taught for almost 15 years; his description of the experience is rather remarkable. Though Smith says he had always believed in God, "I had had no direct personal encounter with God of the sort that bhakti yogis, Pentecostals, and born-again Christians describe. The Good Friday Experiment changed that," Smith said, several decades after the experiment. Many of the other individuals who received psilocybin that day felt the same way—the same could not be said for controls.

Turning Off

Such a response alludes to one of the main problems that continue to dog psychedelic experiment: blinding. If half of a group of people involved in a study with a psychedelic feel a slight tingling sensation and the other half believe they are cultivating a personal relationship with God, the idea of control and blinding goes out the window. Other methodologic problems began to arise (eg, participant bias due to the subject-expectancy effect, lack of objectivity on the part of researchers, inadequate follow-up), and it soon became clear that, though roughly 1,000 papers on psychedelics were published between the early 1950s and the late 1960s—involving approximately 40,000 test subjects to treat a laundry list of conditions that included depression, alcoholism, obsessive-compulsive disorder, and end of life anxiety—many of them had not been well designed and could not be held up to proper scrutiny.[18(pp44,45)] As noted in Chapter 1, methodologic difficulties continue to be an issue with studies involving psychedelics, with proper blinding being the most significant challenge.

Methodologic scruples were soon overshadowed by more pressing and cultural concerns. As the 1960s progressed, Leary became increasingly famous as he encouraged a generation of young people to use psychedelics in uncontrolled settings and "turn on, tune in, drop out." Though he considered himself the "high priest" of psychedelics, he soon became just one guru among many as the countercultural movement continued to spread. This led to a moral panic among concerned parents, politicians, and authorities by the mid-1960s and would not subside for nearly a decade.

Concurrently, new regulations, including the 1962 Kefauver-Harris Amendment noted earlier and the Drug Abuse Control Amendments of 1965, made it more difficult for researchers to access psychedelics. The former requires firms to prove that a drug is safe and provide evidence of efficacy for the intended use. The latter, which went into effect in 1966, banned the possession of psychedelics and identified them as controlled substances, meaning that a license was needed to manufacture or distribute them (possession of LSD would not be criminalized until yet another amendment to the Food, Drug, and Cosmetic Act was passed in 1968). These restrictions, in conjunction with the growing ferocity of the reaction against psychedelics and the counterculture movement, led Sandoz to announce that they would end production of Indocybin and Delysid in August of 1965.

Though the CSA of 1970 is oftentimes blamed for making research into psychedelics (and cannabis) too cumbersome, it did not come out of the blue. The first bricks in the wall that would long obstruct psychedelic research were laid in the 1960s as organizations such as the U.S. Food and Drug Administration (FDA) were given more authority to regulate the use of drugs. It's worth noting that psychedelics had nothing to do with the initial push to better regulate pharmaceutical companies. Instead, they were put in place after thalidomide—which was used as a sedative and for morning sickness and was approved in West Germany during the late 1950s and early 1960s—was shown to cause severe birth defects. Due to inadequate human testing, this connection was not established until thousands of children had been affected.[27]

A Shortcut to Mystical Experiences

As the obstacles to psychedelic research were being instituted, debate continued among philosophers and theologians about the use of psychedelics to evoke mystical experiences or, in the phrasing of the time, spiritual awakenings. According to some, psychedelics could only offer an ersatz experience lacking the full magnitude of a spontaneous mystical experience or one induced by non-psychedelic means (eg, fasting, self-flagellation, transcendental meditation).[25(pp15-32)] Smith, who had participated in the Good Friday Experiment, disagreed. In his 1964 essay, "Do Drugs Have Religious Import?" he argued, "Given the right set and setting, the drugs can induce religious experiences that are indistinguishable from such experiences that occur spontaneously."[25(p20)]

As more people experimented with psychedelics, Smith's tone began to change. His 1967 essay, "Psychedelic Theophanies and the Religious Life," which first appeared in the liberal Protestant journal *Christianity and Crisis*, is a notable departure from his position only 3 years prior. While he begins with a clear affirmation ("Psychedelic experiences can be religious") and states that psychedelic experiences can result in religious experiences and even theophanies (ie, encounters with visible/sensible manifestations of the divine), the essay is indicative of a widespread change among academicians who had been very enthusiastic and optimistic about psychedelics. While clinical researchers may have begun to doubt whether their therapeutic value was worth the dangers associated with uncontrolled use, Smith's concern was more that their use was being cheapened. He did not see how a "psychedelic movement" could survive if it lacked a clear-eyed social program, felt no bounds to moral or legal restraints, and did nothing to prepare individuals for the psychedelic experience. On the last point, Huston was particularly damning, alluding to Jesus' advice about not casting pearls before swine—either "the subject will be damaged, or the significance of the experience will be missed, and the encounter trivialized."[25(pp41,42)]

By the end of the 1960s, Smith was not alone in feeling disillusioned with the state of what he described as the "psychedelic movement," as the drugs were regularly being used without the level of respect they deserved. Instead, they became nothing more than inebriants. As federal regulations were enacted to disrupt bootleg manufacturing and distributing operations and laws were passed to criminalize personal drug use, the vast majority of the medical community shied away from psychedelic drugs and quietly swept more than a decade of research under the rug.

Conclusion: Psychedelic Research After 1970

The prohibition of psychedelics did not begin with the passage of the CSA. The regulatory environment had been changing for nearly a decade, and the medical community had been souring on psychedelics for nearly as long. Whatever optimism had existed at the start of the 1960s had essentially evaporated by the time the CSA was enacted. As Chapter 4 explores in greater detail, the legislation did not explicitly prohibit the use of illicit drugs in research; it simply introduced so much red tape that studies became prohibitively time consuming and resource intensive. Moreover, stigmas about the use of these drugs persisted for decades, further discouraging their study.

Psychedelic research continued into the 1970s at Spring Grove in Maryland. The last sanctioned dose of psilocybin at that facility was administered in 1977; it would be more than two decades until the drug was legally administered in the United States again.[28] By the 1980s and very early 1990s, research had come to a standstill. Rick Strassman's work on the physiologic effects and self-reports of individuals who had received DMT in controlled settings during the 1990s was a notable exception, but his work did not attract significant attention, nor did it jump-start the psychedelic renaissance.

This would have to wait until 2006. The year saw the publication of Francisco Moreno and colleagues' work in treating obsessive-compulsive disorder with psilocybin, as well as Roland Griffiths and colleagues' paper on psilocybin and mystical-type experience, which was loosely based on the Good Friday Experiment. Since that time, the floodgates have opened and dozens of studies on LSD, psilocybin, mescaline, and other psychedelics have been published. The second half of this book (Chapters 8-20) will be an examination of these studies.

REFERENCES

1. Heinrich M, Mah J, Amirkia V. Alkaloids used as medicines: structural phytochemistry meets biodiversity-an update and forward look. *Molecules*. 2021;26(7):1836. doi:10.3390/molecules26071836
2. Etkin NL. *Edible Medicines: An Ethnopharmacology of Food*. University of Arizona Press; 2007:5-13.
3. Booth M. *Opium: A History*. St. Martin's Press; 1996:68-69.
4. Hofmann A. *LSD: My Problem Child*. Multidisciplinary Association for Psychedelic Studies (MAPS); 2009.
5. Goutarel R, Gollnhofer O, Sillans R. Pharmacodynamics and therapeutic applications of iboga and ibogaine (Gladstone WJ, trans). *Psychedelic Monogr Essays*. 1993;6:71-111.
6. Barker SA. N, N-Dimethyltryptamine (DMT), an endogenous hallucinogen: past, present, and future research to determine its role and function. *Front Neurosci*. 2018;12:536. doi:10.3389/fnins.2018.00536. PMID: 30127713; PMCID: PMC6088236.
7. Jay M. *Mescaline: A Global History of the First Psychedelic*. Yale University Press; 2021.
8. Prentis DW, Morgan FP. Anhalonium lewinii (mescal buttons). A study of the drug, with especial reference to its physiological action upon man, with report to experiments. *Ther Gnz*. 1895;11(9). Accessed May 21, 2024. https://collections.nlm.nih.gov/bookviewer?PID=nlm:nlmuid-101751140-bk
9. Ellis H. Mescal: a new artificial paradise. *Contemp Rev*. 1898;73:130-141. Accessed on May 21, 2024. https://www.samorini.it/doc1/alt_aut/ek/ellis-mescal-a-new-artificial-paradise.pdf
10. Friesen P. Psychosis and psychedelics: historical entanglements and contemporary contrasts. *Transcult Psychiatry*. 2022;59(5):592-609. doi:10.1177/13634615221129116. PMID: 36300247; PMCID: PMC9660273.
11. Haarmann T, Rolke Y, Giesbert S, Tudzynski P. Ergot: from witchcraft to biotechnology. *Mol Plant Pathol*. 2009;10(4):563-577. doi:10.1111/j.1364-3703.2009.00548.x
12. Valenstein ES. *The War of the Soups and the Sparks: The Discovery of Neurotransmitters and the Dispute Over How Nerves Communicate*. Columbia University Press; 2005.
13. Schiff PL. Ergot and its alkaloids. *Am J Pharm Educ*. 2006;70(5):98. doi:10.5688/aj700598

14. Packer S. Jewish mystical movements and the European ergot epidemics. *Isr J Psychiatry Relat Sci*. 1998;35(3):227-239; discussion 240-241. PMID: 9803689.
15. Muraresku BC. *The Immortality Key: The Secret History of the Religion with No Name*. St. Martin's Press;2020:1-36.
16. Arthur G. Historical profile Henry Hallett Dale. *Lancet*. 2016;15:1013. Accessed January 12, 2024. https://www.thelancet.com/pdfs/journals/laneur/PIIS1474-4422(16)30167-3.pdf
17. Holze F, Vizeli P, Ley L, et al. Acute dose-dependent effects of lysergic acid diethylamide in a double-blind placebo-controlled study in healthy subjects. *Neuropharmacology*. 2021;46(3):537-544. doi:10.1038/s41386-020-00883-6
18. Pollan M. *How to Change Your Mind: What the New Science of Psychedelics Teaches Us About Consciousness, Dying, Addiction, Depression, and Transcendence*. Penguin Books; 2019.
19. Petranker R, Anderson T, Farb N. Psychedelic research and the need for transparency: polishing Alice's looking glass. *Front Psychol*. 2020;11:1681. doi:10.3389/fpsyg.2020.01681. PMID: 32754101; PMCID: PMC7367180.
20. Zafar R, Siegel M, Harding R, et al. Psychedelic therapy in the treatment of addiction: the past, present and future. *Front Psychiatry*. 2023;14:1183740. doi:10.3389/fpsyt.2023.1183740. PMID: 37377473; PMCID: PMC10291338.
21. Rucker JJH, Iliff J, Nutt DJ. Psychiatry & the psychedelic drugs. Past, present & future. *Neuropharmacology*. 2018;142:200-218. doi:10.1016/j.neuropharm.2017.12.040. PMID: 29284138.
22. Smart RG, Storm T, Baker EFW, Solursh L. A controlled study of lysergide in the treatment of alcoholism: the effects on drinking behavior. *Q J Stud Alcohol*. 1966;27(3):469-482.
23. Lowe H, Toyang N, Steele B, et al. The therapeutic potential of psilocybin. *Molecules*. 2021;26(10):2948. doi:10.3390/molecules26102948. PMID: 34063505; PMCID: PMC8156539.
24. Doblin R. Dr. Leary's Concord Prison Experiment: a 34-year follow-up study. *J Psychoactive Drugs*. 1998;30(4):419-426. doi:10.1080/02791072.1998.10399715. PMID: 9924845.
25. Smith H. *Cleansing the Doors of Perception: The Religious Significance of Entheogenic Plants and Chemicals*. Jeremy P. Tarcher/Putnam; 2000.
26. Doblin R. Pahnke's "Good Friday experiment": a long-term follow-up and methodological critique. *J Transpers Psychol*. 1991;23(1):1-28. Accessed April 16, 2024. https://www.atpweb.org/jtparchive/trps-23-91-01-001.pdf
27. Kim JH, Scialli AR. Thalidomide: the tragedy of birth defects and the effective treatment of disease. *Toxicol Sci*. 2011;122(1):1-6. doi:10.1093/toxsci/kfr088. Erratum in: *Toxicol Sci*. 2012;125(2):613. PMID: 21507989.
28. Richards WA. *Sacred Knowledge: Psychedelics and Religious Experience*. Columbia University Press; 2015:4.

4

Regulations

With the exception of ketamine, the psychedelics discussed in this book are viewed as almost entirely illicit by the federal government, largely due to a key piece of legislation known as the Controlled Substances Act of 1970 (CSA). More than just creating the legal framework that has regulated the manufacture, distribution, prescription, and use of drugs in the United States for over 50 years, the CSA was a watershed moment in the history of the United States because it transformed the criminal justice system, further criminalizing drug use and providing the legal framework for a decades-long War on Drugs that continues to have significant impact in terms of human and financial costs. A full discussion of the social and political ramifications of the War on Drugs is beyond the scope of this book, but it should be noted that the federal government is believed to have spent more than $1 trillion in funding said war since 1971.[1] Perhaps more alarming is the fact that states cumulatively spend $182 billion annually to incarcerate close to 2 million Americans for drug-related offenses.[2]

Although it is not my intention to diminish the devastation that the War on Drugs has had on communities throughout the United States and beyond, nor to deny how the criminalization of drug use has been destabilizing to urban communities, particularly minorities, the focus of this book is on the science of psychedelics, so this chapter will examine how regulations have affected the scientific community by preventing research into psychedelic drugs via cumbersome regulations created by the CSA. Psychedelics are classified as Schedule I drugs, which imposes severe restrictions on their use, hampers scientific research, and consequently leads to the lack of clinical evidence which legitimizes the restrictions, further contributing to lack of clinical evidence. This cycle has frustrated attempts to study the therapeutic value of these drugs for decades. It has also left clinicians without solid information to discuss the risks and benefits of using psychedelics with patients, who may then conduct their own research and be exposed to misinformation that severely downplays the risks of psychedelics and encourages reckless behaviors.

The Controlled Substances Act of 1970

Title II of the Comprehensive Drug Abuse Prevention and Control Act of 1970, more commonly known as the Controlled Substances Act of 1970 (CSA), was enacted to establish federal regulations overseeing the manufacture, distribution, import, export, and use of drugs. The act also fulfilled the United States' obligation to comply with the Single Convention on Narcotic Drugs, a treaty strongly supported by the United States that was originally ratified by the United Nations in 1961 but has since been amended many times to address an international need to restrict the use, manufacture, and distribution of specific drugs.[3,4] For example, psychedelics like psilocybin, lysergic acid diethylamide (LSD), and mescaline were reclassified as Schedule I substances (meaning they are subject to the strictest restrictions) in 1967.[5]

Domestically, the CSA created a five-tier classification system based on a multidimensional framework that considers accepted medical use, abuse potential, and harmfulness. Within this system, the five schedules of substances are numbered I-V. Drugs within Schedule I are considered to be the most harmful, to have the highest abuse potential, and to possess *no accepted medicinal use*. Consequently, they have no indications, cannot be prescribed, and clinicians are prohibited from using them off-label. Drugs within schedules II, III, IV, and V have progressively lower potentials for abuse and dependence. They also pose progressively fewer risks to patients (see Table 4.1).[6]

Most of the drugs discussed in this book fall under Schedule I, including psilocybin, LSD, *N*, *N*-dimethyltryptamine (DMT), mescaline, ibogaine, and 3,4-methylenedioxymethamphetamine (MDMA). Ketamine is a Schedule III drug with accepted medical uses, including in psychiatry. It is also regularly used in so-called ketamine clinics to treat depressive disorders.

TABLE 4.1 Drug Scheduling

Schedule	Definition	Examples
Schedule I	Drugs with no currently accepted medical use and a high potential for abuse.	Cannabis, **N, N-Dimethyltryptamine (DMT)**, heroin, **ibogaine, lysergic acid diethylamide (LSD)**, mescaline, 3,4-methylenedioxymethamphetamine (MDMA), **peyote, psilocybin**
Schedule II	Drugs with a high potential for extreme psychological or physical dependence, as well as abuse. Drugs of this class pose significant dangers to users and the public.	Amphetamine, cocaine, fentanyl, methadone, morphine, opium, oxycodone
Schedule III	Drugs with a moderate to low potential for physical and psychological dependence. The risk of abuse is higher than drugs within Schedule IV but lower than drugs in Schedule II.	Anabolic steroids, buprenorphine, dronabinol, **ketamine**
Schedule IV	Drugs with a low potential for abuse and low risk of physical or psychological dependence	Alprazolam, chloral hydrate, clobazam, flunitrazepam, modafinil, propoxyphene
Schedule V	Drugs with a lower potential for abuse than Schedule IV drugs. This class of drugs often consists of preparations containing limited quantities of certain narcotics.	Epidiolex (cannabidiol), pregabalin, pyrovalerone

Bold denotes a drug described in this book.
Source: United States Drug Enforcement Administration. Drug scheduling. Accessed May 9, 2024. https://www.dea.gov/drug-information/drug-scheduling

There are ongoing efforts to reclassify some of these drugs, particularly MDMA. Although there have been several successful phase 3 trials involving MDMA's use in the treatment of posttraumatic stress disorder (PTSD), the US Food and Drug Administration (FDA) has determined that more studies are needed before taking action.

Enforcement, Rescheduling, and Descheduling

Since being established in 1973, the Drug Enforcement Agency (DEA) has been in charge of enforcing and regulating the CSA, although the power to determine the scheduling of substances falls on both the FDA and the DEA.[3] When determining if a drug should be *rescheduled* (defined as when the schedule of a drug is changed) or *descheduled* (defined as when a drug is removed entirely from the list of substances regulated by the CSA), eight factors are considered.[7] They are:

1. The drug's potential for abuse
2. Scientific evidence of its pharmacology
3. The current state of knowledge with respect to the drug
4. The drug's known pattern of abuse
5. The significance, duration, and scope of abuse
6. Potential risks to public health
7. The psychic or physiologic dependence liability of the drug
8. Whether the drug is a precursor of a substance already covered by the CSA

When descheduling or rescheduling a drug, the FDA is responsible for the evaluation of relevant data and then submits their findings to the DEA. The DEA then makes a final proposal for descheduling or rescheduling based on said evidence. The DEA, the Department of Health and Human Services, or an interested party may also submit a petition to remove, add, or change the schedule of a substance. Final approval is then issued by the US Attorney General.[3] It should be noted that this is a simplified description of the procedures involved in rescheduling/descheduling drugs and that the process is far more complex due to the potential for judicial review, the need to comply with international treaties, and politics.[8]

Criticism of Rescheduling and Descheduling Processes

There have been numerous criticisms of the processes required to either reschedule or deschedule a drug, the most common and logical being that the restrictions on Schedule I drugs make it difficult to conduct research that could demonstrate a drug's clinical utility. In a way, the absence of evidence becomes evidence of absence—or rather inefficacy.

Additionally, potential risks to public health become more apparent for highly restricted drugs because those who choose to use said drugs necessarily cannot do so in clinical or controlled settings. Instead, these drugs are very often used in unsafe settings, increasing the *perceived risk* of the drug, even if the drug's *inherent risk* is quite low. For example, the illicit use of MDMA in dance clubs has been frequently reported by law enforcement agencies since at least the 1980s. In this setting, MDMA can enhance feelings of euphoria, empathy, and connectivity to others within such closed settings. However, one of the well-documented adverse effects of MDMA is hyperthermia, which can lead to significant complications, especially if one is in a hot and humid environment—like the center of a dance club. In some cases, complications following MDMA use at large festivals have led to death.[9] Conversely, within a clinical setting, hyperthermia has been a well-documented adverse event, but similar complications never arise since there are proper treatment and life support systems in place.[10]

Similarly, the acute effects of psychedelics can lead patients to behave in an erratic or reckless fashion, exposing them to significant risks. These risks can be virtually eliminated with proper support from therapists who have been trained to guide patients through psychologically difficult scenarios and to administer antianxiety medications (typically a benzodiazepine) either upon patient request or should a clear clinical need present itself. In extreme situations, the session can be terminated via the administration of an atypical antipsychotic to disrupt activity at $5\text{-}HT_{2A}$ receptors. These precautions are discussed with the patient on the day of the dosing session, as well as in preparatory sessions that occur before dosing. In an uncontrolled setting, patients may receive absolutely no instructions about what to expect and may have limited or no support systems, although they are under the influence of the drug.

It is worth noting that despite these physical and psychological concerns, as well as the dangers of use in an uncontrolled setting, virtually all the psychedelics have demonstrated a good safety profile as they are considered to be relatively nontoxic. In other words, the potential risks to public health arise from illicit use.

Decline in Clinical Studies

Even after CSA was enacted, it did not simply end research into psychedelics. In fact, scientific papers continued to be published into the 1970s, though new research effectively grounded to a halt (see Figure 4.1). The logistical headache of procuring and securing Schedule I drugs became too cumbersome for researchers. Until recently, obtaining these drugs was extremely time-consuming and resource intensive and could take several years of filling out tedious paperwork and jumping through administrative hoops to get approval to run a preclinical trial.[11] Resource-strapped organizations simply cannot afford the arduous process, and even institutions with resources to spare have been reluctant to invest significant amounts of funding into a line of inquiry that may take years or even decades to bear fruit—if it does so at all.

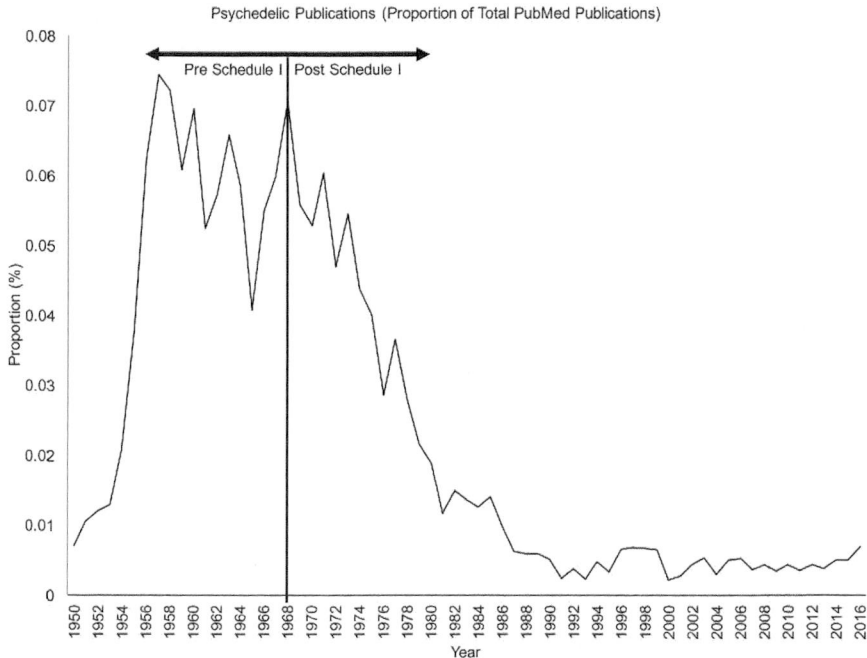

Figure 4.1 Decline in publications about psychedelics following the classification of psychedelics as Schedule I drug by the UN. (Source: Rucker JJH, Iliff J, Nutt DJ. Psychiatry & the psychedelic drugs. Past, present & future. *Neuropharmacology*. 2018;142:200-218. doi:10.1016/j.neuropharm.2017.12.040. PMID: 29284138.)

Additionally, the reputation of psychedelics (and marijuana) had been tarnished due to excessive recreational use by members of the counterculture in the second half of the 1960s and was in many ways blamed for the anarchy of the era. At the very least, they were seen as a catalyzing agent that led many to (in the words of Timothy Leary) "turn on, tune in, drop out," and all the exciting research that had been conducted in the 1950s and early 1960s was eventually buried as serious researchers turned their backs on these drugs.[12]

This decline in legitimacy continues to hover over the reputation of psychedelics even today. Many institutions are concerned that greenlighting a study involving psychedelics will be perceived as a tacit endorsement of their recreational use, though this stigma has been eroded over the last two decades due to the work of hundreds of courageous and diligent researchers at institutions like New York University, Johns Hopkins, and the University of California Los Angeles (just to name a few). Though the barriers continue to exist and entrenched beliefs about long-discredited studies continue to color debate,[1] more and more institutions, private firms, and venture capitalists have been convinced by preliminary clinical evidence that these drugs will soon have established medicinal uses.

Requirements for Clinical Studies

Should researchers have adequate funding and the blessing of an institution or private company to study a Schedule I drug, they must first obtain a license from the DEA to conduct research on the drug and obtain a controlled substance registration at the state level.[13] Researchers must also get approval from an institutional review board (IRB) to ensure the trial complies with established research ethics, and this process alone can take several years. Researchers will then have to apply for an Investigational New Drug number from the FDA, which works with research teams to ensure studies comply with existing regulations.

Should clinical trials commence, the National Institute of Drug Abuse (NIDA) will procure the actual drugs, typically from a private company with a Schedule I license to manufacture said drug. Site visits by the DEA to the facility where the study is taking place will occur before the study commences. Unannounced site audits from federal authorities will also occur to ensure the drug is being securely stored and that all laboratory equipment is up to code.

Breakthrough Status

In recent years, several drugs discussed in this book have been designated as breakthrough therapies by the FDA. According to the FDA, breakthrough therapy designation is designed "to expedite the development and review of drugs that are intended to treat a serious condition and preliminary clinical evidence indicates that the drug may demonstrate substantial improvement over available therapy on a clinically significant endpoint(s)."[14]

Obtaining breakthrough status is no easy feat, as clinical evidence must be presented to the FDA and—as explained above—it can take several years to gather the necessary clinical evidence. Moreover, the evidence must demonstrate a clear advantage over available therapies in treating a disease, disorder, or symptoms associated with a disorder. Of

---

[1] A 2002 study published in the journal *Science* claimed that MDMA was highly neurotoxic. Within the press, this resulted in reports about MDMA causing "holes in the brain." Though the study was retracted in 2003 because 9 of the 10 participants were mistakenly given methamphetamine (not MDMA!), the error did not receive nearly enough attention from the press, and even some physicians continue to believe the original story about the dangers of MDMA. Similarly, a study published in the 1960s famously claimed that LSD causes chromosomal damage. This did not survive scrutiny and was fully discredited in the early 1970s. Still, many educated people continue to believe it even in 2024.

the drugs covered in this book, ketamine, MDMA, LSD, and psilocybin have been granted breakthrough designation by the FDA.

Drugs that obtain breakthrough therapy are eligible for fast-track designation features, guidance on drug development, and organizational commitment.[14]

Decriminalization and Legalization

The term *decriminalization* frequently arises in any discussion about drug policy. Decriminalization refers to the removal of criminal sanctions for the possession of specific drugs (typically up to a specific amount), but drugs may still be seized, and offenders may still incur civil penalties or be required to seek treatment for problematic use. Individuals who grow, manufacture, or sell drugs that have been decriminalized can still face criminal penalties. To reiterate, decriminalization does not allow drugs to be used, sold, or manufactured/grown without penalty. *Legalization* means that the use of a drug is permitted under law, typically with some restrictions (eg, minimum age to purchase, maximum amount allowed in a single purchase). Legalization may also entail the creation of a regulated market for the drug.

Decriminalization is part of a larger discussion of drug policy and mass incarceration that goes well beyond the scope of this book. Central to the argument is that vast amounts of resources are dedicated to enforcing the criminalization of drugs that could be put to use in better ways. Domestically, decriminalization as a policy promotes redirecting resources away from law enforcement and the construction, maintenance, and staffing of penitentiaries. Resources are instead directed toward preventing problematic drug use and providing treatment to individuals with substance use disorders. It should be stressed that those who favor decriminalization are not always advocates for legalization.

In 2020, Oregon became the first state to decriminalize psilocybin after voters approved Ballot Measure 109.[15] The resultant therapeutic paradigm supports adult use, and it will be described in the following section.

As of this writing, the following cities have decriminalized at least one entheogenic plant:

■ 2019
- Denver, CO (psilocybin)
- Oakland, CA (psilocybin and peyote)

- **2020**
  - Santa Cruz, CA (psilocybin)
  - Ann Arbor, MI (all entheogens)
  - Washington, DC (psilocybin, mescaline, and ayahuasca)
- **2021**
  - Washtenaw County, MI (psilocybin, mescaline, and ayahuasca)
  - Somerville, MA (all entheogens)
  - Cambridge, MA (all entheogens)
  - Northampton, MA (all entheogens)
  - Seattle, WA (all entheogens)
  - Arcata, CA (all entheogens)
  - Easthampton, MA (all entheogens)
  - Detroit, MI (all entheogens)
  - Port Townsend, WA (all entheogens)
- **2022**
  - Hazel Park, MI (all entheogens)
  - San Francisco, CA (all entheogens)
- **2023**
  - Ferndale, MI (all entheogens)
  - Jefferson County, WA (all entheogens)
  - Berkeley, CA (all entheogens)
  - Minneapolis, MN (all entheogens)
  - Portland, ME (all entheogens)

Voters in Colorado passed a ballot initiative legalizing the use of "healing centers" to administer psilocybin, mescaline, ibogaine, and DMT under supervised conditions. The preliminary rules regarding the therapeutic use of these drugs were released in early 2024, but as of this writing, the finalized framework has yet to be published.[16] Of note, the initiative also decriminalized the possession, sharing, and cultivation of these four drugs among adults over the age of 21.

Supported Adult Use

Supported adult use began in Oregon starting in 2023 following the passage of Ballot Measure 109 in 2020. "Supported adult use" is a treatment paradigm referring to the legalized administration of psilocybin in supportive facilitates. Adults (referred to as "clients" in the statute) are now allowed to legally purchase mushrooms from licensed cultivators and to consume them in licensed facilities under the care of a certified facilitator.[17] Facilitators must be licensed by the Oregon Health Authority.[18]

"Psilocybin services" need not be administered by a medical doctor under Oregon law, nor do clients need to have any diagnosable condition. Facilitators have the freedom to determine if psilocybin services are appropriate, given the client's familial and personal background. They also have the freedom to determine the dose.[17]

What is currently required is that clients meet with a licensed facilitator for a preparatory session. They must complete forms providing their personal information and ensuring informed consent. Safety and support plans, as well as transportation plans to and from the facility, are also drafted. Integration sessions are optional, though the facilitator is required to check on the client within 72 hours.[19]

At present, psilocybin services are expensive (a single session is said to have cost $3,000), and there are only a handful of facilities licensed to administer these services.[15] However, this is an experiment playing out in real time, and many within the medical community are nervous that the administration of these drugs by inexperienced individuals (even if they are licensed by the state) could lead to incidents where individuals engage in reckless behaviors or are abused, exploited, or otherwise harmed by bad or incompetent actors. In addition, there is concern that these individuals may not fully comprehend the impact of these substances and lack sufficient experience to respond appropriately in crises. More importantly, if enough of these incidents occur, we could see another freeze on psychedelic research.

That said, these drugs have been administered by shamans, guides, and other folk healers for thousands of years who do not practice or even believe in Western medicine. Though there is significant trepidation surrounding the launch of Oregon's program based on our belief that only medical professionals are capable of caring for those who wish to use these drugs, we may be surprised by the outcome of this pilot program—though the results remain to be seen.

Religious Freedom

Although the United States has favored a largely punitive approach to illicit drug use for decades, there have been exemptions for individuals who are using substances for religious purposes. The story of the Native American Church (NAC) and its use of peyote, a cactus containing the classic psychedelic mescaline, is informative and presents a stark contrast to the kind of prohibitionism that has been described throughout this chapter. (For more about the pharmacology of mescaline, see Chapter 12.)

History of Religious Peyote Use

Archaeological evidence of peyote use in North America dates back to at least 4000 BCE.[20(p34)] Use appears to have continued uninterrupted for several millennia, as early European accounts from the 16th century suggest that ceremonial peyote use was relatively common among the cultures stretching from central Mexico to what is today Texas, which represent the limits of peyote's natural habitat. In addition to religious and ceremonial use, peyote was a part of several indigenous armamentaria for more acute medical problems, including minor injuries like burns, wounds, and snakebites. Traditional use of peyote was largely suppressed by the Spanish conquistadors beginning in the 16th century, particularly in the more accessible regions of Mexico, but the tradition was kept alive by cultures further away from the administrative apparatus of New Spain.[20(pp33-49)]

It does not appear that peyote use was common among indigenous peoples who resided in the more northern portions of the Great Plains or east of the Mississippi River prior to European contact. However, as these individuals were forcefully relocated to Indian Territory (modern-day Oklahoma) following the passage of the Indian Removal Act of 1830, as well as numerous wars, they were introduced to peyote. The spread of what became known as the "peyote cult" accelerated in the aftermath of the American Civil War.[20(pp53-75)]

As historian Mike Jay describes in his book, *Mescaline: A Global History of the First Psychedelic*, this emerging religion was "pan-Indian, drawing on the shared traditions of formerly hostile peoples obliged to live cheek by jowl."[20(p59)] Over time, this "pan-Indian" ceremony led by a "roadman" and involving the administration of peyote in a tipi became standardized, and a syncretistic religion developed that included elements of Christianity and traditional Native American theologies. Though variations arose and continue to persist between different roadmen, one of the many tenets of the religion is that the peyote cactus is itself a teacher with a unique spirit and that ingestion of peyote allows for direct communion with a monotheistic Great Spirit.[21] Quanah Parker, a Comanche leader who played a crucial role in the formal creation of the NAC, evidently once claimed, "The white man goes into his church house and talks *about* Jesus, but the Indian goes into his tipi and talks *to* Jesus."[20(p72)]

The trade of peyote was first banned in Oklahoma in 1886 due to the religion's growing popularity in conjunction with the belief that peyote was being used as an intoxicant or deliriant. As the peyote religion spread, so did the efforts to prohibit its use. In response, representatives from multiple tribes signed a charter of incorporation of the NAC in 1918 as a means to preserve their freedom to use peyote as a sacrament. Though the NAC has repeatedly had to fight for their religious liberty over many decades, their right to use peyote has been enshrined by several landmark pieces of legislation. The two most important are the American Indian Religious Freedom Act of 1978, which recognizes that, though peyote is a Schedule I drug under the CSA, members of the NAC have legal protections to use the plant, and the American Indian Religious Freedom Act Amendments of 1994, enacted to enforce the provisions of the 1978 law.[20(pp103-128)]

The Religious Freedom Restoration Act

In 1993, the federal government enacted the Religious Freedom Restoration Act, which prohibits the federal government from unreasonably interfering with or burdening an individual's right to exercise their religion. This act has successfully been used as a means to argue that the DEA should allow for a religious exemption to the CSA that applies to groups beyond the NAC. In 2020, the DEA issued a guidance document on the subject, stipulating that exceptions can be granted if parties can demonstrate that the use of scheduled drugs is sincere and religious in nature and that the lack of exemption results in a substantial burden.[22]

Conclusion

The regulatory environment that governs the use, distribution, and production of psychedelic drugs is changing rapidly, as public interest in psychedelic medicine soars and more policymakers question the wisdom of strictly prohibiting and criminalizing this class of drugs. However, as drugs are rescheduled or decriminalized and views on psychedelics soften in general, we run the risk of allowing the pendulum to swing in the opposite direction. Many people may adopt the misguided belief that they can be safely used in uncontrolled environments or without supervision. This is not the case.

Clinicians should be willing to respond to patients' curiosity about psychedelics with an honest discussion about the risks and benefits of these drugs. We should neither reflexively belittle them because they are currently classified as Schedule I substances nor incautiously celebrate their potential without acknowledging their dangers. Ideally, we should have enough knowledge about these drugs to allow our patients to make informed and well-founded decisions.

REFERENCES

1. Farber D. Introduction. In: Farber D, ed. *The War on Drugs: A History*. New York University Press; 2022:1-13.
2. Sawyer W, Wagner P. Mass incarceration: the whole pie 2024. Prison Policy Initiative. Published March 14, 2024. Accessed May 9, 2024. https://www.prisonpolicy.org/reports/pie2024.html
3. Ortiz NR, Preuss CV. Controlled Substance Act. 2023 Mar 24. *In: StatPearls* [Internet]. StatPearls Publishing; 2024. PMID: 34662058. Accessed May 3, 2024.
4. Booth M. *Cannabis: A History*. Picador; 2003:249-250.
5. Nutt D. Psychedelic drugs-a new era in psychiatry? *Dialogues Clin Neurosci*. 2019;21(2):139-147. doi:10.31887/DCNS.2019.21.2/dnutt. PMID: 31636488; PMCID: PMC6787540.
6. United States Drug Enforcement Administration. Drug scheduling. Accessed May 9, 2024. https://www.dea.gov/drug-information/drug-scheduling
7. Drug Enforcement Agency. The Controlled Substances Act. Accessed May 2, 2024. https://www.dea.gov/drug-information/csa
8. Bloomberg S, Harriman A, Pennington S. Re/descheduling marijuana through administrative action. *Oklahoma Law Rev*. 2024;76:517-573. Accessed May 3, 2024. https://digitalcommons.law.ou.edu/olr/vol76/iss3/2
9. Ridpath A, Driver CR, Nolan ML, et al. Illnesses and deaths among persons attending an electronic dance-music festival—New York City, 2013. *Morb Mortal Wkly Rep. 2014*;63(50):1195-1198. PMID: 25522087; PMCID: PMC5779530.
10. Colcott J, Guerin AA, Carter O, Meikle S, Bedi G. Side-effects of MDMA-assisted psychotherapy: a systematic review and meta-analysis. *Neuropsychopharmacology*. 2024;49(8):1208-1226. doi:10.1038/s41386-024-01865-8. PMID: 38654146.
11. Rucker JJH, Iliff J, Nutt DJ. Psychiatry & the psychedelic drugs. Past, present & future. *Neuropharmacology*. 2018;142:200-218. doi:10.1016/j.neuropharm.2017.12.040. PMID: 29284138.
12. Pollan M. *How to Change Your Mind: What the New Science of Psychedelics Teaches Us About Consciousness, Dying, Addiction, Depression, and Transcendence*. Penguin Books; 2019:57-58.
13. Howk H. Controlled substance licensing requirements. Wolters Kluwer. Published February 2, 2024. Accessed May 10, 2024. https://www.wolterskluwer.com/en/expert-insights/controlled-substance-registration-requirements
14. U.S. Food and Drug Administration. Breakthrough therapy. Last modified January 4, 2018. Accessed May 3, 2024. https://www.fda.gov/patients/fast-track-breakthrough-therapy-accelerated-approval-priority-review/breakthrough-therapy
15. Baker M. A new era of psychedelics in Oregon. *New York Times*. Updated October 25, 2023. Accessed May 10, 2024. https://www.nytimes.com/2023/10/23/us/oregon-psychedelic-mushrooms.html
16. Willard K. Colorado releases draft regulations for psychedelic 'healing center' facilitators. KDVR website. Updated March 12, 2024. Accessed May 10, 2024. https://kdvr.com/news/local/colorado-releases-draft-regulations-for-psychedelic-healing-centers/
17. Prichep D. In Oregon, psilocybin treatment is an experiment in real time. National Public Radio website. Published February 28, 2024. Accessed May 10, 2024. https://www.npr.org/2024/02/28/1234012939/in-oregon-psilocybin-treatment-is-an-experiment-in-real-time

18. Frost A. Oregon psilocybin rules shape who can provide and access care. Oregon Public Broadcasting website. Updated June 9, 2022. Accessed May 10, 2024. https://www.opb.org/article/2022/06/09/oregon-psilocybin-rules-shape-who-can-provide-and-access-care/
19. Oregon Health News Blog. Psilocybin 101: what to know about Oregon's psilocybin services. Published April 12, 2023. Accessed May 10, 2024. https://covidblog.oregon.gov/psilocybin-101-what-to-know-about-oregons-psilocybin-services/
20. Jay M. *Mescaline: A Global History of the First Psychedelic*. Yale University Press; 2021.
21. Doesburg-van Kleffens M, Zimmermann-Klemd AM, Gründemann C. An overview on the hallucinogenic peyote and its alkaloid mescaline: the importance of context, ceremony and culture. *Molecules*. 2023;28(24):7942. doi:10.3390/molecules28247942
22. Drug Enforcement Administration. Diversion Control Division. Guidance Document. Published November 20, 2020. Accessed May 9, 2024. https://www.deadiversion.usdoj.gov/GDP/(DEA-DC-5)(EO-DEA-007)(Version2)RFRA_Guidance_(Final)_11-20-2020.pdf

5
The Psychedelic Experience

Psychedelics produce profound changes in perception, mood, emotion, and even cognition. There is extensive literature documenting the effects of psychedelics, ranging from the appearance of vivid and kaleidoscopic visions, synesthesia, and enhanced feelings of empathy with other beings, as well as out-of-body and near-death experiences (NDEs), ego dissolution, oceanic boundlessness, and oneness with the universe. These experiences can be revelatory, ineffable, and life-changing, as well as quite varied. For example, if two very similar people are given the same dose of a psychedelic in the same setting, they may report dramatically different experiences. Consequently, attempting to describe the sensory content of a psychedelic experience with full fidelity will necessarily fall short—it is too varied, and, in many cases, words may be inadequate tools to accurately describe the subjective effects.

In addition to alterations in sensory perception, mood, and emotion, psychedelics at moderate or high doses are known to occasion mystical-type experiences, which are characterized by, among other things, a greater sense of unity or interconnectivity, ego dissolution, oceanic boundlessness, sacredness, and profound feelings of awe or peace.[1] These kinds of experiences are not solely caused by psychedelics; they can also occur spontaneously or following any number of actions capable of inducing a nonordinary state of consciousness (NOSC). However, part of what makes psychedelics so unique and invaluable is that they have shown remarkable consistency in inducing such states.

Similar to the tremendous differences one may observe in sensory content while under the influence of psychedelics, the specifics of each mystical-type experience are also unique. Despite this, researchers have observed several elements of mystical experiences that are not only common but can be assessed for their level of completeness using self-report measures and clinician-administered scales. The two most common are the Mystical Experience Questionnaire (MEQ) and Hood's Mysticism Scale (M-scale). Evidence suggests a positive correlation between the completeness of a mystical experience and the therapeutic value of psychedelics, suggesting that these experiences are central to the treatment's efficacy and clinical outcomes. Meanwhile, alterations in sensory perception are of secondary importance from a clinical perspective.

Onset, Peak, and Comedown Experiences

The effects of orally administered classic psychedelics (psilocybin, lysergic acid diethylamide [LSD], mescaline), ayahuasca (which contains *N, N*-dimethyltryptamine [DMT]), ibogaine, and 3,4-methylenedioxymethamphetamine (MDMA) are felt gradually. Time of onset may vary not only for each substance but also between individuals. In most cases, the effects are felt within 30 to 60 minutes. MDMA, psilocybin, and LSD tend to be felt sooner, while mescaline and ibogaine's effects tend to take the longest to become discernable. Similarly, peak effects of psychedelics tend to occur within 90 minutes following administration, though the peak effects of mescaline and ibogaine may not be felt for as long as 2 hours. The total duration of effect is far more varied (see Table 5.1).

Unlike orally administered psychedelics, ketamine is administered intravenously, while esketamine (Spravato) is administered as a nasal spray within a clinical setting. DMT is frequently administered intravenously when used in clinical settings. Outside of a clinical setting, ketamine may be snorted or smoked, while DMT is most commonly smoked. Both have a very rapid onset, with peak effects experienced immediately. The total duration for the former is usually no more than 60 minutes while the latter is typically no more than 30 minutes.

The pharmacology of each drug will be discussed at length in their respective chapters.

TABLE 5.1 Approximate Onset, Peak Experience, and Total Duration of a Moderate Dose of Orally Administered Psychedelics

Drug	Onset (min)	Time Until Peak Reached (min)	Total Duration of Effect (h)
Psilocybin	30	60-90	4-6
LSD	30	60-90	8-12
Ayahuasca	30	90	4-6
Mescaline	60	120	10-12
Ibogaine	60	120	12-28[a]
MDMA	40	75-125	3-6

LSD, lysergic acid diethylamide; MDMA, 3,4-methylenedioxymethamphetamine.
[a]The effects of ibogaine come in three distinct phases, as noted in Chapter 15. The above consists of a 4- to 8-hour oneiric phase followed by a more introspective phase that lasts for 8 to 20 hours. The third phase is more of an aftereffect characterized by a heightened sense of awareness and sleep problems, and it may persist for up to 72 hours.

Sensory Effects

Though psychedelics can cause alterations in the perception of all five senses, the visual effects are the most pronounced. Interestingly, the individual may experience this with their eyes open or closed. Synesthesia, meaning when sensory information is experienced via multiple sensory faculties (eg, seeing music or tasting color), is also another common sensory experience.

In most cases, individuals do not believe these visions to be part of ordinary reality, resulting in what was often referred to in the early 20th century as "double consciousness" or *état mixte* (or, in the phrasing of Leuner, the "reflective ego remnant"[2]).[3] This unique state of mind allows one to experience the illusions and remain aware of the fact that they do not exist in objective reality.

Open-Eye Visualizations

When the eyes are open, individuals commonly report noticing that colors are more vivid or intense, even at low doses of psychedelics. Additionally, individuals may perceive a sense of movement in their peripheral visual fields, inanimate and stationary objects may appear to pulsate or breathe, patterns may blur, and halo effects may be apparent. Individuals may also exhibit exaggerated pareidolia, a phenomenon where one unconsciously imposes a pattern on stimuli, usually visual. For example, a person may believe that a boulder resembles the profile of a person or that a cloud looks like an animal. Palinopsia (a trailing effect), micropsia, and macropsia may also occur at moderate doses.

At higher doses, intricate geometric patterns may be superimposed over one's field of vision. Full-blown hallucinations are possible even when one's eyes are open.

Closed-Eye Visualizations

Closed-eye visualizations may range from speckles of color and light to vivid and intricate geometric patterns. These visualizations are often characterized as arabesques or containing motifs from Mexico, Central America, South America, or Africa. In some cases, there seems to be a strong cultural influence over these visualizations. For example, the use of iboga may result in closed-eye visualizations that feel African in nature, whereas peyote may induce visualizations that are reminiscent of the American Southwest or Mexico. The term *elementary hallucinations* refers to these kinds of patterns. Alternatively, *complex hallucinations* refer to more elaborate structures, including vast landscapes or cities.[4]

At high enough doses of certain psychedelics, especially DMT and ketamine, a dissociative state can occur that blurs the distinction between open-eye and closed-eye visualizations.

Emotional Effects

Psychedelics tend to have a positive impact on mood when administered in a controlled and safe setting. Individuals may also report an intensification of emotions and find themselves overwhelmed by giddiness, a feeling of communal love, the need to grin or laugh, a sense of playfulness, and childlike wonder. Many individuals report feeling as though they are seeing the world again through the eyes of a child. Positive mood is even more pronounced with entactogens like MDMA, further promoting prosocial behaviors.[4]

Individuals may also feel anxious, afraid, or paranoid, especially if they fear losing control. In most cases, these negative feelings will pass with support from guides but can become quite intense, especially among psychedelic-naive patients.

Nonordinary States of Consciousness

Psychedelics are one means of producing NOSCs. This term is preferred over "altered state of consciousness" because it places greater emphasis on the fact that these states are not merely alterations of "ordinary" consciousness, but rather represent unique emotional, psychological, and cognitive states. In addition, they are distinct from the experiential repertoire of consciousness as we experience it on a day-to-day basis. NOSCs can also be induced through deep meditation, hypnosis, certain forms of breathwork, sensory deprivation, fasting, shamanistic drumming, and physical movements like yoga or some forms of dance.

NOSCs are typically characterized as being transient in nature and producing a shift in perspective that is both external and internal. In other words, individuals do not simply see an interpersonal problem or other conflict with "fresh eyes" or a more objective view; rather, NOSCs appear to allow one to scrutinize one's own ego and construction of self as if from the perspective of a more impartial observer. As Chapter 7 will explore, there are neurologic correlates to this phenomenon involving disruption of the default mode network (DMN), which has been referred to as the "biological substrate of the Freudian ego."[5] It is associated with moral decision-making, counterfactual thinking, self-consciousness, and mental time travel (ie, the capacity to reconstruct a personal narrative from episodic memories and to anticipate future events).[5]

NOSCs are also associated with mystical experiences. Although entry into an NOSC is not sufficient for a mystical experience, it does seem to be necessary.

Mystical Experiences

Mystical experiences have been reported with and without the use of substances for thousands of years across various cultures. In some cases, mystical sects have sprouted from established religious traditions following the mystical experience of a prophet, saint, or guru. Some of the most well-known mystic sects include Sufism and Kabbalism, which exist within the religious framework of Islam and Judaism, respectively. It is worth emphasizing that mystical traditions and experiences are not limited to a single religion, sect, dogma, ideology, or spiritual practice, but the notion that they all share a "common core" of features is controversial among some religious scholars.[1] It should also be noted that the most central element to this "common core" is less about spiritual insights, which may not occur at all during a mystical experience, and more about the experience of unity.[1]

In most cases, mysticism is grounded in the metaphysical belief that there exists a spiritual realm and that this realm is accessible to mortals via a variety of practices that promote asceticism and turning away from the material world via fasting, meditation, prayer, contemplating the divine, and yoga. These practices allow one to attain a state of purity or enlightenment, as well as ecstasy or *wajd* (a Sufi term to describe spiritual joy) that allows for union and communication directly with the spiritual realm and, in some cases, the divine.

Although there were many philosophers and ancient scientists who could be described as mystics (eg, Plotinus, Avicenna, Maimonides, Blaise Pascal), finding such individuals became a rarity following the age of Enlightenment with the rise of the natural sciences and materialism. It was not until the end of the 19th century and the work of American psychologist and philosopher William James that mystical experiences were afforded credence within the burgeoning field of psychology. Rather than simply ignore mystical experiences or write them off as being indicative of psychosis, James thought they were worthy of consideration, representing the actualization of a type of consciousness that fell outside the norm. In his book, *The Varieties of Religious Experience*, James notes, "Our normal waking consciousness . . . is but one special type of consciousness, whilst all about it, parted from it by the flimsiest of screens, there lie potential forms of consciousness entirely different."

In James' view, there are four elements that make up the mystical experience: ineffability, a noetic quality, transiency, and passivity. To elaborate, the noetic quality refers to the sense of both authority and revelation to the experience, where it is not felt simply as a dream or hallucination, but as though a universal truth is being unveiled. Rene Daumal alternatively referred to it as *certainty*.[6] Transiency refers to how the experience is of brief duration, while ineffability describes how the experience is beyond conveyance through conventional language. Finally, passivity refers to how one feels as though the mystical experience is happening to them and that their will is held in abeyance. It may also be experienced as a form of surrender to a more powerful force.[7]

For Walter Stace, who was writing in the 1950s and 1960s, the conceptualization of the mystical experience shifted, with the central element becoming unity. Moreover, Stace believed that mystical experiences could be described as *introvertive* or *extrovertive*, with the former involving a state where the boundaries between one's own consciousness and the consciousness of a higher power dissolve, suggesting a transcendental consciousness permeating the universe.

Introvertive mystical experiences may also involve an experience of unity devoid of content that is sometimes referred to as "the void."[1] Extrovertive experiences perceive a unifying force coursing through oneself and others, but a sense of autonomy or self is maintained. Of note, both experiences are unifying, though the introvertive force is in many ways more complete.

Stace also provided nine characteristics of all mystical experiences[8]:

1. Internal unity
2. External unity
3. Abolition of spatiotemporal limits (often referred to as "oceanic boundlessness")
4. Inner subjectivity
5. Objectivity and reality (ie, noetic quality)
6. Sacredness
7. Peace and joy
8. Paradoxicality
9. Ineffability

Stace's framework has since been used to create Hood's 32-item M-Scale and the 43-item MEQ. The latter is based on Stace's work but also owes its genesis to Walter Pahnke's Good Friday Experiment, which was discussed in Chapter 3. Both continue to enjoy wide usage, with the M-Scale being used in the landmark study of psychedelics and mystical-type experiences published by Griffiths and colleagues in 2006. The authors describe the use of the M-Scale in the following manner: "A total score and three empirically derived factors are measured: interpretation (corresponding to three mystical dimensions described by Stace (1960): noetic quality, deeply felt positive mood, and sacredness); introvertive mysticism (corresponding to the Stace dimensions of internal unity, transcendence of time and space, and ineffability); and extrovertive mysticism (corresponding to the dimension of the unity of all things)."[9]

The latter scale, which is also referred to as the Pahnke-Richards MEQ, has also been used in several more recent studies. The original model was based on Pahnke's work. For Pahnke, unity was also believed to be central to the mystical experience, noting that "Even if all the other categories are represented, such an experience must be considered as close to, but not strictly the same as the most complete mystical experience by our definition."[10] Pahnke noted nine distinct categories similar to the ones noted earlier in his dissertation.[10] They were:

1. Unity
2. Transcendence of time and space

3. Deeply felt positive mood
4. Sense of sacredness
5. Objectivity and reality
6. Paradoxicality
7. Alleged ineffability
8. Transiency
9. Persisting positive changes in attitude and behavior

To achieve a "complete" mystical experience, participants had to score 60% of the maximum score or higher in each of the subcategories noted previously, with a score of 60% of the maximum score or higher for the unity subcategory being necessary.[11] More recent versions of the MEQ (eg, the MEQ30) have been developed but have not significantly strayed from this conceptual model.[11]

During Pahnke's Good Friday Experiment, approximately 30% to 40% of those who were given psilocybin had a complete mystical experience. These results did not change at a 6-month follow-up or even a 25-year follow-up. Individuals in the psilocybin group also continued to report persistent positive changes in attitude due to the mystical experience even many decades later, while controls reported no such effects.

In Griffiths' 2006 study (briefly described in Chapter 3), which modified and improved upon Pahnke's original experiment, 60% of participants who were given psilocybin met the criteria for a complete mystical experience.[12] Additional studies by Griffiths have confirmed that psilocybin can occasion mystical-type experiences (see Chapter 9 for details).[1]

Furthermore, mystical experiences are tied to enduring improvements in mood, attitude, and behaviors, indicating that the strength of the mystical experience or degree of completeness is of therapeutic importance. In other words, *the experience itself has therapeutic value*. Although the question of whether mystical experiences can be reducible to neural processes (to be explored in Chapter 7) remains an open question, attributing the benefits of psychedelics simply to activity at certain receptors is a form of pharmacologic reductionism and, more importantly, inaccurate.

Organic Mystical Experiences and Psychedelic-Induced Mystical Experiences

In many cultures, particularly those that are rooted in mysticism, individuals may dedicate years attempting to induce an NOSC and be rewarded with a mystical experience, epiphany, or theophany.

Consequently, many practitioners of these extremely demanding disciplines may regard psychedelics as being a kind of shortcut to mysticism and may consider psychedelic-induced NOSCs to be artificial. They feel that there is no shortcut to the path of enlightenment since all mystical practices must endure the ardors of the path, which is a necessary part of attaining enlightenment.[13]

Despite the belief among many traditional mystics that psychedelic-induced NOSCs are not genuine, researchers utilizing the MEQ and M-Scale found that they are extremely similar, if not the same.[1] These parallels are not only in reference to phenomenological experience but also refer to the neural bases of mystical experiences.

Near-Death Experiences and Psychedelic-Induced Near-Death Experiences

There are also parallels between some psychedelic experiences and NDEs, which are a distinct type of mystical experience frequently described by people who are on the verge of death. These experiences are centered on out-of-body experiences, feelings of surrender and peace, travel through a void or tunnel, bright lights, autobiographical review ("life flashing before one's eyes"), interactions with sentient beings, and approaching a point of no return.[14] With the exception of reaching a point of no return, these same elements are frequently reported following the administration of ibogaine, higher doses of ketamine, and either smoked or intravenous DMT.

The phenomenological similarities between DMT and NDEs were measured by Timmermann and colleagues using a variety of scales (including the MEQ). Although there are significant disparities between NDEs and the DMT experience, the authors did find similarities in scores when measuring for degree of unitive experience and the sense of joy produced by the experience.[15] A review of written reports by Martial and colleagues found semantic similarities between psychedelics and NDEs, with ketamine producing the most pronounced similarities.[16] Of note, experiences pertaining to specific drugs will be described in greater detail in their respective chapters.

Subjective Differences Between the Psychedelics

With the exception of DMT, the effects of classic psychedelics are phenomenologically similar. A study by Ley and colleagues that used a randomized, double-blind, placebo-controlled cross-over model when comparing the acute effects of mescaline, LSD, and psilocybin found that participants ($n = 32$) had difficulty distinguishing among the three, even though more than half (63%) of the participants reported previous psychedelic use. Despite their prior use, only 48.4% correctly identified that they had received a 200-mg dose of psilocybin, 53.3% were able to correctly identify that they had received a 500-mg dose of mescaline, while 58.1% were able to correctly identify that they had received a 100-µg dose of LSD during the study. Following the study, all three groups (psilocybin, mescaline, and LSD) were better at correctly identifying the drug they had received (78.1%, 81.2%, and 68.7%, respectively).[17]

The other psychedelics have some notable differences in subjective effects that will be briefly outlined here.

Ayahuasca

The subjective effects of ayahuasca are distinct, but similar to other tryptamine psychedelics like psilocybin or LSD. One major difference is that individuals who take part in ayahuasca ceremonies regularly report interactions with sentient beings that introduce themselves as the spirits of plants from the armamentarium of South America's folk healers. This is also common in peyote ceremonies. Consequently, individuals will speak of these plants as helpers and guides not in the sense that they induce a state where one is receptive to instruction; rather, they will afford the spirits of these plants a sense of agency and even wisdom. It is not a conceptual model that is easily harmonized with rationalist or materialist metaphysics.

N, N-dimethyltryptamine

The subjective effects of DMT when ingested outside of the context of ayahuasca are dramatically dose dependent. Smaller doses may be similar to the effects of mescaline, LSD, or psilocybin, but larger doses tend to induce "breakthrough" experiences. These are likened to being transported to another dimension or universe. While in this dissociative state, individuals describe a hyperrealistic environment filled with vivid geometric patterns that may or may not be populated by sentient beings. These breakthrough periods often last no more than 15 or 20 minutes, during which individuals are largely unresponsive to external stimuli.[18]

Ketamine

The effects of ketamine are also more stepwise than linear. At low doses, the effects of ketamine are similar to alcohol while larger doses can lead to dissociative experiences. In some cases, these experiences can result in individuals feeling as though they have been transported to another dimension in a manner akin to DMT. As noted previously, the subjective effects of ketamine are also similar to NDEs.[19]

Ibogaine

The acute effects of ibogaine tend to induce what is often described as a "waking dream" that is intensely autobiographical. (On account of the strongly oneiric [dream-like] effects, ibogaine is sometimes referred to as a "oneirophrenic" drug.) Visual effects are most intense when the individual's eyes are closed and may be suppressed when their eyes are open. The content of these visual effects tends to involve interactions with personifications of Jungian archetypes, deceased loved ones, and plant spirits, especially the spirit of the iboga plant. Autobiographic review is commonly reported.[20]

Entactogens

The effects of entactogens like MDMA are distinct from other psychedelics, largely because they rarely produce the same kind of intense visualizations. Rather, individuals report positive changes in emotion and mood that may result in euphoria, reduced anxiety, and increases in introspection and prosocial behaviors. This class of drugs also tends to reduce the fear of emotional injury and decreases one's psychological defenses, resulting in a state of mind that is more empathetic, compassionate, and trusting of others. This is believed to be clinically relevant because it facilitates the exploration of traumatic memories within the context of posttraumatic stress disorder (PTSD) and beyond. According to the Multidisciplinary Association for the Psychedelic Studies' manual for MDMA-assisted psychotherapy in the treatment of PTSD, "Research participants have said that being able to successfully process painful emotions during MDMA-assisted psychotherapy has given them a template for feeling and expressing pain that has changed their relationship to their emotions."[21]

Individuals under the acute influence of MDMA and other entactogens (such as methylenedioxyamphetamine [MDA] or 2,5-dimethoxy-4-ethylthiophenethylamine [2C-T-2]) may also experience anxiety, paranoia, overwhelming emotions, and vivid recollection of traumatic or difficult memories. However, these challenging experiences can be avoided or mitigated in a supportive and/or clinical environment. Working through these challenges may also catalyze breakthroughs and assist the therapeutic process.[22]

There is some evidence that personality may influence the subjective effects of entactogens. A pooled analysis of 10 randomized, double-blind, placebo-controlled, cross-over studies conducted by Studerus and colleagues found some correlations between certain personality traits and the subjective experience of MDMA. In particular, they found that individuals with a higher score on the "openness to experience" trait felt a greater sense of "closeness" and "oceanic boundlessness," while also reporting higher scores of "visionary restructuralization." Individuals with a higher score of "neurotic" traits reported more unpleasant or anxious reactions.[23]

Increased Suggestibility

Individuals may become more receptive to foreign ideas while under the influence of psychedelics and shortly after administration. Those who score high in trait conscientiousness are particularly sensitive to psychedelic-induced suggestibility.[24] There are two distinct forms of suggestibility that are relevant here and have been observed with psychedelics.

In the first case, the psychedelic experience can be influenced by suggestion and expectation. For example, a person who is primed to think that a specific psychedelic will induce a highly autobiographical experience where one's life "flashes before their eyes" is more likely to experience that phenomenon than an uninfluenced individual. Similarly, if a group of individuals are all experiencing the effects of a psychedelic, they may all claim to experience a shared illusion after one member of the group vocalizes the content of their vision.

Second, individuals appear to be far more open to suggestion in the aftermath of a psychedelic experience. This can be beneficial from a therapeutic perspective, particularly if an individual has been diagnosed with a substance use disorder, eating disorder, or obsessive-compulsive disorder, and is being encouraged by their therapist, friends, and family to make positive changes to their life. It can help drive these changes, resulting in the disruption of pathologic patterns.[24]

Conversely, increased suggestibility can also be exploited by those who may wish to take advantage of individuals via indoctrination. Even without sinister intent, individuals can be tacitly encouraged to accept new metaphysical beliefs to explain their psychedelic experience or to endorse philosophies, concepts, and therapeutic models that reflect the beliefs of the therapist but would normally be heavily scrutinized by the patient. Other ethical concerns surrounding the administration of psychedelics are covered in the following chapter.

Hallucinogen Persisting Perception Disorder

Finally, it should be noted that some individuals have reported persistent effects following the use of psychedelic drugs, with the fifth edition of the *Diagnostic and Statistical Manual of Mental Disorders* (DSM-5-TR) estimating a prevalence of 4.2% among those who have used psychedelic drugs.[25] Hallucinogen Persisting Perception Disorder (HPPD), as it is known, is more common among polydrug users and has a lower rate of prevalence among individuals participating in psychedelic-assisted psychotherapy, though the occurrence is a possibility. Unfortunately, not enough studies have been performed to determine risk factors.

According to DSM-5-TR, diagnostic criteria include:

1. Following the acute effects of a psychedelic, the individual reexperiences the kinds of alterations in perception that characterize the psychedelic experience (eg, visions of geometric shapes, increased vividness of color, macropsia and micropsia, halo effects).
2. The reexperiencing of these perceptual effects causes distress or impairment.
3. The reexperiencing of these perceptual effects is not attributable to a medication or another medical condition or mental disorder.

There are two subtypes of HPPD. Type 1 is characterized by brief "flashbacks," whereas type 2 is more chronic, with reports of symptoms lasting years.[26]

Conclusion

People who are struggling with depression, substance abuse, anxiety, or other symptoms of mental illness do not feel as though these pathologies can easily be separated from their personalities. They contextualize these symptoms and incorporate them into their personal narratives. A person with negative thoughts about themselves or the world—a symptom in both depressive disorders and PTSD—will earnestly believe things like "the world is a bad place" or "I am unworthy." These views need to be challenged, and psychedelic-assisted psychotherapy facilitates a level of introspection that makes this possible. Such a feat is not accomplished due to the physiologic effects of the drug alone; it is due to the interactive effects between the drug, the setting, the mindsets of the patient, and the therapist's interventions. In other words, psychedelic-assisted psychotherapy bridges the fields of psychotherapy and pharmacotherapy, producing robust results in patients with a host of difficult-to-treat conditions.

As mentioned earlier, the psychedelic experience is a crucial part of psychedelic-assisted psychotherapy. Although recreational users may be attracted to these drugs because of their ability to enhance mood or produce brilliant visualizations, their ability to occasion mystical experiences via NOSCs appears to be their principal value from a therapeutic or ceremonial perspective. The insights gained during these experiences appear to be one of the primary sources, if not *the* primary source, of their tremendous therapeutic promise.

REFERENCES

1. Barrett FS, Griffiths RR. Classic hallucinogens and mystical experiences: phenomenology and neural correlates. *Curr Top Behav Neurosci*. 2018;36:393-430. doi:10.1007/7854_2017_474. PMID: 28401522; PMCID: PMC6707356.
2. Passie T, Guss J, Krähenmann R. Lower-dose psycholytic therapy—a neglected approach. *Front Psychiatry*. 2022;13:1020505. doi:10.3389/fpsyt.2022.1020505. PMID: 36532196; PMCID: PMC9755513.
3. Jay M. *Mescaline: A Global History of the First Psychedelic*. Yale University Press; 2021:133.
4. Swanson LR. Unifying theories of psychedelic drug effects. *Front Pharmacol*. 2018;9:172. doi:10.3389/fphar.2018.00172. PMID: 29568270; PMCID: PMC5853825.
5. Carhart-Harris RL, Friston KJ. REBUS and the anarchic brain: toward a unified model of the brain action of psychedelics. *Pharmacol Rev*. 2019;71(3):316-344. doi:10.1124/pr.118.017160. PMID: 31221820; PMCID: PMC6588209.
6. Daumal R. Two psychedelic experiences: a fundamental experiment. *Psychedelic Rev*. 1965;5:40-48. Accessed on April 29, 2024. https://maps.org/wp-content/uploads/2007/11/01540dau.pdf
7. Pollan M. *How to Change Your Mind: What the New Science of Psychedelics Teaches Us About Consciousness, Dying, Addiction, Depression, and Transcendence*. Penguin Random House; 2019:69-75.
8. Maclean KA, Leoutsakos JM, Johnson MW, Griffiths RR. Factor analysis of the Mystical Experience Questionnaire: a study of experiences occasioned by the hallucinogen psilocybin. *J Sci Study Relig*. 2012;51(4):721-737. doi:10.1111/j.1468-5906.2012.01685.x. PMID: 23316089; PMCID: PMC3539773.
9. Griffiths RR, Richards WA, McCann U, Jess R. Psilocybin can occasion mystical-type experiences having substantial and sustained personal meaning and spiritual significance. *Psychopharmacology (Berl)*. 2006;187(3):268-283.
10. Pahnke WM. *Drugs and Mysticism: An Analysis of the Relationship Between Psychedelic Drugs and the Mystical Consciousness*. Dissertation. Harvard University; 1963:83. Accessed April 29, 2024. https://maps.org/images/pdf/books/pahnke/walter_pahnke_drugs_and_mysticism.pdf
11. Barrett FS, Johnson MW, Griffiths RR. Validation of the revised Mystical Experience Questionnaire in experimental sessions with psilocybin. *J Psychopharmacol*. 2015;29(11):1182-1190. doi:10.1177/0269881115609019. PMID: 26442957; PMCID: PMC5203697.
12. Griffiths RR, Richards WA, McCann U, Jesse R. Psilocybin can occasion mystical-type experiences having substantial and sustained personal meaning and spiritual significance. *Psychopharmacology (Berl)*. 2006;187(3):268-283; discussion 284-292. doi:10.1007/s00213-006-0457-5. PMID: 16826400.
13. Smith H. *Cleansing the Doors of Perception: The Religious Significance of Entheogenic Plants and Chemicals*. Penguin Putname;2000, 33-43.
14. Long J. Near-death experience. Evidence for their reality. *Mo Med*. 2014;111(5):372-380. PMID: 25438351; PMCID: PMC6172100.

15. Timmermann C, Zeifman RJ, Erritzoe D, Nutt DJ, Carhart-Harris RL. Effects of DMT on mental health outcomes in healthy volunteers. *Sci Rep. 2024*;14:3097. doi:10.1038/s41598-024-53363-y
16. Martial C, Cassol H, Charland-Verville V, et al. Neurochemical models of near-death experiences: a large-scale study based on the semantic similarity of written reports. *Conscious Cogn.* 2019;69:52-69. doi:10.1016/j.concog.2019.01.011. PMID: 30711788.
17. Ley L, Holze F, Arikci D, et al. Comparative acute effects of mescaline, lysergic acid diethylamide, and psilocybin in a randomized, double-blind, placebo-controlled cross-over study in healthy participants. *Neuropsychopharmacology.* 2023;48(11):1659-1667. doi:10.1038/s41386-023-01607-2
18. Michael P, Luke D, Robinson O. An encounter with the other: a thematic and content analysis of DMT experiences from a naturalistic field study. *Front Psychol.* 2021 16;12:720717. doi: 10.3389/fpsyg.2021.720717. PMID: 34975614; PMCID: PMC8716686.
19. Kolp E, Friedman HL, Krupitsky E, et al. Ketamine psychedelic psychotherapy: focus on its pharmacology, phenomenology, and clinical applications. In: Wolfson P, Hartelius G, eds. *The Ketamine Papers: Science, Therapy, and Transformation.* Multidisciplinary Association for Psychedelic Studies; 2016: 97-197.
20. Brown TK. Ibogaine in the treatment of substance dependence. *Curr Drug Abuse Rev.* 2013;6(1):3-16. doi:10.2174/15672050113109990001. PMID: 23627782.
21. Mithoefer MC. *A Manual for MDMA-Assisted Psychotherapy in the Treatment of Post-traumatic Stress Disorder.* Multidisciplinary Association for Psychedelic Studies; 2017:13-14. Accessed April 24, 2024. https://maps.org/wp-content/uploads/2022/05/MDMA-Assisted-Psychotherapy-Treatment-Manual-V8.1-22AUG2017.pdf
22. Zaretsky TG, Jagodnik KM, Barsic KM, et al. The psychedelic future of post-traumatic stress disorder treatment. *Curr Neuropharmacol.* 2024;22;636-735. doi:10.2174/1570159X22666231027111147
23. Studerus E, Vizeli P, Harder S, Ley L, Liechti ME. Prediction of MDMA response in healthy humans: a pooled analysis of placebo-controlled studies. *J Psychopharmacol.* 2021May;35(5):556-565. doi:10.1177/0269881121998322. PMID: 33781103; PMCID: PMC8155734.
24. Carhart-Harris RL, Kaelen M, Whalley MG, Bolstridge M, Feilding A, Nutt DJ. LSD enhances suggestibility in healthy volunteers. *Psychopharmacology (Berl).* 2015;232(4):785-794. doi:10.1007/s00213-014-3714-z. PMID: 25242255.
25. Vis PJ, Goudriaan AE, Ter Meulen BC, Blom JD. On perception and consciousness in HPPD: a systematic review. *Front Neurosci.* 2021;15:675768. doi:10.3389/fnins.2021.675768. PMID: 34456666; PMCID: PMC8385145.
26. Halpern JH, Lerner AG, Passie T. A review of hallucinogen persisting perception disorder (HPPD) and an exploratory study of subjects claiming symptoms of HPPD. *Curr Top Behav Neurosci.* 2018;36:333-360. doi:10.1007/7854_2016_457. PMID: 27822679.

6
Psychedelic-Assisted Psychotherapy

The focus of this book is on psychedelic substances, but psychotherapy plays a crucial role in enhancing the therapeutic value of these drugs. The "set and setting" during a psychedelic experience have a tremendous amount of influence on the subjective experience of the patient, and so does the level and quality of support with which they are provided. Consequently, trained therapists are integral and necessary components of psychedelic-assisted psychotherapy. More than just providing a supportive and welcoming environment that is conducive to the patient's embrace of the psychedelic experience, therapists must know how to serve as effective guides.

The phrase "set and setting" has a great deal of significance within the world of psychedelic research and often extends into cannabis culture as well. There is a good reason for this, as these are two of three determining factors that can affect a psychedelic experience within the clinic—the third being "support." To review, *set* refers to the mindset of the patient, meaning their personality, level of intelligence, current mood, expectations about psychedelics, and concern about past or upcoming events. The therapist's mindset is important, as well. *Setting* refers to the physical, emotional, and social environment in which the person finds themselves. Finally, *support* refers to support systems in place before, during, and after the administration of the psychedelic.

This chapter will provide a brief overview of the elements of psychedelic-assisted psychotherapy. Though best practices have not been established by any formal agency or organization, basic protocols for the administration of psychedelics have been established over the course of several decades. That said, it should be noted that each drug discussed in this book is unique and that there are subtle (and sometimes less than subtle) differences between their subjective effects, even among the classic, serotonergic psychedelics like lysergic acid diethylamide (LSD) and psilocybin. Of note, many clinics (run by mental health as well as nonmental health practitioners) offer ketamine therapy without psychotherapy, though there are also ketamine clinics where psychotherapy is an integral part of the treatment plan.

Psychedelics in the Clinic

As described in Chapter 3, psychedelics have been used in experimental psychiatry for decades. Although mescaline was often seen as a clinical curiosity that (even into the 1950s) was thought to induce temporary psychosis, the growing popularity of LSD within the medical community throughout that decade revealed that psychedelics had several clinical applications.[1]

Despite recognition of psychedelics' potential utility, there remained a lack of appreciation for how set and setting could influence the contours of the psychedelic experience. Researchers would provide minimal preparatory remarks about the nature of the drug, administer a moderate or large dose, and then leave the individual alone in a sterile examination room with a bed and a few other pieces of furniture, oftentimes for hours on end. In some cases, even restraints were used.[2] Psychedelic researcher William Richards' recollection of his first experience with psilocybin in Germany in 1963 illustrates this experience quite well. As he wrote in his 2016 book, *Sacred Knowledge*, the study took place in "a rather dim and drab basement room, just large enough for a cot, an end table, and a chair."[3(ppxvii-xx)] Although restraints were not used in his case, his tone is still colored by astonishment about how he received no guidance or preparation and that he had virtually no human contact of any kind throughout the experience (a psychiatric resident evidently came in at one point to test his knee reflexes).[3(pixx)] Though Williams still managed to have what could be described as a mystical-type experience, the literature from the 1950s and even into the

1960s is replete with stories of participants responding to such hostile elements with anxiety, hostility, and terror.

As the administration of psychedelics became more humane, two distinct and far more effective paradigms arose to administer psychedelics in the clinic: the psycholytic paradigm and psychedelic-assisted psychotherapy.[4] In the psycholytic model, a relatively small dose of the psychedelic drug is administered. According to Bravo and Grob, "The psychedelics were seen as drugs that could weaken an individual's psychological defenses, thus releasing unconscious material and heightening emotional responsiveness for a patient in psychoanalytically oriented psychotherapy."[5] Psycholytic therapy was far more popular on the European continent, with leading figures like Hanscarl Leuner of Germany continuing his therapeutic work with psychedelics into the 1980s.[4] However, within the United States, this treatment modality has been out of favor since the 1950s.

Psychedelic-assisted psychotherapy is notably different from the psycholytic paradigm because patients receive moderate to large doses of classic psychedelics like LSD or psilocybin. As described in Chapter 3, this paradigm was developed by psychiatrists Abram Hoffer and Humphrey Osmond (who coined the term "psychedelic") in the late 1950s in Saskatchewan. It usually includes a dyadic structure across three phases: pretreatment seasons, treatment sessions, and posttreatment sessions. The two therapists (typically but not necessarily a male-female dyad) should be present during all phases, but it is especially important for both therapists to be present during treatment sessions.[6] Psychiatric work being conducted with drugs like psilocybin, LSD, ibogaine, 3,4-methylenedioxymethamphetamine (MDMA), and mescaline follows this model, which will be outlined in the remainder of this chapter. It should be noted that one distinction between the use of drugs like MDMA and classic psychedelics like psilocybin or LSD is that the former often involves substantial and sustained interactions between patients and therapists, whereas the latter may not involve a lot of direct interactions between patient and therapists until the session is coming to close (oftentimes within the last hour or so).[6] This is due to the different subjective effects of these drugs.

Creating the Right Set

"Set" refers to the patient's mindset. The effects of psychedelic drugs can be unpredictable, especially in psychedelic-naive individuals. Consequently, clinicians should strive to establish a therapeutic alliance with the patient over the course of multiple pretreatment sessions so they can become trusted guides during the psychedelic experience. Meetings prior to the dosing session should involve a discussion of the patient's personal and medical background, what (if any) medications they are currently taking, any experience with psychedelics, what they hope to gain from the treatment, and any concerns or anxieties they have about using psychedelics.[5]

As the establishment of a therapeutic alliance is what is crucial, one should not limit themselves to a set number of hours or meetings. All patients are different. Some may need more hours of preparation, while others may need less. However, for reference, the technique of ketamine-assisted psychotherapy developed by Krupitsky involves at least 5 to 10 hours of psychotherapy before the administration of ketamine.[7] Meanwhile, Horton and colleagues found in their review of 11 trials with psilocybin that the mean number of sessions was 3.31 (±1.44), and the average total time dedicated to these preparatory sessions was approximately 6 hours.[6]

Therapists may choose to give patients reading material or instructions prior to the dosing session. Some therapists believe that dietary restrictions, abstinence from sex and intoxicants, and daily exercises for the body and mind (eg, meditation and yoga) are also necessary. As an example, Kolp describes a preparatory period of 6 weeks prior to ketamine administration that involves weekly participation in group psychotherapy; a calorie-restricted, whole food plant-based diet; optimal hydration; limited screen time; avoidance of sugar, caffeine, nicotine, alcohol, and other drugs; and a daily regimen of exercise, meditation, and spiritual contemplation.[7]

Creating the Right Setting

As noted previously, "setting" refers to the patient's environment while they are experiencing the acute effects of the psychedelic. Patients should feel psychologically free to speak openly and honestly without judgment, and they should also feel at ease within the physical space that they occupy. Consequently, psychedelics should be administered in rooms that are above all else private, quiet, and comfortable. Comfort refers to the temperature in the room, the lighting, the furniture, and even the aesthetics. As noted earlier, best practices indicate that there should be two therapists during sessions, and each should engage in empathetic and active listening during sessions.

As outlined by the Multidisciplinary Association for Psychedelic Studies' (MAPS) manual for MDMA-assisted psychotherapy in treating posttraumatic stress disorder (PTSD), furniture should include a sofa or futon, as well as chairs for therapists.[i] Patients should also have access to blankets and pillows. With respect to aesthetics, MAPS recommends fresh flowers and artwork that avoids powerful or negative imagery. In addition, the manual notes "The setting should be more similar to a comfortably furnished living room than a medical facility."[8] Amenities should include high-quality snacks, a stereo, video recording equipment, and medical equipment (including rescue medications to relieve anxiety [eg, benzodiazepines] or in extreme cases a 5-HT$_{2A}$ antagonist like olanzapine [Zyprexa] or perhaps ketanserin when working with classic psychedelics).[9] A nearby area should be available to accommodate the patient—and a significant other, if desired—should they want to stay the night.[8]

In most cases, patients are equipped with eyeshades and headphones connected to the stereo. A playlist with classical or ambient music has become standard, and songs typically do not have lyrics. Should any song in the playlist include singing, it should be performed in a language that is unfamiliar to the patient and not a song with which they are familiar so as to avoid introducing content or themes that might distract them. The goal of the music is to draw the patient inward, and Zaretsky and colleagues report that many patients feel as though music has a central therapeutic function in psychedelic-assisted psychotherapy.[2]

Providing the Right Support

Therapists should have received training in facilitating psychedelic-assisted psychotherapy, which includes didactic instruction on the nuances of psychedelic experiences and potential adverse events, as well as ways to minimize, mitigate, or resolve negative reactions. Additionally, training should center on providing a nondirective and supportive setting with an empathic, nonjudgmental presence. The goal is to facilitate a more introspective experience and to respect patients' innate capacity to heal. Therapists may also provide physical reassurance

---

[i] The MAPS manual is an excellent resource that goes into detail about best practices when administering MDMA and PTSD, but many of the lessons are universal for any psychedelic. The manual can be downloaded for free: https://maps.org/wp-content/uploads/2022/05/MDMA-Assisted-Psychotherapy-Treatment-Manual-V8.1-22AUG2017.pdf

and reality orientation.[6] Other forms of support either before or after treatment sessions may include conventional therapies like motivational enhancement therapy (MET), cognitive-behavioral therapy (CBT), supportive-expressive group therapy, and eclectic psychotherapeutic intervention.[6]

Should the patient experience somatic manifestations of trauma, therapists may guide the patient using breathing techniques, and may use therapeutic touch when appropriate, or focused bodywork to ameliorate these issues. A discussion of the potential use of touch should occur during preparation sessions to unambiguously understand the patient's level of comfort with touch (see "Consent Agreements" section). Any form of touch during the treatment session should be preceded by proper communication and notice, as well as respect for the patient's autonomy and vulnerabilities while under the influence of psychedelic drugs. Any touch that is explicitly sexual or colored by sexual connotations is categorically unethical and abusive. Although it is not always encouraged that clinicians instigate therapeutic touch, withholding touch may be countertherapeutic in some instances or even perceived as neglectful by the patient. Therapists ought to always put the needs of the patient first in these situations.

Therapists should also be familiar with the patient's social support network and consider if and how these individuals can be of assistance. In some cases, it can be as little as providing transportation to and from the clinic following a session. In other cases, a member of the support system may come to pretreatment or integrative sessions to help with the healing process within a clinical setting. They may then use the lessons they learned to provide additional support outside of the clinic. In some cases, therapists may even feel it appropriate to invite a loved one into the therapeutic session close to its end. As noted earlier, some patients may benefit from an overnight stay with a significant other.

Posttreatment and Integration

Following treatment sessions, patients should undergo at least one posttreatment session to speak about their experience in detail and reflect upon its significance. Therapists should use this opportunity to assist patients in processing the experience in a manner that leads to lasting therapeutic effects. Integration sessions should occur between treatment sessions if psychedelics are to be administered multiple times. Posttreatment sessions can also explore the implications of the treatment, especially after several weeks or months.[2]

Consent Agreements

The effects of psychedelic drugs can be difficult to explain or comprehend, especially if the patient has never used them before. Their unique effects can also complicate the informed consent process. Given that no government agencies have approved the use of psychedelics in the psychedelic-assisted psychotherapy paradigm, there are no formal guidelines for practitioners at this time. However, informed consent is vital to the ethical practice of medicine, and therapists should make a good-faith effort to abide by the spirit of medical ethics even in the absence of established protocols or prescriptive guidelines.

Marks and colleagues contend that any informed consent involving psychedelics must address seven distinct elements: "(1) The potential for acute and chronic perceptual disturbances, (2) possible personality changes and altered metaphysical beliefs, (3) the role of limited physical touch, (4) the potential for patient abuse or coercion, (5) the role and risks of data collection, (6) relevant clinician discourses, and (7) interactive patient education and comprehension assessment."[10]

To comply with these various elements, clinicians should make good-faith efforts to inform patients about the full range of effects of psychedelics. There should be special emphasis on the fact that these drugs are unique and go beyond alterations in sense perception. Particularly if the patient has a mystical-type experience, the subjective effects can be profound and even life-changing. This may significantly change the way they perceive the world. Another potential risk to be discussed is that some individuals may experience chronic perceptual disturbances (hallucinogen-persisting perception disorder [HPPD]) following the use of psychedelics (see Chapter 5). In addition to these potential long-term effects, patients may be more suggestible following the use of psychedelics in the weeks or months following administration and should know to be vigilant against the possibility of exploitation—including by therapists.

To avoid unwanted touch, clinicians and patients should agree upon and document the types of reassuring or therapeutic touch to which the patient consents. Marks and colleagues provide one example of a simplified system using colors that patients may employ to signify the level of touch with which they are comfortable. For example, they may say "red" to convey that they no longer wish to be touched or "green" to convey that they have consented to the touch as discussed prior to the session.

Should the patient be involved in a clinical trial, they should be fully aware of any data that will be collected. If the practitioner has any affiliation with a pharmaceutical company that is sponsoring the trial, that information should be disclosed as well.

It is absolutely vital that patients fully understand the full scope of risks associated with psychedelic-assisted psychotherapy, and it is up to clinicians to proactively provide unbiased information so that patients can make fully informed decisions about their health.

Scalability

As one considers the level of care and investment of time that therapists must make with each patient, it becomes very clear that psychedelic-assisted psychotherapy can be very resource intensive, especially if the treatment involves multiple sessions where psychedelics are administered. Facilities would have to adapt because the protocols outlined above would be demanding on individual personnel, as therapists would be expected to remain with participants for 8 hours or more and would likely have difficulty seeing other patients on those days. However, it could be argued that conventional treatment modalities require more time and resources over the long run and that psychedelic-assisted psychotherapy is more efficient because remission of some disorders may be achieved with only a handful of sessions (compared to hours upon hours of therapy and regular calibrations of medications). The acute demand for specific personnel for an entire day presents a challenge for the scalability of psychedelic-assisted psychotherapy, given the current framework of our medical system.

It should be reiterated that this criticism pertains to psychedelic-assisted psychotherapy and that there may be other paradigms involving psychedelic drugs that may be less resource intensive but still effective. This will no doubt be an area of future research, as institutions and private companies seek novel and more efficient ways to ensure certified therapists are providing psychedelic-assisted psychotherapy without detracting resources from existing health care systems.

Conclusion

Though an often-underappreciated element of psychedelic-assisted psychotherapy, particularly in the media, therapists play a vital role in catalyzing insights and focusing on the subjective effects of psychedelic drugs to optimize their therapeutic value. Well before the clinical use of psychedelics started in earnest during the 1950s and 1960s, the role of the guide was seen as essential to the psychedelic experience. It was simply played by a shaman, healer, or roadman. In many ways, therapists should see themselves as an extension of this tradition while being firmly grounded in the scientific world.

REFERENCES

1. Jay M. *Mescaline: A Global History of the First Psychedelic*. Yale University Press; 2019:169-198.
2. Zaretsky TG, Jagodnik KM, Barsic KM, et al. The psychedelic future of post-traumatic stress disorder treatment. *Curr Neuropharmacol*. 2024;22:636-735. doi:10.2174/15701 59X22666231027111147
3. Williams RA. *Sacred Knowledge: Psychedelics and Religious Experiences*. Columbia University Press; 2015.
4. Passie T, Guss J, Krähenmann R. Lower-dose psycholytic therapy—a neglected approach. *Front Psychiatry*. 2022;13:1020505. doi:10.3389/fpsyt.2022.1020505. PMID: 36532196; PMCID: PMC9755513.
5. Bravo G, Grob C. Shamans, sacraments, and psychiatrists. *J Psychoactive Drugs*. 2012;21(1):123-128. doi:10.1080/02791072.1989.10472149
6. Horton DM, Morrison B, Schmidt J. Systematized review of psychotherapeutic components of psilocybin-assisted psychotherapy. *Am J Psychother*. 2021;74(4): 140-149. doi:10.1176/appi.psychotherapy.20200055. PMID: 34293927.
7. Kolp E, Friedman HL, Krupitsky E, et al. Ketamine psychedelic psychotherapy: focus on its pharmacology, phenomenology, and clinical applications. In: Wolfson P, Hartelius G, eds. *The Ketamine Papers: Science, Therapy, and Transformation*. Multidisciplinary Association for Psychedelic Studies; 2016:97-197.
8. Mithoefer MC. *A Manual for MDMA-Assisted Psychotherapy in the Treatment of Post-traumatic Stress Disorder*. Multidisciplinary Association for Psychedelic Studies; 2017:13-14. Accessed April 24, 2024. https://maps.org/wp-content/uploads/2022/05/MDMA-Assisted-Psychotherapy-Treatment-Manual-V8.1-22AUG2017.pdf
9. Becker AM, Klaiber A, Holze F, et al. Ketanserin reverses the acute response to LSD in a randomized, double-blind, placebo-controlled, crossover study in healthy participants. *Int J Neuropsychopharmacol*. 2023;26(2):97-106. doi:10.1093/ijnp/pyac075. PMID: 36342343; PMCID: PMC9926053.
10. Marks M, Brendel RW, Shachar C, Cohen IG. Essentials of informed consent to psychedelic medicine. *JAMA Psychiatry*. 2024;81(6):611-617. doi:10.1001/jamapsychiatry.2024.0184. PMID: 38598209.

7
How Psychedelics Affect the Brain

Though each psychedelic discussed in this book has a unique pharmacology and mechanism of action, there are some generalizations that can be made when it comes to how these drugs affect the brain. This chapter provides an overview of these shared effects, while the unique mechanisms of action for each drug will be covered in their respective chapters. In particular, this chapter describes the primary site (5-HT$_{2A}$) of drug action for classic psychedelics, the brain regions affected by psychedelics (particularly the default mode network [DMN]), how psychedelics are believed to affect global brain functioning, and more importantly how all of these drugs appear to open what are known as critical periods for social reward learning.

As a reminder, "classic psychedelics" include psilocybin, lysergic acid diethylamide (LSD), mescaline, N,N-dimethyltryptamine (DMT). Entactogens such as 3,4-methylenedioxymethamphetamine (MDMA), oneirogens such as ibogaine, and dissociative anesthetics such as ketamine (collectively known as "atypical psychedelics") have distinct mechanisms of action at receptor sites that will be covered in their respective chapters, though there are some overlaps with the classic psychedelics that will be the focus of this chapter.

The notion that consciousness can be explained entirely by the activity of neural networks is based on metaphysical assumptions that are commonly known as physicalism. The view presented later is not meant to be an endorsement of a purely physicalist model but rather a more modest and evidence-based contention that conscious experience is mediated through the activity in the brain. In other words, there are clear neural correlates to lived experience. When these correlates are altered, consciousness itself is altered.

Primary Target Receptor: 5-HT$_{2A}$

Classic or serotonergic psychedelics possess a structural similarity to serotonin (5-hydroxytryptamine [5-HT]). Serotonin plays numerous roles in the central nervous system (CNS), peripheral nervous system, and enteric nervous system. Serotonin is the natural ligand of a family of G protein–coupled receptors that mediate both excitatory and inhibitory neurotransmission. There are seven types of serotonin receptors, as well as several subtypes.

One such subtype, 5-HT$_{2A}$, is the primary target of serotonergic psychedelics, where they act as agonists. Said activity is believed to be responsible for the preponderance of these drugs' effects. This is evidenced by the fact that the subjective effects of psychedelics can be blunted or eliminated with the administration of 5-HT$_{2A}$ antagonists such as ketanserin.[1]

5-HT$_{2A}$: Distribution and Activation

5-HT$_{2A}$ receptors are expressed throughout the body and widely distributed throughout the parts of the CNS that are central to cognition, executive functions, memory, and emotional regulation.[2] 5-HT$_{2A}$ receptors are expressed in all laminae of the neocortex (especially layers I, IV, and V) and are particularly high in the claustrum, frontal and temporal cortices, the reticular nucleus of the thalamus, ventral tegmental area, locus coeruleus, amygdala, and DMN.[3] Many of these brain areas are associated with stress responses, and stress has been shown to increase the expression of 5-HT$_{2A}$ receptors.[4] Moreover, these receptors are highly expressed in the visual cortex, which may help explain why perceptual changes associated with psychedelics are most saliently visual.[5]

Crucially, 5-HT$_{2A}$ receptors are also highly expressed at dendrites of pyramidal neurons in layer V of the prefrontal cortex, which is connected to the amygdala, ventral tegmental area, and nucleus accumbens.[1]

The presence of 5-HT_{2A} receptors on pyramidal neurons, interneurons, and glial cells in the hippocampus, amygdala, and neocortex has been confirmed by morphologic and double immunofluorescence analyses.[2]

Activation of 5-HT_{2A} receptors results in the release of glutamate, α-amino-3-hydroxy-5-methyl-4-isoxazolepropionic acid (AMPA) potentiation, and the increase of brain-derived neurotrophic factor (BDNF). BDNF activates tropomyosin-related kinase B (TrkB) receptors, as well as one of the signaling pathways of mammalian target of rapamycin complex 1 (mTORC1).[6] Of note, preclinical studies have suggested that stimulation of 5-HT_{1A} may also activate a cascade involving AMPA, BDNF, and mTOR signaling.[7] Activation of these pathways is associated with increased synaptogenesis and neuroplasticity, which, when paired with psychotherapy, are believed to be the primary therapeutic avenue through which psychedelic medicines operate.[7]

In the case of MDMA, serotonergic activity occurs via two routes. Firstly, it demonstrates a weak affinity for 5-HT_{1A}, 5-HT_{2A}, and 5-HT_{2C} receptors, as well as a stronger affinity for 5-HT_{2B} receptors. Though weak, agonism at 5-HT_{2A} is responsible for any visual disturbances and can be blocked by ketanserin, a selective 5-HT_{2A} antagonist.[8] Secondly, MDMA binds to serotonin transporters (SERTs), leading to inhibition of serotonin reuptake and an increase in extracellular serotonin.

The administration of classic psychedelics results in the downregulation of 5-HT_{2A} receptors. Tachyphylaxis, which Buchborn and colleagues define as, "in-between-session tolerance occurring at repeated short-interval application," is a prominent feature of all classic psychedelics and one of the reasons why they have limited abuse potential.[9] The decline in subjective effects with repeated administration is very pronounced but temporary. While it is true that upregulation of 5-HT_{2A} receptors is associated with increased stress and that downregulation of 5-HT_{2A} receptors results in reduced activity in the medial prefrontal cortex (mPFC) and amygdala—which are both pathologically hyperactive in depressive disorders, anxiety disorders, and trauma- and stressor-related disorders such as posttraumatic stress disorder (PTSD)—the transient nature of the downregulation makes it an uncompelling mediator for the therapeutic effects of psychedelics.[10,11]

Consciousness and the Hierarchical Brain

Though neuroscience is perhaps decades away from explaining consciousness entirely, if indeed that is possible at all, several organizing principles of the mind have been proposed that seem to be corroborated by clinical evidence. One such principle is that the mind is adaptive and that beliefs are constantly and unconsciously being updated to improve the precision of our predictive capabilities. Carhart-Harris and Friston describe this model of predictive coding further, writing that "the brain instantiates, within its hierarchical architecture, best-guess statistical approximations (generative models) of the causes of its sensorium based on Bayesian principles of empirically informed belief updating."[5] To put it more straightforward: The brain is wired to reduce its own prediction errors.

To do so, the brain relies upon an established hierarchy. According to Carhart-Harris and Friston and their REBUS (RElaxed Beliefs Under pSychedelics) model, signaling from sensory epithelia represents the lowest level of this hierarchy, neuronal populations of superficial pyramidal cells represent the middle levels of the hierarchy, and deep pyramidal cells sit at the top of this hierarchy.[5] The relay of sensory input travels in a bottom-up direction, while higher levels work in a top-down manner to instantize the input. "The recurrent neuronal message passing (ie, neuronal dynamics) tries to minimize the amplitude of prediction errors at each and every level of the hierarchy, thereby furnishing the best explanation for sensory input at multiple levels of hierarchal abstraction," write Carhart-Harris and Friston.[5] Precision of posterior beliefs (priors) is experienced subjectively and intuitively as felt confidence. The greater the precision, the greater the experience of confidence.

One of the peculiarities of this top-down system is that high-level priors can override sensory inputs that are considered aberrant. As one example that was referred to in the late Daniel Dennett's book, *Consciousness Explained*, we all have a blind spot.[12] This is not a metaphor. You have a blind spot, I have a blind spot, and anyone else reading this book has a blind spot because a portion of each eye has no photoreceptors at the site of the optic nerve.

Though we do not regularly perceive this blind spot, it can be revealed through a simple experiment. Close one eye, and then look at the cross in Figure 7.1 while holding the page about 10 in from your open eye (you may need to adjust the distance between your eye and the book).

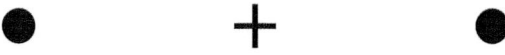

Figure 7.1 The blind spot illusion reveals that the brain "fills in" the portion of the eye without photoreceptors. (Taken from Daniel Dennett's *Consciousness Explained*.)

When your left eye is closed, the black circle on the left disappears. When your right eye is closed, the right circle disappears.

This phenomenon represents something far more profound than a blind spot, of course. Instead of being an area within your field of vision that is discernibly incapable of perception, it is instead presented within your conscious mind as a continuation of its surroundings. This is a salient reminder that consciousness is not a passive experience. Consciousness is an active, rigorously organized process that is mediated through the CNS. "In our present context," philosopher Thomas Metzinger wrote, "a fruitful way of looking at the human brain, therefore, is as a system which, even in ordinary waking states, constantly hallucinates at the world, as a system that constantly lets its internal autonomous simulational dynamics collide with the ongoing flow of sensory input, vigorously dreaming at the world and thereby generating the content of phenomenal experience."[13]

The Default Mode Network and Compression

Within the hierarchy of the brain, the DMN occupies the top position. This network consists of four strongly interconnected brain regions: the precuneus, mPFC, posterior cingulate cortex (PCC), and angular gyrus.[14] *The DMN is a resting-state network, meaning that it experiences increased activity when individuals are not performing tasks, and that activity in the network decreases when task-dependent attention is demanded.*[14] The DMN is activated when your thoughts turn inward and more introspective. These metacognitive activities have been described as "species-defining" processes, including moral reasoning, counterfactual thinking, and self-consciousness.[5] The DMN has also been described (somewhat loosely) as the neural equivalent of the Freudian ego.[5]

Given the DMN's position at the top of the hierarchy, its priors are given more weight than priors from lower rungs of the hierarchy. They are also central to the construction of one's identity or ego. More than simply being overweighted within the conscious mind, the priors of the DMN compress bottom-up signals to the point that they lose any influence over consciousness and become virtually imperceptible.[5] This becomes problematic when the priors of the ego become pathologic, resulting in maladaptive coping mechanisms to trauma or stress, which can lead to rumination and thought suppression.[15] It can also prevent the infiltration of new information and the establishment of new priors. In other words, the DMN becomes a closed loop where problematic patterns are repeated, and pathologies thrive.

Alterations in Functional Connectivity

When individuals enter into non-ordinary states of consciousness (NOSC), particularly while under the influence of classic psychedelics, they also experience alterations in functional connectivity between brain regions. This can be conceived as an increase in entropy within the brain. Carhart-Harris defines entropy as, "A dimensionless quality that is used for measuring uncertainty about the state of a system, but it can also imply physical qualities, where high entropy is synonymous with high disorder."[16] Higher states of entropy within the brain are characterized by increased randomness, disorder, unpredictability, and disruptions in top-down cognitive processing.[14]

While in this state, there is an increased synchronization of regions responsible for processing sensory information (eg, the visual cortex, precuneus, and postcentral gyrus) and desynchronization of the DMN.[17] The more intensive the decoupling of the DMN from other brain networks, the greater the sense of ego dissolution.[17] Psychedelics appear to be capable of causing such a disruption to the DMN through their primary mechanism of action at the 5-HT$_{2A}$ receptor.

When the DMN is disrupted, the high-level priors described earlier relax their imperium over consciousness, leading to a temporary "flattening" of the brain's rigid hierarchies and a heightened state of plasticity. This flattening of the hierarchy allows for more bottom-up signaling to become part of one's conscious experience, leading to some of the most unique subjective effects of psychedelics and mystical experiences, including ego dissolution, a sense of unity with others or the universe, vivid autobiographical recall, and near-death-like experiences.

Additionally, the signals from the lower rungs of the system become more perceptible and are recognized within conscious experience. Consequently, pathologic priors become subject to greater scrutiny, and this capacity for insight while the subjective effect of the drug is at its peak, when coupled with psychotherapy, can grant patients a level of introspection on their condition that would otherwise be difficult to achieve. As the effects of the drug wear off, consciousness returns to its ordinary state, but the patient retains the insights gained during the psychedelic experience.

Alterations in functional connectivity may also lead to a disruption in cortico-striatal-thalamo-cortical (CSTC) pathway. Within this pathway, the thalamus plays the role of gatekeeper and filters sensory information as it is passed on to the cerebral cortex. Psychedelics appear to reduce gating by the thalamus, which may explain some of the subjective effects of these drugs. This process is also mediated through agonist activity at 5-HT$_{2A}$ receptors.[6]

As proposed by Barrett and colleagues, yet another potential mechanism of action of psychedelics involves disruptions of cortical networks by activating receptors in the claustrum.[18] Since the claustrum has a high density of both 5-HT$_{2A}$ receptors and κ-opioid receptors, this could potentially be a target for both classic psychedelics and ibogaine, which is a κ-opioid receptor agonist.[19]

Classic psychedelics also reduce the reactivity of the amygdala, which is responsible for emotional processing, interpreting stimuli, and releasing distress signals should it perceive said stimuli to be potentially dangerous. Studies have found that psilocybin, LSD, and ayahuasca attenuate the amygdala's sensitivity to threatening visual stimuli, indicating that classic psychedelics can reduce fear responses triggered by negative or traumatic associations with stimuli.[6] Restoration of functional connectivity between the amygdala and ventromedial prefrontal cortex, which exhibits top-down inhibitory control over the amygdala in normal conditions, has also been reported following the administration of psilocybin and could have clinical relevance to individuals with depressive disorders and anhedonia.[20]

To summarize, the activity of classic psychedelics at 5-HT$_{2A}$ receptors decreases connectivity within several parts of the brain, which is experienced as a destabilization of reinforced patterns of thinking and behaving. In individuals who are trapped in pathologic cycles—whether it involves problematic substance use, excessive rumination, obsessions and compulsions, inability to process trauma, negative thoughts about oneself, or unhealthy coping mechanisms—these disruptions in ordinary neural pathways and increased cortical plasticity correspond with heightened introspection and many of the subjective experience associated with psychedelics and mystical-type experiences (eg, ego dissolution, near-death experiences). With the assistance of therapists before, during, and after the psychedelic session, patients can develop a means of adjusting and correcting these pathologic patterns.

The Reopening of Critical Windows

One question that has puzzled researchers for several years is why classic psychedelics and other drugs such as ibogaine, ketamine, and MDMA all seem to have similar effects in terms of their abilities to improve mood, reduce the severity of PTSD, and help treat substance use disorders despite having distinct mechanisms of action. Research pioneered by Gül

Dölen of John Hopkins University has potentially shed some light on the matter and suggested that all these drugs open what are known as critical periods for social reward learning by conferring a state of metaplasticity in neurons within certain brain regions. Although "neuroplasticity" is a somewhat nebulous word to begin with, and "metaplasticity" is even murkier, it is being used here to denote a state where neurons are more receptive to stimuli that induce plasticity. Authors of the study note that this is a naturally occurring phenomenon that happens during specific periods of brain development, where "increased malleability of synaptic, circuit, and behavioral modifications" respond to "ethologically relevant stimuli."[21]

Through the use of mouse models, Dölen's team has found that classic psychedelics, as well as ibogaine, ketamine, and MDMA, all demonstrate the capacity to reopen the critical period for social reward learning, though the duration correlated with the acute subjective effects of each psychedelic. For ketamine, the acute effects last for approximately 30 to 120 minutes, and the critical period remains open for 48 hours. For psilocybin and MDMA, the acute effects last for 3 to 6 hours, while the critical window remains open for 2 weeks. For LSD and ibogaine, the acute effects are 8 to 10 hours and 36 to 72 hours, respectively, while the critical window remains open for 3 weeks and 4 weeks, respectively.[21]

Perhaps most notably, the research team has suggested that the psychedelics they studied—including classic psychedelics, ibogaine, ketamine, and MDMA—share a common mechanism that is downstream from their initial targets (ie, 5-HT$_{2A}$ receptors for classic psychedelics, κ-opioid receptors for ibogaine, *N*-methyl-D-aspartate [NMDA] receptors for ketamine, and SERTs for MDMA). This mechanistic convergence occurs at the level of DNA transcription of the extracellular matrix (ECM). They write, "Psychedelics act at a diverse array of binding targets...to trigger a downstream signaling response that leads to activity-dependent...degradation of the ECM, which in turn is the permissive event that enables metaplasticity."[21]

A Note on Microdosing

This book is largely focused on psychedelic-assisted psychotherapy, which, as noted in previous chapters, is a treatment modality that relies on a few moderate or large doses of psychedelics coupled with several weeks or months of psychotherapy. The clinical evidence discussed throughout this book is based, solely almost if not entirely, on this treatment paradigm. Microdosing, which involves the regular use of psychedelics at doses low enough to have a pharmacologic effect without notable subjective effects, stands outside of this paradigm. According to Beaton and colleagues, the microdoses for LSD are typically 6 to 20 µg, while the doses for dried psilocybin mushrooms are 0.2 to 0.5 g. Microdoses are self-administered every 3 days for 1 to 2 months.[22]

At present, there is weak, largely observational and anecdotal evidence to support its efficacy, with the majority of available literature indicating that individuals feel that the practice increases creativity, productivity, and mood and that it diminishes anxiety and depressive symptoms.[22] For individuals who are not struggling with a diagnosable mental illness but are seeking to try a new wellness routine, this seems like an attractive (albeit illegal) option, especially given the amount of media attention psychedelics and microdosing have both enjoyed. This brings up concerns about how much of the self-reported effects are due to the drugs versus a placebo effect.

Of the few controlled studies published, the results have been largely underwhelming. Cavanna and colleagues found that microdosing psilocybin failed to produce notable improvements in creativity or performance. In fact, participants' performance suffered in some cases because of the subjective effects of the mushrooms. The study's randomized, double-blind placebo-controlled design involved an active dose of 0.5 g psilocybin and 34 participants over the course of 3 weeks, which included 1 week of psilocybin treatment (administered on Wednesday and Friday) and 1 week of placebo separated by 1 week without measurement.[23]

Beyond concerns about efficacy and legal issues, microdosing may also adversely affect cardiovascular function via persistent 5-HT_{2B} stimulation. While the association between microdosing and valvular heart disease (VHD) has not become a serious public health concern, there is evidence that persistent use of 5-HT_{2B} agonists such as ergotamine, pergolide, MDMA, and especially fenfluramine/phentermine (fen-phen) can cause VHD.[24,25] Symptoms of VHD include shortness of breath and weakness. It can also cause sudden cardiac death. Classic psychedelics (eg, LSD, psilocybin, mescaline, DMT) are 5-HT_{2B} agonists.

Conclusion

It would be a mistake to close this chapter with the impression that there is a substantial understanding of the pharmacology of psychedelics. While researchers have a general idea as to how they can disrupt the cortical networks that dominate ordinary states of consciousness, we are only just beginning to understand how to make use of these extremely powerful tools to help patients. Researchers are also still working to fully elucidate the pharmacologic targets of these drugs; to better understand the pharmacologic nuances of each drug; the relationship between subjective effects and therapeutic outcomes; and how to best offer psychological support before, during, and after dosing.

It is an exciting time, no doubt, but it is also a time to be weary of hubris and to tread lightly as clinical trials progress.

REFERENCES

1. Vollenweider FX, Kometer M. The neurobiology of psychedelic drugs: implications for the treatment of mood disorders. *Nat Rev Neurosci.* 2010;11(9):642-651. doi:10.1038/nrn2884. PMID: 20717121.
2. Zhang G, Stackman RW Jr. The role of serotonin 5-HT2A receptors in memory and cognition. *Front Pharmacol.* 2015;6:225. doi:10.3389/fphar.2015.00225. PMID: 26500553; PMCID: PMC4594018.
3. Nichols DE. Psychedelics. *Pharmacol Rev.* 2016;68(2):264-355. doi:10.1124/pr.115.011478. Erratum in: *Pharmacol Rev.* 2016;68(2):356. PMID: 26841800; PMCID: PMC4813425.
4. Murnane KS. Serotonin 2A receptors are a stress response system: implications for post-traumatic stress disorder. *Behav Pharmacol.* 2019;30(2 and 3):151-162. doi:10.1097/FBP.0000000000000459. PMID: 30632995; PMCID: PMC6422730.
5. Carhart-Harris RL, Friston KJ. REBUS and the anarchic brain: toward a unified model of the brain action of psychedelics. *Pharmacol Rev.* 2019;71(3):316-344. doi:10.1124/pr.118.017160. PMID: 31221820; PMCID: PMC6588209.
6. Zaretsky TG, Jagodnik KM, Barsic KM, et al. The psychedelic future of post-traumatic stress disorder treatment. *Curr Neuropharmacol.* 2024;22;636-735. doi:10.2174/1570159X22666231027111147
7. Fukumoto K, Fogaça MV, Liu RJ, et al. Medial PFC AMPA receptor and BDNF signaling are required for the rapid and sustained antidepressant-like effects of 5-HT1A receptor stimulation. *Neuropsychopharmacology.* 2020;45(10):1725-1734. doi:10.1038/s41386-020-0705-0. PMID: 32396921; PMCID: PMC7419563.
8. Liechti ME, Saur MR, Gamma A, Hell D, Vollenweider FX. Psychological and physiological effects of MDMA ("Ecstasy") after pretreatment with the 5-HT(2) antagonist ketanserin in healthy humans. *Neuropsychopharmacology.* 2000;23(4): 396-404. doi:10.1016/S0893-133X(00)00126-3. PMID: 10989266.
9. Buchborn T, Lyons T, Knöpfel T. Tolerance and tachyphylaxis to head twitches induced by the 5-HT2A agonist 25CN-NBOH in mice. *Front Pharmacol.* 2018;9:17. doi:10.3389/fphar.2018.00017. PMID: 29467649; PMCID: PMC5808243.
10. Vargas AS, Luís Â, Barroso M, Gallardo E, Pereira L. Psilocybin as a new approach to treat depression and anxiety in the context of life-threatening diseases—a systematic review and meta-analysis of clinical trials. *Biomedicines.* 2020;8(9).331. doi:10.3390/biomedicines8090331. PMID: 32899469; PMCID: PMC7554922.
11. Urban MM, Stingl MR, Meinhardt MW. Mini-review: the neurobiology of treating substance use disorders with classical psychedelics. *Front Neurosci.* 2023;17:1156319. doi:10.3389/fnins.2023.1156319. PMID: 37139521; PMCID: PMC10149865.
12. Dennett D. *Consciousness Explained.* Back Bay Books; 1991:323-325.
13. Metzinger T. *Being No One: The Self-Model Theory of Subjectivity.* The MIT Press; 2003:52.
14. Gattuso JJ, Perkins D, Ruffell S, et al. Default mode network modulation by psychedelics: a systematic review. *Int J Neuropsychopharmacol.* 2023;26(3):155-188. doi:10.1093/ijnp/pyac074. PMID: 36272145; PMCID: PMC10032309.

15. Barba T, Buehler S, Kettner H, et al. Effects of psilocybin versus escitalopram on rumination and thought suppression in depression. *BJPsych Open*. 2022;8(5):e163. doi:10.1192/bjo.2022.565. PMID: 36065128; PMCID: PMC9534928.
16. Carhart-Harris RL, Leech R, Hellyer PJ, et al. The entropic brain: a theory of conscious states informed by neuroimaging research with psychedelic drugs. *Front Hum Neurosci*. 2014;8:20. doi:10.3389/fnhum.2014.00020. PMID: 24550805; PMCID: PMC3909994.
17. Timmermann C, Bauer PR, Gosseries O, et al. A neurophenomenological approach to non-ordinary states of consciousness: hypnosis, meditation, and psychedelics. *Trends Cogn Sci*. 2023;27(2):139-159. doi:10.1016/j.tics.2022.11.006. PMID: 36566091.
18. Barrett FS, Krimmel SR, Griffiths RR, Seminowicz DA, Mathur BN. Psilocybin acutely alters the functional connectivity of the claustrum with brain networks that support perception, memory, and attention. *Neuroimage*. 2020;218:116980. doi:10.1016/j.neuroimage.2020.116980. PMID: 32454209; PMCID: PMC10792549.
19. Köck P, Froelich K, Walter M, Lang U, Dürsteler KM. A systematic literature review of clinical trials and therapeutic applications of ibogaine. *J Subst Abuse Treat*. 2022;138:108717. doi:10.1016/j.jsat.2021.108717. PMID: 35012793.
20. Mertens LJ, Wall MB, Roseman L, Demetriou L, Nutt DJ, Carhart-Harris RL. Therapeutic mechanisms of psilocybin: changes in amygdala and prefrontal functional connectivity during emotional processing after psilocybin for treatment-resistant depression. *J Psychopharmacol*. 2020;34(2):167-180. doi:10.1177/0269881119895520. PMID: 31941394.
21. Nardou R, Sawyer E, Song YJ, et al. Psychedelics reopen the social reward learning critical period. *Nature*. 2023;618(7966):790-798. doi:10.1038/s41586-023-06204-3. PMID: 37316665; PMCID: PMC10284704.
22. Beaton B, Copes H, Webb M, Hochstetler A, Hendricks PS. Accounting for microdosing classic psychedelics. *J Drug Issues*. 2019;50(1):1-12. doi:10.1177/0022042619871008
23. Cavanna F, Muller S, de la Fuente LA, et al. Microdosing with psilocybin mushrooms: a double-blind placebo-controlled study. *Transl Psychiatry*. 2022;12(1):307. doi:10.1038/s41398-022-02039-0. PMID: 35918311; PMCID: PMC9346139.
24. Droogmans S, Cosyns B, D'haenen H, et al. Possible association between 3,4-methylenedioxymethamphetamine abuse and valvular heart disease. *Am J Cardiol*. 2007;100(9):1442-1445. doi:10.1016/j.amjcard.2007.06.045. PMID: 17950805.
25. Wadden TA, Berkowitz RI, Silvestry F, et al. The fen-phen finale: a study of weight loss and valvular heart disease. *Obes Res*. 1998;6(4):278-284. doi:10.1002/j.1550-8528.1998.tb00350.x. PMID: 9688104.

8

Potential Clinical Indications

So far, this book has focused on the potential benefits of psychedelic medicines, their history of use around the world, and how regulations have been put into place that have made it difficult to study their potential use in various disorders. Later chapters that discuss specific drugs will describe how they have been used historically or within a clinical setting to treat said disorders. This chapter focuses on the disorders themselves and provides information about their epidemiology, etiology, and course. The conditions included within this chapter are affective disorders, anxiety disorders, obsessive-compulsive and related disorders, trauma- and stressor-related disorders, eating disorders, and substance use disorders. It also features a discussion of their use in palliative care and, more importantly, suicidality.

To avoid redundancy and the need to dedicate portions of individual chapters to describing the basics of these conditions, this chapter provides an overview of all the potential indications of psychedelics. In addition to avoiding redundancy, there is significant overlap among the conditions that psychedelic medicines are believed to treat, and this subject matter serves as a companion to the previous chapter. As noted before, classic psychedelics, which target serotonergic pathways (particularly 5-HT_{2A}), can improve symptoms associated with many anxiety and mood disorders.[1] Subsequent chapters will delve further into describing the mechanisms of action of these drugs, as well as how they affect the pathophysiology of specific psychiatric conditions.

Another reason to discuss all these disorders in one chapter is to highlight how interconnected many of these psychiatric conditions are. Although mental illnesses are strictly categorized and organized as per the *Diagnostic and Statistical Manual of Mental Disorders (DSM-5-TR)*, clinicians recognize that many patients exhibit symptoms that do not strictly fall under one particular diagnosis and are along a spectrum, which makes it often difficult to pinpoint a particular disorder. Their pathologies exist along multiple dimensions that may implicate several disorders even if they only meet the criteria for one. (As a common example, diagnoses of substance use disorders and trauma- and stress disorders tend to coexist because individuals frequently develop the former as a means of self-medicating to cope with the latter.) By including all these disorders in one place, readers will gain an appreciation of how mental illness can be conceptualized in a broader manner.

Before describing these conditions, it should be noted that, as of this writing, the Food and Drug Administration (FDA) has not approved the use of any psychedelic covered in this book for psychiatric purposes except esketamine (an isomer of ketamine marketed under the name Spravato), which was approved for use in 2019 for the treatment of treatment-resistant depression and as crisis intervention for patients with suicidal thoughts or actions.[2]

Affective Disorders

Affective disorders (or mood disorders) are a broad class of conditions that include bipolar disorders, major depressive disorder (MDD), cyclothymia, and premenstrual dysphoric disorders, among others. Individuals with these conditions struggle to exert control over their mood, which in some cases can make them feel helpless and despondent.

Bipolar Disorders

Bipolar disorders are characterized by cycling between manic (or hypomanic) and depressive episodes. Manic episodes are characterized by a persistent elevation in mood and an inflated sense of self, as well as symptoms that include increased loquaciousness, racing thoughts, reckless or disinhibited behaviors (hypersexuality and promiscuity, impulsive travel, excessive spending, etc), hyperintense goal-oriented activity, weight changes, insomnia, and a low tolerance for frustration. Symptoms must persist for at least 1 week for the majority of the day, every day, to qualify as a manic episode. A hypomanic episode is less intensive and less protracted than a manic episode, lasting more than four consecutive days but less than seven.

With bipolar I disorder, individuals experience episodes of mania, as well as episodes of depression, which may precede or follow the manic episode. They may also experience hypomanic episodes. With bipolar II disorder, there is at least one episode of hypomania, as well as at least one depressive episode, but no manic episode. Diagnostically, this represents the primary difference between bipolar I disorder and bipolar II disorder. Cyclothymic disorder is a less severe form of bipolar disorder defined by alternating episodes of hypomania and depression. Bipolar disorders are estimated to affect approximately 2.4% of the global population.[3] Bipolar disorder is chronic, with a remitting and relapsing course, but it is manageable with treatment.

There is a strong genetic component in bipolar disorders, but environmental elements and psychosocial stressors have been implicated in the etiology of the disorders as well. Disease pathologies may also be associated with neurophysiologic anomalies, including deficits in neural plasticity and dendritic spine loss, as well as disruptions in neuronal interconnectivity, mitochondria dysfunction, neuroinflammation, excessive oxidative stress, hyperactive apoptosis, and epigenetic changes that affect histone and DNA methylation.

Clinical trials with classic psychedelics like psilocybin and lysergic acid diethylamide (LSD) have typically excluded individuals with a personal or family history of bipolar disorders, largely due to concerns that psychedelics may induce a manic episode (ie, a Treatment Emergent Affective Switch) and lead to increasingly impulsive or reckless behaviors. However, the literature on the subject is not as robust as one might assume. A review by Gard and colleagues found only 17 published case studies between 1966 and 2021 where a psychedelic (including psilocybin, LSD, ayahuasca, or N,N-dimethyltryptamine [DMT]) may have precipitated a manic episode. Two of those cases involved an individual who may have had a prior diagnosis of bipolar disorder, and five cases involved an individual with a family history of bipolar disorder. The authors note that polysubstance use was involved in 5 of the 17 cases and that repeated use of psychedelics within a short period of time occurred in 9 of the 17 cases.[4]

Individuals with bipolar disorders who have used psychedelics report a relatively low incidence of mood switch. An online survey conducted between October 2020 and January 2021 involving 541 individuals with bipolar disorders claimed that psilocybin use was more beneficial than harmful.[5]

Given the difficulty in treating bipolar disorders and their effect on patient quality of life, as well as the self-reports of improvements in quality of life following the use of psychedelics, more clinical research into the effects of psychedelics in patients with bipolar disorders seems warranted, especially in conjunction with other medications like mood stabilizers. This will likely be an area of more intensive research in the coming years. However, until these studies are conducted, clinicians should continue to screen for a personal or family history of bipolar disorder.

Major Depressive Disorder

MDD can occur alone or as part of bipolar disorder. When it occurs alone, it is also known as *unipolar depression*. MDD is characterized by protracted symptoms that include, but are not limited to, depressed mood, diminished interest in or difficulty in deriving pleasure from virtually all activities (anhedonia), changes in weight (increases or decreases), changes in sleep patterns (insomnia or hypersomnia), fatigue, difficulties with concentration, feelings of emptiness, low energy, loss of libido, low frustration tolerance, hopelessness, and thoughts of suicide. Symptoms must be present for at least 2 weeks and represent a change from previous functioning.

The prevalence of MDD is estimated to be twice as high in women as in men.[6] It is also believed to be highest among young adults aged 18 to 25 years, followed by adolescents aged 12 to 17. Data from the 2015 to 2020 National Survey on Drug Use and Health indicates a prevalence of 17.2% and 16.9%, respectively.[7] Overall, the lifetime prevalence of MDD was estimated to be 11.1% in low-income countries and 14.6% in high-income countries prior to the COVID-19 pandemic.[8] As of 2017, the global average was estimated to be 13.2%.[8] However, this rate is not as constant as once thought, and upward of 50% of MDD cases are preceded by a precipitating event.[9] Consequently, widespread cataclysms can lead to significantly higher rates, as became evident during the height of the COVID-19 pandemic in 2020. During the lockdowns in the spring of that year, surveys found that the estimated global prevalence of MDD climbed as high as 27.1%.[10]

MDD can also occur without a precipitating event, as its etiology is heterogeneous and multifactorial, frequently involving dysfunction in neurotransmitters like serotonin, noradrenaline, γ-aminobutyric acid (GABA), glutamate, and neurotrophic factors, as well as their corresponding pathways. It may also involve dysfunction in the hypothalamic-pituitary-adrenal (HPA) axis, the immune system, cellular stress mechanisms, and the endocannabinoid system. Genetics and epigenetic factors appear to also play a role, as do social and environmental factors.[11]

Given the heterogeneity of MDD, it has proven to be an extremely difficult condition to treat, and its course is varied. An estimated 40% of patients experience symptom improvement within 3 months of onset, and 80% of patients experience symptom improvement within 1 year of symptom onset.[12(p165)] Treatment most commonly consists of a combination of psychotherapy and psychopharmaceuticals (eg, selective serotonin reuptake inhibitors [SSRIs], serotonin-norepinephrine reuptake inhibitors [SNRIs], tricyclics and tetracyclics) and other modalities including brain stimulation techniques. For some patients, depressive symptoms may abate and never return. For others, conventional treatment options may not be effective (see "Treatment-Resistant Depression" section), or depressive symptoms may be chronic (see "Persistent Depressive Disorder" section).

Given the heterogeneity of MDD, it is difficult to pinpoint a singular reason psychedelics may be effective treatment options. Despite a satisfactory explanation, studies have shown that patients with MDD have experienced symptom improvement following psychedelic-assisted therapy, especially with classic psychedelics and ketamine.[13]

Treatment-Resistant Depression

Treatment-resistant depression is not a unique condition and is not recognized in DSM-5-TR. It has no formal definition but refers to difficulties in treating depressive disorders and can be said to occur when a patient has experienced little to no response (narrow definition) or an inadequate response (less narrow definition) to one or more trials with antidepressant treatment. Unfortunately, treatment-resistant depression is quite common. Within the narrow definition, it is estimated that treatment-resistant depression occurs in 10% to 30% of patients with MDD.[14] As 40% to 70% of patients respond to treatment, a less narrow definition would suggest that treatment-resistant depression occurs in 30% to 60% of patients.[15]

Psychedelics are not considered first-line treatments for depressive disorders; ergo, they are by definition only to be considered as potential treatments for treatment-resistant depression. This includes esketamine.

As explored in later chapters, numerous other psychedelics have been proposed as a potential treatment for treatment-resistant depression, including psilocybin, LSD, DMT, ayahuasca, mescaline, ibogaine, and 5-methoxy-*N,N*-dimethyltryptamine (5-MeO-DMT).[16,17]

Depression Following a Terminal Diagnosis

Many individuals have significant depression upon being diagnosed with a terminal illness like advanced-stage cancer, oftentimes with comorbid anxiety. Unfortunately, there are not many options for patients. Psychedelic-assisted psychotherapy has proven effective at easing existential crisis and depressive symptoms for many patients who have received a terminal diagnosis.[18]

Persistent Depressive Disorder

Persistent depressive disorder, also known as dysthymia, may be more or less severe than MDD. In diagnosing persistent depressive disorder, symptom severity is secondary; what is of critical importance is the protracted nature of the disturbance, which persists for years. According to DSM-5-TR, a diagnosis of persistent depressive disorder is warranted when the patient experiences a depressed mood for the majority of the day, with symptomatic days outnumbering nonsymptomatic days for at least 2 years in adults and 1 year in children.[12(pp168,169)]

Persistent depressive disorder is believed to occur at roughly the same rate across gender lines, with prevalence in the United States estimated to be approximately 3%.[19] The pathology and treatment for persistent depressive disorder are believed to be similar to MDD, suggesting that psychedelic therapy may be beneficial to those with the disorder.

Anxiety Disorders

Anxiety disorders share a core symptomology, pathophysiology, and etiology, though there is a clear distinction between conditions. For example, a specific phobia is triggered by specific stimuli (eg, enclosed spaces, heights, spiders), while social anxiety disorder is triggered by a broader group of situations (eg, public speaking). Anxiety symptoms tend to revolve around feelings of dread and are accompanied by somatic complaints indicative of a hyperactive autonomic response (see Table 8.1). These symptoms can influence cognition and lead to distortions in perception.

TABLE 8.1 Signs and Symptoms Associated With Anxiety Disorders

Physical Signs	Psychological Symptoms
Trembling, twitching, feeling shaky	Feeling of dread
Backache, headache	Difficulty concentrating
Muscle tension	Hypervigilance
Shortness of breath, hyperventilation	Insomnia
Fatigability	Decreased libido
Startle response	"Lump in the throat"
Autonomic hyperactivity	Upset stomach ("butterflies")
Flushing and pallor	
Tachycardia, palpitations	
Sweating	
Cold hands	
Diarrhea	
Dry mouth (xerostomia)	
Urinary frequency	
Paresthesia	
Difficulty swallowing	

Historically, the cumulative lifetime prevalence of all anxiety disorders in the United States had been 17.2%, while the 12-month prevalence has been 11.1%.[20] The COVID-19 pandemic has had a dramatic effect on both figures, leading to significant increases, and even now these figures continue to fluctuate.[21] At the start of the pandemic, in April 2020, the National Center for Health Statistics (NCHS) and the Census Bureau began collecting data about anxiety and depressive symptoms via the Household Pulse Survey. Their report shows that anxiety and depressive symptoms (not to be confused with a diagnosis of either an anxiety disorder or a mood disorder) have remained elevated since 2020.[22]

The causes of anxiety disorders are heterogeneous, involving genetic, psychological, and environmental components that can lead to dysfunctions in autonomic reactions with increased sympathetic tone and catecholamine release. In addition to being associated with hyperactivity in the limbic system, as well as the temporal cerebral cortex, anxiety states may correlate with neuroinflammation and aberrations in neurotransmitter signaling, resulting in increases in excitatory neurotransmitters (including increased dopaminergic activity) and decreased signaling of inhibitory neurotransmitters, particularly GABA.[23]

Depending on severity, impairment can be severe, oftentimes leading to significant disruptions in one's social life, as well as familial, occupational, or academic duties. Most anxiety disorders tend to be chronic in nature; though they are treatable, patients may go through extended periods of remission.[24]

Classic psychedelics and nonclassic psychedelics have both been used to treat anxiety disorders with promising results.

Generalized Anxiety Disorder

Generalized anxiety disorder involves excessive worry about everyday life circumstances, events, or conflicts. Symptoms oftentimes fluctuate and frequently overlap with other medical or psychiatric disorders (particularly depressive and other anxiety disorders). According to the World Health Organization's World Mental Health Survey, the lifetime and 12-month prevalences of generalized anxiety disorder in the United States are 5.7% and 3.1%, respectively.[25] Women are believed to experience the disorder approximately twice as often as men.[20]

Social Anxiety Disorder

Social anxiety disorder is a nonrational fear of public situations often associated with panic attacks. It is estimated that over 12% of people in the United States may be affected by symptoms at some point in their lifetimes, with the 12-month prevalence being 6.8%.[25] It is equally common in men and women.[25]

Panic Disorder

Panic disorder is characterized by spontaneous panic attacks, the symptoms of which are outlined in Table 8.2. Within the United States, panic disorder is believed to have 12-month and lifetime prevalences of 2.7% and 4.7%, respectively, with women being more frequently affected than men.[25]

Anxiety Following a Terminal Diagnosis

Many individuals have significant anxiety upon being diagnosed with a terminal illness, like advanced-stage cancer, and may oftentimes experience comorbid depression as well. Unfortunately, there is a dearth of options available to ameliorate patients' distress. Psychedelic-assisted psychotherapy has proven effective at easing end-of-life anxiety symptoms for many patients.[18]

TABLE 8.2 Signs and Symptoms Associated With Panic Disorder

Recurrent unexpected panic attacks (focal fear lasting a few minutes) with ≥4 of:

1. Palpable heart pulsations or tachycardia
2. Diaphoresis
3. Jitteriness
4. Sensations of shortness of breath or smothering
5. Suffocating feelings
6. Chest pain
7. Queasy, upset stomach
8. Dizziness or vertigo
9. Hot flushes or chilliness.
10. Numbness or tingling
11. Detachment from oneself or reality
12. Worries about losing control ("freaking out")
13. Worries about death

These attacks must cause either persistent worry about future attacks or a maladaptive behavioral change to evade future attacks.

(Panic attacks can be present in anxiety and other disorders. In panic disorder, they are otherwise unprovoked.)

Obsessive-Compulsive and Related Disorders

Obsessive-compulsive and related disorders are a category within DSM-5-TR that includes the more well-known obsessive-compulsive disorder (OCD), as well as body dysmorphic disorder (BDD), among others.

Obsessive-Compulsive Disorder

Symptoms of OCD include obsessions and compulsions that are oftentimes accompanied by ritualization. An obsession is a recurrent and intrusive thought, feeling, idea, or sensation. Obsessions associated with OCD are very often tied to notions of contamination (eg, "This is dirty") or recurrent doubts (eg, "Did I turn off the stove?"). In contrast, a compulsion is a purposeful, standardized, and repeated behavior that a person feels obligated to perform as a consequence of the obsession. Common compulsions include hand washing, counting, tapping, or avoiding (eg, not walking through certain doors). An individual with OCD may have an obsession, a compulsion, or both.

The etiology of OCD is neuropsychiatric, with strong genetic components.[i] Various functional brain imaging studies have shown increased activity (eg, metabolism and blood flow) in the frontal lobes, the basal ganglia (especially the caudate), the thalamus, and the cingulum of individuals with OCD.[26] Additionally, computed tomographic (CT) and magnetic resonance imaging (MRI) studies have found bilaterally smaller caudates in those with OCD.[27] Meanwhile, cognitive and neuropsychiatric tests have found increased cognitive rigidity and impairment in executive functioning.[28]

The lifetime prevalence of OCD in the general population is estimated to be 2.3%, while the 12-month prevalence is believed to be 1.2%.[29] As many as 90% of patients with OCD have a comorbid condition, such as an anxiety disorder (75.8%), mood disorder (63.3%), impulse control disorder (55.9%), or substance use disorder (38.6%).[29] In addition to having a negative impact on quality of life, OCD is associated with an increased risk of suicidal ideation, especially if compounded by comorbid MDD.[30]

The course of OCD is usually long but variable; some patients experience a fluctuating course, while others experience a constant one, and a minority of individuals have a deteriorating course. A follow-up study lasting over 40 years found that 83% of individuals with OCD experienced improvements in symptoms, but full remission was attained in only 20% of the study's participants.[31] Remission is more likely among those who experience onset in childhood or adolescence.[32]

Studies involving classic psychedelics have shown efficacy in improving symptoms of OCD and appear to be preferred to ketamine or entactogens like 3,4-methylenedioxymethamphetamine (MDMA). Of the classic psychedelics, psilocybin, LSD, ayahuasca, and DMT (in that order) were found to be the most impactful.[33]

---

[i] There is also evidence linking streptococcal-A infection and OCD symptoms, possibly because the initial infection results in an autoimmune disorder affecting the central nervous system (CNS). In addition to symptoms resembling OCD, patients report neurologic abnormalities, regressions in social and emotional development, psychological problems, and a decline in academic performance. The condition is known as pediatric autoimmune neuropsychiatric disorder associated with streptococcal infections (PANDAS).

Body Dysmorphic Disorder

Patients with BDD are preoccupied by a distorted perception (not of delusional proportions) of their body. In some cases, the belief may center on a perceived defect that is specific to one part of the body (eg, nose, ears, calves) or in general.

Veale and colleagues estimate prevalence to be between 1.9% among adults, 2.2% among adolescents, and 3.3% among students, with notably higher rates in different medical settings:

- Adult psychiatric (inpatient): 7.4%
- Adolescence psychiatric (inpatient): 7.4%
- Adult psychiatric (outpatient): 5.8%
- General cosmetic surgery: 13.2%
- Rhinoplasty surgery: 20.1%
- Orthognathic surgery: 11.2%
- Orthodontic/cosmetic dentistry: 5.2%
- Dermatology (outpatient): 11.3%
- Cosmetic dermatology (outpatient): 9.2%
- Acne dermatology: 11.1%[34]

In their 2013 paper, Bjornsson and colleagues found that onset may occur from adolescence through early adulthood, with the most common age of onset between 12 and 13 years and that two-thirds of those who participated in the study had met the diagnostic criteria for BDD by the age of 18. Additionally, the Bjornsson study reported several common comorbidities among participants, some of the most common of which include MDD (75%), substance use disorders (33.9%), OCD (30.6%), and eating disorders (11.7%).[35]

The course of BDD is typically chronic, especially without treatment. In the absence of psychiatric intervention, many patients may make repeated visits to doctors, plastic surgeons, or dermatologists for years, if not decades. Psychotherapy and pharmacotherapy with antidepressants are typically the first lines of treatment. Although plastic surgery may lead to temporary symptom improvement, it frequently fails to resolve the underlying pathology. Psychedelic therapy represents a possible means of resolution, possibly by changing the patient's perspective.

Trauma- and Stressor-Related Disorders

Trauma- and stressor-related disorders arise in the wake of extremely stressful or traumatic events. Though the word "trauma" has been popularized and "de-medicalized," especially on social media platforms, DMS-5-TR adheres to a strict definition of "trauma" in Criterion A for posttraumatic stress disorder (PTSD).[12(pp271-276)] An experience that satisfies Criterion A is necessary but not sufficient for a diagnosis of PTSD. Examples can be found in Table 8.3.

A lesser-known trauma- and stressor-related disorder, adjustment disorder, represents an emotional or behavioral response to one or more identifiable stressors that can be considered out of proportion to the severity of antecedent stressors. These stressors need not be as severe as those listed in Table 8.3 and may include experiences like losing a job, ending a serious relationship, or the death of a friend or relative.

TABLE 8.3 Trauma Clusters and Specific Events

Trauma Cluster	Specific Event
Collective violence	Civilian in a war zone; refugee from a war zone; civilian in a terrorized region; relief worker in a war zone; kidnapping victim
Caused/witnessed bodily harm	Accidentally caused injury or death; purposefully tortured, maimed or killed another; combat experience; saw atrocities; witnessed death/dead body/gruesome injury
Interpersonal violence	Battered by caregiver; witnessed physical fights at home; assault by a noncaregiver
Intimate partner/sexual violence	Rape; sexual assault; battered by spouse/partner; stalked; traumatic event to loved one; private event; other event
Accident/injuries	Child with serious illness; natural disaster; life-threatening illness; toxic chemical exposure; auto accident; other life-threatening accident
Other traumas	Unexpected death of loved one; mugged or threatened with a weapon; human-caused disaster

Stress exposure is universal, and trauma exposure that satisfies Criterion A is also quite common, with average rates across the United States estimated to be 82.7%.[36] In marginalized communities, exposure may be upward of 90%.[37] Despite the regular occurrence of stressful and even traumatic events, most individuals do not develop trauma- and stressor-related disorders. Why some people are resilient, while others are not, continues to be a question that is central to the pathology and treatment of trauma- and stressor-related disorders.

Adjustment disorder is believed to have a lifetime prevalence of between 1% and 2% of the population.[38] The lifetime prevalence of PTSD in the United States is estimated to be 6.9%.[36]

Posttraumatic Stress Disorder

PTSD centers on dysfunctions in neural systems devoted to fear conditioning and fear extinction.[39] All vertebrates respond to perceived dangers with a stress response (ie, the fight-flight-freeze response) that involves activation of the sympathetic nervous system. With PTSD, the response becomes overactive following trauma, resulting in the core symptoms of the disorder: intrusive thoughts, memories, or dreams about the traumatic event; "flashbacks"; difficulty remembering the event; exaggerated startle responses; and avoidance of stimuli associated with the event. Patients with PTSD frequently have psychiatric comorbidities like MDD, anxiety disorders, and substance abuse disorders. Additionally, patients with PTSD frequently struggle with medical conditions associated with substance abuse disorders (eg, heart disease, liver disease, memory loss) and instability in housing, occupations, and relationships.

Studies into the pathophysiology of PTSD have revealed that the dysfunction correlates with structural components of the central nervous system (CNS)—including the amygdala, thalamus, hippocampus, HPA axis, and medial prefrontal cortex, among others—and several neurotransmitters and hormones, including epinephrine, norephedrine, and cortisol.[40]

Current treatment options like prolonged exposure therapy, cognitive behavioral therapy, and psychopharmacology do typically lead to symptom improvement, but many patients never manage to achieve full remission. Veterans oftentimes have the most difficulty finding symptom relief, with a recent review finding that approximately two-thirds of veterans continue to exhibit PTSD symptoms even after receiving treatment.[41]

Preliminary trials have shown that many patients experience rapid and sustained symptom improvement when treated with MDMA. Following a randomized, placebo-controlled phase 3 trial with MDMA-assisted psychotherapy, Mitchell and colleagues found that 86.5% (45 of 52) of participants in the MDMA group reported a clinically meaningful improvement in symptoms after 18 weeks, 71.2% (37 of 52) no longer met DMS-5 criteria for PTSD, and 46.2% (24 of 52) met remission criteria.[42] Concerns about "functional unblinding" have been raised as a response to these exceptional results, since most patients in the active arm of the study knew they received the drug and most of those in the control arm knew they received placebo. As noted elsewhere, this was one of the reasons why an advisory panel for the FDA voted in June 2024 against approving MDMA for the treatment of PTSD and why the FDA ultimately voted against approving it 2 months later.

Research has indicated that classic psychedelics like psilocybin may assist in the treatment of PTSD symptoms, but the body of evidence to understand the risks and benefits of using these drugs for trauma- and stressor-related disorders remains small.[43]

Adjustment Disorder With Anxiety

Like PTSD, adjustment disorder results from a strong and dysfunctional emotional or behavioral response to a stressful life event. Adjustment disorder is a unique condition that does not stem from the exacerbation of a preexisting condition, and patients with adjustment disorder experience clinically significant impairment that interferes with their ability to fulfill their occupational, academic, or social duties. Symptoms may include depressive, reckless, or anxious behaviors. Anxious symptoms may include palpitations, jitteriness, and agitation, but do not meet the definition of an anxiety disorder as per DMS-5-TR. Depending on the nature of the stressor, adjustment disorder can be either transient or chronic, but it is self-resolving once the stressor or its consequences have been eliminated. A diagnosis of adjustment disorder is often appropriate for patients struggling to cope with a terminal diagnosis.

Interventions to help patients resolve adjustment disorder (due to existential duress or otherwise) are urgently needed, largely because of the association between the disorder and both self-harm and suicide.[38] Unfortunately, there are relatively few treatment options available due to lack of research into the condition. Psychedelics could be one option.

Eating Disorders

The defining features of all eating disorders are abnormal eating patterns and pathologic relationships with food. Disorders including anorexia nervosa, bulimia nervosa, and binge eating disorder can impair psychological, social, academic, and/or occupational functioning while also seriously affecting one's physical health. Patients with these disorders frequently substitute healthy or normal pursuits with preoccupations surrounding food and weight, and they often justify these preoccupations with society's tacit and explicit endorsements of beauty standards that celebrate thinness or lionize the cosmetics of fitness over athletic performance (ie, appreciating an athlete's physique instead of their ability to excel in a given sport).

It should be emphasized that many individuals with eating disorders not only have a toxic relationship with food but also with exercise (known as dysfunctional exercise), which can precede, maintain, or exacerbate eating disorder pathology. Exercise is generally recognized as being health promoting, but excessive exercise can lead to acute injuries like sprains, stress fractures, and heat stroke. When individuals have low energy availability, as is the case when they severely restrict calorie intake over long periods of time, the risk of acute injuries and cardiovascular complications increases.[44]

Psychedelic-assisted psychotherapy with drugs like MDMA, ketamine, psilocybin, ayahuasca, and ibogaine may help patients develop healthy beliefs about their body image, process trauma, and normalize reward processing.[45]

Anorexia Nervosa

The term "anorexia nervosa" (often shortened to just "anorexia") is derived from the Greek word *anorexia*, meaning "loss of appetite," and the Latin word *nervosa*, meaning "of nervous origin." The condition is characterized by a pathologic and self-induced need to starve oneself, an obsession with thinness and fear of being overweight, and the presence of medical signs and symptoms that result from malnutrition. Anorexia is typically accompanied by a distortion of body image, where one perceives themselves as being heavier than they actually are. It may be accompanied by binging and purging behaviors or a relentless need to exercise and appear fit. Perfectionist or obsessional personality traits are common in both subtypes.[46] They may be very successful academically, socially, or (if adults) professionally.

There are two subtypes of anorexia—food restricting and binge eating/purging—that occur with near-equal frequency. In the former, caloric restrictions are extreme. Many individuals may consume only 300 to 500 calories per day. The latter is characterized by rigorous dieting with alternating cycles of binge eating and purging episodes.

In females, the onset of anorexia typically occurs between 14 and 18 years of age, with the highest incidence rate occurring around 15 years of age.[47] Menopause appears to be another trigger for anorexia.[47] In males, onset appears to be most common in the age range of 11 to 20 years.[48] van Eeden and colleagues estimate lifetime prevalence to be between 0.1% and 3.6% in females and 0.0% and 0.3% in males.[47] Frequent comorbidities of anorexia include anxiety disorders, seasonal affective disorder, substance use disorders, and oppositional defiant disorder.[49] A history of trauma is also common.[50] The rate of suicide among individuals with anorexia is believed to be more than 6 times greater than the general population.[51]

The course of anorexia varies. By some estimates, approximately half of surviving individuals with the disorder recover, 30% experience symptom improvement, and 20% experience chronic symptoms without notable improvement.[52] Current therapies include inpatient hospitalization, psychotherapy, and pharmacotherapy with antidepressants, especially in patients with comorbid MDD. However, given the high rate of suicidality among individuals with anorexia, more treatment options (especially fast-acting ones) are needed.

Bulimia nervosa

Bulimia nervosa (often shortened to just "bulimia") is a condition where binge eating occurs alongside compensatory and potentially unhealthy methods of preventing weight gain. Unlike anorexia, individuals with bulimia may maintain a normal body weight. However, in both anorexia and bulimia, the patient possesses a morbid fear of fatness, a relentless drive for thinness (or both), and typically has a severely distorted body image.

There are two subtypes of bulimia: the purging subtype and the nonpurging subtype. In the former, individuals may induce vomiting or use laxatives or emetics to compensate for binging behaviors. In the latter, individuals will use extreme regimens of diet and exercise to prevent weight gain, potentially leading to acute injuries or cardiovascular problems. Patients with the purging subtype of bulimia also put themselves at risk of medical complications, including hypokalemia from vomiting or laxative abuse and hypochloremic alkalosis. Gastric and esophageal tears may also occur, though these complications are rare.

Patients with bulimia, and those with anorexia, tend to be high achievers and respond to societal pressures that pertain to their appearance, particularly with respect to body size. One distinction is that patients with bulimia may be more extroverted, irascible, and impulsive than patients with anorexia. There is a high rate of comorbid mental disorders among patients with bulimia. Hudson and colleagues estimate a lifetime prevalence to be the following:

- MDD: 31%
- Bipolar disorders: 18.5%
- Seasonal affective disorder: 22.1%
- Anxiety disorders: 49.9%
  - Social phobia: 20.3%
  - Specific phobia: 36.7%
  - Panic disorder: 11.1%
- PTSD: 26.5%
- Substance use disorder: 19.3%
- Attention-deficit hyperactivity disorder (ADHD): 20.0%
- Oppositional defiance disorder: 24.4%
- Conduct disorder: 29.0%[49]

Individuals may initiate stimulant use as a means to control weight and appetite, as many stimulants are appetite suppressants, and later develop a problematic relationship with these drugs.

The lifetime prevalence of bulimia has declined in recent years, but lifetime prevalence is still estimated to be up to 3% in females and over 1% in males, though some estimates place incidence rates to be significantly higher among females than males, with ratios as high as 26:1.[47] Onset is often later than that of anorexia, occurring more frequently in early adulthood (early 20s), especially among females.

Recovery is more common among patients with bulimia than anorexia, with more than half of patients experiencing full or partial remission.[53] Unfortunately, the disorder is likely to persist for over 12 months in more than half of patients.[54] They tend to show improvement with treatment, which typically includes psychotherapy and pharmacotherapy with antidepressants. Though less severe than anorexia, elevated rates of suicidality (including ideation, attempts, and completions) have been reported among patients with bulimia.[55]

Binge Eating Disorder

Binge eating disorder is characterized by regularly occurring episodes of binging, which is defined as both eating an abnormally large amount of food over a short period of time and feeling a lack of control during the binging episode. In addition to quantity and feelings of being overly full, DSM-5-TR notes that individuals with the disorder eat when not physically hungry; eat when alone; and feel distress, guilt, or shame about the binging episodes. Some patients with the disorder may be obese, while others may be able to ostensibly control their weight through dieting behavior.

Binge eating disorder typically begins in adolescence or early adulthood but can also begin in later adulthood. Global lifetime prevalence is believed to be higher in women (0.6%-1.8%) than in men (0.3%-0.7%), and common comorbidities include mood disorders (70%), substance use disorders (68%), anxiety disorders (59%), borderline personality disorder (49%), and PTSD (32%).[56] More than one in five individuals with binge eating disorder report at least one suicide attempt.[56]

Remission is more common in binge eating disorder than in anorexia nervosa or bulimia nervosa, but the course can be chronic.[57] The most common pharmacotherapy options are SSRIs or antiepileptic drugs. Successful psychotherapeutic options will avoid focusing on weight loss and more on the pathologic association to food, which may be grounded in low self-esteem, perfectionism, or trauma. Psychedelic-assisted therapy may be beneficial in helping patients better understand and resolve their problematic relationship with food.

Substance Use Disorders

Substance use disorders have a strong psychosocial component that can be influenced by a variety of factors, including socioeconomic status, genetics, race, personal history, and neurobiology. Although individuals ultimately have agency over their actions, the aforementioned factors can heavily influence the probability of whether or not an individual develops a problematic relationship with one or multiple substances.

The use of illicit drugs is extremely common. Approximately half of the US population 12 years of age and older have used an illicit substance at least once in their lifetimes: 46.9% have tried marijuana, 15.0% have tried cocaine, 5.9% have tried methamphetamine, and 2.3% have tried heroin.[58] According to the Centers for Disease Control and Prevention (CDC), about 14.5% of persons aged 12 or older were estimated to have had a substance use disorder in 2019.[59] The CDC also reported that more than 109,000 people in the United States died due to a drug overdose in 2022.[60] Overdose deaths have been climbing consistently since 1999.[61]

With respect to media coverage of overdoses, there tends to be an intense focus on opioids, which have been responsible for the majority of deaths. What often goes unmentioned is that an additional 99,000 deaths were attributable to alcohol in 2020 alone, representing approximately 3% of all deaths in the United States for that year (statistics for more recent years were not available).[62] Though this figure represents a significant jump of 25% from the number of alcohol-related deaths in 2019 and could be considered an outlier, it's important to note that the annual mean change in alcohol-related deaths climbed at a rate of 2.2% between 1999 and 2017.[62] As was so often the case, the pandemic did not create new problems; it merely exacerbated existing ones.

Illicit substance abuse affects multiple areas of functioning and can exacerbate comorbid psychiatric conditions. The inverse is also true; many psychiatric conditions, especially severe and persistent mental illnesses, can exacerbate substance use disorders. Unfortunately, there is a very high rate of comorbidity in addition to the potential for bidirectionality, especially for anxiety, bipolar, psychotic, and depressive disorders, as well as borderline and antisocial personality disorders.[63]

According to DSM-5-TR, the signs and symptoms of substance use disorders are characterized by a maladaptive pattern of substance use, leading to clinically significant impairment or distress. Individuals with substance use disorders experience cravings, engage in drug-seeking behaviors, and will frequently be intoxicated in situations where it may be physically hazardous to themselves or others (eg, driving an automobile or operating a machine) or where intoxication will disrupt their ability to competently perform tasks, schoolwork, or occupational demands. Evidence of tolerance (an increase in the amount of the problematic substance to achieve the desired level of intoxication) and withdrawal syndromes upon cessation will also be present.

As subsequent chapters will explore, studies have been conducted indicating that psychedelics may help individuals with the following substance use disorders:

- Alcohol use disorder
- Stimulant use disorder
- Cocaine use disorder
- Tobacco use disorder
- Opioid use disorder
- Cannabis use disorder

Classic psychedelics may not completely eliminate cravings or withdrawal symptoms, but patients often come away from sessions involving psychedelic-assisted therapy reawakened to the possibilities beyond compulsive drug use. This change in perspective seems to be what gives them the strength to stop using drugs. Ibogaine appears to have a unique mechanism of action that will be explored in Chapter 13.

Palliative Care

Existential anxiety and/or depressive symptoms frequently occur in individuals following a terminal diagnosis. In one way, there is nothing pathologic about either condition. Coming to terms with death is very difficult. However, in some cases, it can interfere with one's daily functioning and become a drain on one's quality of life. Psychedelic-assisted psychotherapy has repeatedly demonstrated some efficacy in quelling existential anxiety and/or depression, oftentimes by providing patients with a mystical-like experience that brings them a sense of peace.

Suicidality

Suicidality is not a recognized condition in DSM-5-TR. Instead, suicidality may result due to a wide variety of factors that may be social, psychological, or even neurobiological. It may occur with or without the presence of a diagnosed mental illness, and even though mental illness may increase the risk of suicide, it is still a poor indicator of suicidality. Among individuals with a previous suicide attempt—which is often considered to be one of the best predictors of future suicide completion—only between 3% and 5.4% of people will complete suicide.[64] Unfortunately, suicide rates have experienced an upward trajectory in the United States for the last 25 years.[65]

On account of the rising number of individuals who complete suicide, the difficulty in treating patients who express suicidal intentions, and the overall lack of options when treating patients who feel as though nothing will work for them, mental health professionals need treatment options with better outcomes.

Given psychedelics' ability to change patient perspectives, provide novel insights, improve depressive symptoms, and induce mystical-type experiences, psychedelic medicines may offer some hope. According to a systematic review, there does not seem to be a severe danger of suicidality when psychedelics are used in a clinical setting. However, the evidence to support the claim that psychedelic medicines can benefit suicidal patients is weak, and more studies will need to be conducted.

Conclusion

This chapter was meant to provide readers with background knowledge of the many conditions that psychedelic medicines may potentially treat. In the coming chapters, we will move beyond the theoretical framework and examine the findings of preclinical and clinical studies involving specific psychedelics.

REFERENCES
1. Lowe H, Toyang N, Steele B, et al. Psychedelics: alternative and potential therapeutic options for treating mood and anxiety disorders. *Molecules*. 2022;27(8):2520. doi:10.3390/molecules27082520. PMID: 35458717; PMCID: PMC9025549.
2. U.S. Food and Drug Administration. FDA approves new nasal spray medication for treatment-resistant depression; available only at a certified doctor's office or clinic. Published March 5, 2019. Accessed February 20, 2024. https://www.fda.gov/news-events/press-announcements/fda-approves-new-nasal-spray-medication-treatment-resistant-depression-available-only-certified
3. Merikangas KR, Jin R, He JP, et al. Prevalence and correlates of bipolar spectrum disorder in the world mental health survey initiative. *Arch Gen Psychiatry*. 2011;68(3):241-251. doi:10.1001/archgenpsychiatry.2011.12. PMID: 21383262; PMCID: PMC3486639.
4. Gard DE, Pleet MM, Bradley ER, et al. Evaluating the risk of psilocybin for the treatment of bipolar depression: a review of the research literature and published case studies. *J Affect Disord Rep*. 2021;6:100240. doi:10.1016/j.jadr.2021.100240
5. Morton E, Sakai K, Ashtari A, Pleet M, Michalak EE, Woolley J. Risks and benefits of psilocybin use in people with bipolar disorder: an international web-based survey on experiences of 'magic mushroom' consumption. *J Psychopharmacol*. 2023;37(1):49-60. doi:10.1177/02698811221131997. PMID: 36515370; PMCID: PMC9834328.
6. Pedersen CB, Mors O, Bertelsen A, et al. A comprehensive nationwide study of the incidence rate and lifetime risk for treated mental disorders. *JAMA Psychiatry*. 2014;71(5):573-581. doi:10.1001/jamapsychiatry.2014.16. PMID: 24806211.
7. Goodwin RD, Dierker LC, Wu M, Galea S, Hoven CW, Weinberger AH. Trends in U.S. depression prevalence from 2015 to 2020: the widening treatment gap. *Am J Prev Med*. 2022;63(5):726-733. doi:10.1016/j.amepre.2022.05.014. PMID: 36272761; PMCID: PMC9483000.
8. Merikangas KR, Rihmer Z. Mood disorders: epidemiology. In: Sadock BJ, Sadock VA, Ruiz P, eds. *Comprehensive Textbook of Psychiatry*. 10th ed. Wolters Kluwer; 2017:1613-1618.
9. Flint J. The genetic basis of major depressive disorder. *Mol Psychiatry*. 2023;28(6):2254-2265. doi:10.1038/s41380-023-01957-9. PMID: 36702864; PMCID: PMC10611584.
10. COVID-19 Mental Disorders Collaborators. Global prevalence and burden of depressive and anxiety disorders in 204 countries and territories in 2020 due to the COVID-19 pandemic. *Lancet*. 2021;398(10312):1700-1712. doi:10.1016/S0140-6736(21)02143-7. PMID: 34634250; PMCID: PMC8500697.
11. Athira KV, Bandopadhyay S, Samudrala PK, Naidu VGM, Lahkar M, Chakravarty S. An overview of the heterogeneity of major depressive disorder: current knowledge

and future prospective. *Curr Neuropharmacol.* 2020;18(3):168-187. doi:10.2174/1570159X17666191001142934. PMID: 31573890; PMCID: PMC7327947.
12. American Psychiatric Association. *Diagnostic and Statistical Manual on Mental Disorders.* 5th ed. The American Psychiatric Association; 2013.
13. Ko K, Kopra EI, Cleare AJ, Rucker JJ. Psychedelic therapy for depressive symptoms: A systematic review and meta-analysis. *J Affect Disord.* 2023;322:194-204. doi:10.1016/j.jad.2022.09.168. Erratum in: *J Affect Disord.* 2024;348:409. PMID: 36209780.
14. Al-Harbi KS. Treatment-resistant depression: therapeutic trends, challenges, and future directions. *Patient Prefer Adherence.* 2012;6:369-388. doi:10.2147/PPA.S29716. PMID: 22654508; PMCID: PMC3363299.
15. Khan A, Brown WA. Antidepressants versus placebo in major depression: an overview. *World Psychiatry.* 2015;14(3):294-300. doi:10.1002/wps.20241. PMID: 26407778; PMCID: PMC4592645.
16. Bosch OG, Halm S, Seifritz E. Psychedelics in the treatment of unipolar and bipolar depression. *Int J Bipolar Disord.* 2022;10(1):18. doi:10.1186/s40345-022-00265-5. PMID: 35788817; PMCID: PMC9256889.
17. Reckweg JT, van Leeuwen CJ, Henquet C, et al. A phase 1/2 trial to assess safety and efficacy of a vaporized 5-methoxy-N,N-dimethyltryptamine formulation (GH001) in patients with treatment-resistant depression. *Front Psychiatry.* 2023;14:1133414. doi:10.3389/fpsyt.2023.1133414. PMID: 37409159; PMCID: PMC10319409.
18. Yu CL, Yang FC, Yang SN, et al. Psilocybin for end-of-life anxiety symptoms: a systematic review and meta-analysis. *Psychiatry Investig.* 2021;18(10):958-967. doi:10.30773/pi.2021.0209. PMID: 34619818; PMCID: PMC8542741.
19. Kessler RC, Berglund P, Demler O, Jin R, Merikangas KR, Walters EE. Lifetime prevalence and age-of-onset distributions of DSM-IV disorders in the National Comorbidity Survey Replication. *Arch Gen Psychiatry.* 2005;62(6):593-602. doi:10.1001/archpsyc.62.6.593. Erratum in: *Arch Gen Psychiatry.* 2005;62(7):768. Merikangas, Kathleen R [added]. PMID: 15939837.
20. Merikangas KR, Eun JD. Epidemiology of anxiety disorders. In: Sadock BJ, Sadock VA, Ruiz P, eds. *Comprehensive Textbook of Psychiatry.* 10th ed. Wolters Kluwer; 2017:1731-1736.
21. World Health Organization. COVID-19 pandemic triggers 25% increase in prevalence of anxiety and depression worldwide. Published March 2, 2022. Accessed February 20, 2024. https://www.who.int/news/item/02-03-2022-covid-19-pandemic-triggers-25-increase-in-prevalence-of-anxiety-and-depression-worldwide
22. Centers for Disease Control and Prevention. Anxiety and depression: Household Pulse Survey. Updated February 23, 2024. Accessed March 1, 2024. https://www.cdc.gov/nchs/covid19/pulse/mental-health.htm
23. Shin LM, Liberzon I. The neurocircuitry of fear, stress, and anxiety disorders. *Neuropsychopharmacology.* 2010;35(1):169-191. doi:10.1038/npp.2009.83. PMID: 19625997; PMCID: PMC3055419.
24. Kimmel RJ, Roy-Byrne P. Clinical features of the anxiety disorders. In: Sadock BJ, Sadock VA, Ruiz P, eds. *Comprehensive Textbook of Psychiatry.* 10th ed. Wolters Kluwer; 2017:1722-1730.
25. The WHO World Mental Health Survey Consortium. Prevalence, severity, and unmet need for treatment of mental disorders in the World Health Organization World Mental Health Surveys. *JAMA.* 2004;291:2581-2590.
26. Graybiel AM, Rauch SL. Toward a neurobiology of obsessive-compulsive disorder. *Neuron.* 2000;28(2):343-347. doi:10.1016/s0896-6273(00)00113-6. PMID: 11144344.
27. Parmar A, Sarkar S. Neuroimaging studies in obsessive compulsive disorder: a narrative review. *Indian J Psychol Med.* 2016;38(5):386-394. doi:10.4103/0253-7176.191395. PMID: 27833219; PMCID: PMC5052949.
28. Stein DJ, Lochner C. Obsessive-compulsive and related disorders. In: Sadock BJ, Sadock VA, Ruiz P, eds. *Comprehensive Textbook of Psychiatry.* 10th ed. Wolters Kluwer; 2017:1785-1798.

29. Ruscio AM, Stein DJ, Chiu WT, Kessler RC. The epidemiology of obsessive-compulsive disorder in the National Comorbidity Survey Replication. *Mol Psychiatry*. 2010;15(1):53-63. doi:10.1038/mp.2008.94. PMID: 18725912; PMCID: PMC2797569.
30. Albert U, De Ronchi D, Maina G, Pompili M. Suicide risk in obsessive-compulsive disorder and exploration of risk factors: a systematic review. *Curr Neuropharmacol*. 2019;17(8):681-696. doi:10.2174/1570159X16666180620155941. PMID: 29929465; PMCID: PMC7059158.
31. Skoog G, Skoog I. A 40-year follow-up of patients with obsessive-compulsive disorder [see comments]. *Arch Gen Psychiatry*. 1999;56(2):121-127. doi:10.1001/archpsyc.56.2.121. PMID: 10025435.
32. Stewart SE, Geller DA, Jenike M, et al. Long-term outcome of pediatric obsessive-compulsive disorder: a meta-analysis and qualitative review of the literature. *Acta Psychiatr Scand*. 2004;110(1):4-13. doi: 10.1111/j.1600-0447.2004.00302.x. PMID: 15180774.
33. Buot A, Pallares C, Oganesyan A, et al. Improvement in OCD symptoms associated with serotoninergic psychedelics: a retrospective online survey. *Sci Rep*. 2023;13(1):13378. doi:10.1038/s41598-023-39812-0. PMID: 37591906; PMCID: PMC10435518.
34. Veale D, Gledhill LJ, Christodoulou P, Hodsoll J. Body dysmorphic disorder in different settings: a systematic review and estimated weighted prevalence. *Body Image*. 2016;18:168-186. doi:10.1016/j.bodyim.2016.07.003. PMID: 27498379.
35. Bjornsson AS, Didie ER, Grant JE, Menard W, Stalker E, Phillips KA. Age at onset and clinical correlates in body dysmorphic disorder. *Compr Psychiatry*. 2013;54(7):893-903. doi:10.1016/j.comppsych.2013.03.019. PMID: 23643073; PMCID: PMC3779493.
36. Koenen KC, Ratanatharathorn A, Ng L, et al. Posttraumatic stress disorder in the World Mental Health Surveys. *Psychol Med*. 2017;47(13):2260-2274. doi:10.1017/S0033291717000708
37. Gillikin C, Habib L, Evces M, Bradley B, Ressler KJ, Sanders J. Trauma exposure and PTSD symptoms associate with violence in inner city civilians. *J Psychiatr Res*. 2016;83:1-7. doi:10.1016/j.jpsychires.2016.07.027
38. O'Donnell ML, Agathos JA, Metcalf O, Gibson K, Lau W. Adjustment disorder: current developments and future directions. *Int J Environ Res Public Health*. 2019;16(14):2537. doi:10.3390/ijerph16142537
39. Wicking M, Steiger F, Nees F, et al. Deficient fear extinction memory in posttraumatic stress disorder. *Neurobiol Learn Mem*. 2016;136:116-126. doi:10.1016/j.nlm.2016.09.016
40. Kim TD, Lee S, Yoon S. Inflammation in post-traumatic stress disorder (PTSD): a review of potential correlates of PTSD with neurological perspective. *Antioxidants*. 2020;9(2):107. doi:10.3390/antiox9020107
41. Steenkamp MM, Litz BT, Hoge CW, Marmar CR. Psychotherapy for military-related PTSD: a review of randomized clinical trials. *JAMA*. 2015;314(5):489-500. doi:10.1001/jama.2015.8370. PMID: 26241600.
42. Mitchell JM, Ot'alora GM, van der Kolk B, et al. MDMA-assisted therapy for moderate to severe PTSD: a randomized, placebo-controlled phase 3 trial. *Nat Med*. 2023;29(10):2473-2480. doi:10.1038/s41591-023-02565-4. PMID: 37709999; PMCID: PMC10579091.
43. Khan AJ, Bradley E, O'Donovan A, Woolley J. Psilocybin for trauma-related disorders. *Curr Top Behav Neurosci*. 2022;56:319-332. doi:10.1007/7854_2022_366. PMID: 35711024.
44. Quesnel DA, Cooper M, Fernandez-Del-Valle M, Reilly A, Calogero RM. Medical and physiological complications of exercise for individuals with an eating disorder: a narrative review. *J Eat Disord*. 2023;11(1):3. doi:10.1186/s40337-022-00685-9. PMID: 36627654; PMCID: PMC9832767.
45. Calder A, Mock S, Friedli N, Pasi P, Hasler G. Psychedelics in the treatment of eating disorders: rationale and potential mechanisms. *Eur Neuropsychopharmacol*. 2023;75:1-14. doi:10.1016/j.euroneuro.2023.05.008. PMID: 37352816.
46. Halmi KA, Sunday SR, Strober M, et al. Perfectionism in anorexia nervosa: variation by clinical subtype, obsessionality, and pathological eating behavior. *Am J Psychiatry*. 2000;157(11):1799-1805. doi:10.1176/appi.ajp.157.11.1799. PMID: 11058477.
47. van Eeden AE, van Hoeken D, Hoek HW. Incidence, prevalence and mortality of anorexia nervosa and bulimia nervosa. *Curr Opin Psychiatry*. 2021;34(6):515-524. doi:10.1097/YCO.0000000000000739. PMID: 34419970; PMCID: PMC8500372.

48. Jaworski M, Panczyk M, Śliwczyński A, et al. Eating disorders in males: an 8-year population-based observational study. *Am J Mens Health*. 2019;13(4):1557988319860970. doi:10.1177/1557988319860970. PMID: 31268395; PMCID: PMC6610443.
49. Hudson JI, Hiripi E, Pope HG Jr, Kessler RC. The prevalence and correlates of eating disorders in the National Comorbidity Survey Replication. *Biol Psychiatry*. 2007;61(3):348-358. doi:10.1016/j.biopsych.2006.03.040. Erratum in: *Biol Psychiatry*. 2012;72(2):164. PMID: 16815322; PMCID: PMC1892232.
50. Sjögren M, Lichtenstein MB, Støving RK. Trauma experiences are common in anorexia nervosa and related to eating disorder pathology but do not influence weight-gain during the start of treatment. *J Pers Med*. 2023;13(5):709. doi:10.3390/jpm13050709. PMID: 37240879; PMCID: PMC10221645.
51. Suokas JT, Suvisaari JM, Gissler M, et al. Mortality in eating disorders: a follow-up study of adult eating disorder patients treated in tertiary care, 1995-2010. *Psychiatry Res*. 2013;210(3):1101-1106. doi:10.1016/j.psychres.2013.07.042. PMID: 23958333.
52. Steinhausen HC. The outcome of anorexia nervosa in the 20th century. *Am J Psychiatry*. 2002;159(8):1284-1293. doi:10.1176/appi.ajp.159.8.1284. PMID: 12153817.
53. Eddy KT, Tabri N, Thomas JJ, et al. Recovery from anorexia nervosa and bulimia nervosa at 22-year follow-up. *J Clin Psychiatry*. 2017;78(2):184-189. doi:10.4088/JCP.15m10393. PMID: 28002660; PMCID: PMC7883487.
54. Udo T, Grilo CM. Prevalence and correlates of DSM-5-defined eating disorders in a nationally representative sample of U.S. adults. *Biol Psychiatry*. 2018;84(5):345-354. doi:10.1016/j.biopsych.2018.03.014. PMID: 29859631; PMCID: PMC6097933.
55. Yao S, Kuja-Halkola R, Thornton LM, et al. Familial liability for eating disorders and suicide attempts: evidence from a population registry in Sweden. *JAMA Psychiatry*. 2016;73(3):284-291. doi:10.1001/jamapsychiatry.2015.2737. PMID: 26764185.
56. Keski-Rahkonen A. Epidemiology of binge eating disorder: prevalence, course, comorbidity, and risk factors. *Curr Opin Psychiatry*. 2021;34(6):525-531. doi:10.1097/YCO.0000000000000750. PMID: 34494972.
57. Miskovic-Wheatley J, Bryant E, Ong SH, et al. Eating disorder outcomes: findings from a rapid review of over a decade of research. *J Eat Disord*. 2023;11(1):85. doi:10.1186/s40337-023-00801-3. PMID: 37254202; PMCID: PMC10228434.
58. SAMSA. 2022 National Survey on Drug Use and Health (NSDUH) releases, Table 1.1B. Accessed February 26, 2024. https://www.samhsa.gov/data/sites/default/files/reports/rpt42728/NSDUHDetailedTabs2022/NSDUHDetailedTabs2022/NSDUHDetTabsSect1pe2022.htm
59. Lange WR, DePadilla L, Parker E, Holland K. Substance use & substance use disorders. Centers for Disease Control and Prevention. Updated May 1, 2023. Accessed February 26, 2024. https://wwwnc.cdc.gov/travel/yellowbook/2024/additional-considerations/substance-use
60. Tanz LJ, Gladden RM, Dinwiddie AT, et al. Routes of drug use among drug overdose deaths—United States, 2020-2022. *MMWR Morb Mortal Wkly Rep*. 2024;73:124-130. doi:10.15585/mmwr.mm7306a2
61. National Institute of Drug Abuse. Drug overdose death rates. Published June 30, 2023. Accessed February 27, 2024. https://nida.nih.gov/research-topics/trends-statistics/overdose-death-rates
62. White AM, Castle IP, Powell PA, Hingson RW, Koob GF. Alcohol-related deaths during the COVID-19 pandemic. *JAMA*. 2022;327(17):1704-1706. doi:10.1001/jama.2022.4308. PMID: 35302593; PMCID: PMC8933830.
63. Kelly TM, Daley DC. Integrated treatment of substance use and psychiatric disorders. *Soc Work Public Health*. 2013;28(3-4):388-406. doi:10.1080/19371918.2013.774673. PMID: 23731427; PMCID: PMC3753025.
64. Bostwick JM, Pabbati C, Geske JR, McKean AJ. Suicide attempt as a risk factor for completed suicide: even more lethal than we knew. *Am J Psychiatry*. 2016;173(11):1094-1100. doi:10.1176/appi.ajp.2016.15070854
65. Centers for Disease Control and Prevention. Suicide increases in 2021 after two years in decline. Updated September 30, 2022. Accessed February 29, 2024. https://www.cdc.gov/nchs/pressroom/nchs_press_releases/2022/20220930.htm

9

Psilocybin

Psilocybin is a tryptamine alkaloid and prodrug found in hundreds of mushroom species. Its metabolite, psilocin, is known to produce the psychedelic effects associated with psilocybin or "magic" mushrooms. The acute effects include alterations in sensory perception (eg, visual hallucinations, synesthesia), changes in perception, distortions in the sense of time, euphoria, ego dissolution, and even mystical-like experiences. Nausea, anxiety, increased sympathetic activity (especially raised blood pressure and heart rate), and headaches are also frequently experienced. However, nausea is far more common when one consumes raw or dried mushrooms as opposed to synthetic psilocybin.

In the days and weeks following administration of psilocybin, many people report anxiolytic and antidepressant effects, suggesting a transdiagnostic mechanism that may help treat a variety of disorders that extend well beyond mood and anxiety disorders. However, it is currently not clear how the neurophysiologic and therapeutic effects of psilocin are sustained once psilocin has been eliminated from the body; it is only clear that psilocin appears to enhance neuroplasticity and synaptic rewiring for several weeks following administration.[1] Additionally, individuals report subjective experiences associated with the psychedelic experience that profoundly affect them psychologically in the short- and long term, particularly if an individual has a mystical-type experience. What remains an open question is to what degree the mystical-type experience is necessary for psychedelic-assisted psychotherapy to be effective when given with psilocybin.

Even if all the mechanisms of psilocybin-assisted psychotherapy are not fully understood, clinical trials are investigating its potential efficacy in treating many difficult-to-treat conditions, including depressive and substance use disorders, as well as anorexia nervosa, obsessive-compulsive disorder (OCD), and body dysmorphia disorder. It has also been used in palliative care settings to mitigate anxiety and depressive symptoms associated with existential crisis and the fear of death.

As of this writing, psilocybin is considered a Schedule I drug and is not indicated for any condition. However, three distinct formulations of psilocybin have been granted breakthrough therapy designation by the Food and Drug Administration (FDA). Compass Pathways' psilocybin formulation, COMP360, was granted breakthrough therapy designation in 2018 for treatment-resistant depression, followed by Usona Institute in 2019 for major depressive disorder. In 2024, breakthrough therapy designation was also granted to the company Cybin for CYB003, a deuterated psilocybin analogue, which has shown efficacy in treating major depressive disorder.

History

There are hundreds of species of mushrooms that contain psilocybin. The majority of them belong to the genus *Psilocybe*, which appeared well before the emergence of early hominids and enjoys wide distribution across all continents with the exception of Antarctica. There are 21 species of *Psilocybe* known in Asia, 15 in Australia, 6 in Africa, 12 in Europe, 22 in the United States and Canada, 55 in Mexico, and 40 in Central and South America.[2] Given their prevalence, it is extremely likely that early humans encountered these mushrooms well before the launch of written history. Unfortunately, mushrooms are soft-bodied organisms and decompose relatively quickly, making direct evidence of their culinary, ceremonial, or medicinal use by prehistorical humans extremely rare. Consequently, most evidence of their use is based on indirect evidence.

The first indirect evidence of psychedelic mushrooms being consumed was found on the cave walls of the Tassili n'Ajjer in Algeria, dating from 7000 to 5000 BCE. The paintings strongly suggest the use of psychotropic mushrooms, as does a mural from the Spanish archaeological site Selva Pascual, which dates to 6000 to 4000 BCE.[2] Evidence of psilocybin mushroom use is far more common in the Americas, as they were a common feature within many pre-Columbian cultures, and they were widely used for ceremonial and religious purposes. Following the conquest and colonization of the Americas by Europeans, the practice was denounced and prohibited, but managed to survive in small enclaves, particularly in the hinterlands of Mesoamerica.[3]

As noted in Chapters 2 and 3, up until the 20th century, ceremonies involving psychedelic mushrooms were largely kept secret from church and state authorities, as well as from Europeans and their descendants in the Americas. Interestingly, this practice continued until R. Gordon Wasson was welcomed into one such ceremony in 1955.[4] As described in Chapter 3, Wasson published a story about the experience in an issue of *Life* magazine that was published in May 1957.[5] In 1958, Albert Hoffman of Sandoz Pharmaceuticals (also the discoverer of lysergic acid diethylamide [LSD]) isolated psilocybin from a sample of *Psilocybe mexicana* originally obtained by Wasson. Psilocybin was synthesized that same year, and Sandoz briefly began marketing Indocybin, the trade name for synthetic psilocybin starting in 1960.[6]

Psilocybin received significant attention from researchers in the early 1960s, largely for its ability to occasion mystical-type experiences. Systematic investigations into the effects of psilocybin resulted in the "Good Friday Experiment" and the "Concord Prison Experiment." The former involved 20 divinity students from Harvard University, the result of which suggested that psilocybin was capable of producing mystical-like experiences within religious contexts. The latter experiment attempted to see if psilocybin-assisted psychotherapy could be used to reduce rates of recidivism following incarceration. While the lead researcher, Timothy Leary, heralded the study as a success, a reexamination of the data by Rick Doblin later revealed that there was not a significant difference in recidivism rates between the experimental group and the general prison population.[7]

As the 1960s wore on, concern over the recreational use of psychedelics like psilocybin and LSD overshadowed the potential therapeutic uses of these drugs, which led Sandoz in 1965 to discontinue production of Indocybin.[8] In 1967, psilocybin and LSD were classified as Schedule I substances by the United Nations Convention on Drugs.[9] Psilocybin was then designed as a Schedule I drug under the Controlled Substances Act of 1970, though limited research involving psilocybin continued until the late 1970s. William A. Richard had the "dubious distinction" of administering what was believed to have been the last dose of psilocybin to a patient at the Maryland Psychiatric Research Center in 1977.[10] By the 1980s, the idea that psilocybin had any therapeutic potential was considered highly dubious despite the decades of research, which was largely forgotten by all but a handful of independent researchers and psychedelics enthusiasts. During the last quarter of the 20th century, mainstream clinicians typically considered psilocybin to be solely a drug of abuse or mocked as a being a relic of 1960's counterculture.

As explored in Chapter 4, the chilling effect on research has more recently thawed, and renewed interest in psilocybin has led to a myriad of studies about its applications in psychiatry despite prohibition at the federal level. The 2006 paper by Griffiths and colleagues, "Psilocybin Can Occasion Mystical-Type Experiences Having Substantial and Sustained Personal Meaning and Spiritual Significance," is often credited as kickstarting this renaissance of psychedelic research. This groundbreaking research paper, as well as the many trials into the potential uses of psilocybin, is explored in this chapter.

Pharmacology

Psilocybin (4-phosphoryloxy-*N*,*N*-dimethyltryptamine) is a tryptamine alkaloid that is found in the fruiting bodies of hundreds of species of mushrooms in varying concentrations.[11] These mushrooms can be eaten raw, though they are more commonly consumed dried. Psilocybin may also be extracted from mushrooms or created synthetically. Though concentrations of psilocybin vary between samples, 2.5 g of dried mushrooms is believed to be roughly equivalent to 25 mg of psilocybin isolate (either extract or synthetic).[12]

Depending on the dose, the more intense subjective effects tend to last 4 to 6 hours and can be characterized by a spectrum of psychological effects. In small doses, individuals are likely to experience euphoria and minor sensory distortions. In larger doses, psilocybin can induce visionary or mystical-type experiences, ego dissolution, and feelings of unity with others or the universe. These experiences are often accompanied by a sense of ineffability, reverence, peace, joy, or equanimity.[13] The intensity of one's subjective experience is dose dependent and can be influenced by one's prior experience with psychedelics, as well as mental outlook and environmental factors (ie, "set and setting").

Description

The fruiting bodies of mushrooms that contain psilocybin come in a variety of shapes and sizes. Any damage to mushrooms that contain psilocybin will typically result in a blue color at the site of the injury.[14] Concentrations of psilocybin can vary widely from species to species and even from sample to sample.

In their purified state, psilocybin and psilocin are white crystalline powders that can degrade if exposed to light and are more stable in dark, cold, and inert atmospheres.[15] Psilocybin is more stable than psilocin.[16] Psilocybin has a molecular weight of 284.25 g/mol, a melting point of 224 °C, and a water solubility of 2.7 g/L. In contrast, psilocin has a molecular weight of 204.27 g/mol, a melting point of 174.5 °C, and a water solubility of 4.08 g/L.[15]

Route of Administration

Psilocybin-containing mushrooms are taken orally. They can be consumed raw, dried, or steeped in hot water to create tea. As the taste of the mushrooms can be unpleasant, they are sometimes eaten with other foods that might include peanut butter or chocolate. Smoking mushrooms is believed to degrade psilocybin and is not recommended.

In clinical settings, synthetic psilocybin is almost always administered orally. It may be administered as a single fixed dose of 15, 20, 25, or 30 mg, representing very mild, mild, moderate, and moderately high doses, respectively. "Heroic" doses approaching 60 mg have been well tolerated in controlled environments but are rare in a clinical setting.[17] Body weight does not appear to have a significant effect on the subjective effects of psilocybin.[18]

Pharmacokinetics

Psilocybin is a prodrug that is converted into the pharmacologically active psilocin (4-hydroxy-N,N-dimethyltryptamine) following ingestion. Psilocin is structurally akin to serotonin and passes through the blood-brain barrier.

Absorption

Following oral administration, psilocybin is rapidly converted to psilocin via dephosphorylation in the stomach. Any remaining psilocybin is later converted to psilocin through alkaline phosphatase in the intestines, kidneys, or blood. It is estimated that 50% of psilocybin is absorbed through the gastrointestinal tract.[15]

Ley and colleagues found the average C_{max} for a 20-mg psilocybin dose (n = 32) to be 17 ng/mL (range: 9.6-34.0 ng/mL).[19] The average C_{max} for the active metabolite was found to be 70 ng/mL (range: 43-127 ng/mL).[19]

The same authors reported an average T_{max} for psilocybin and psilocin of 2.1 hours (range: 1-5 hours) and 4.4 hours (range: 3-8 hours), respectively.[19] Maximum plasma concentration for a 25-mg dose of psilocybin is believed to be 18.7 to 20 ng/mL with a similar T_{max} (~2 hours).[12]

Bioavailability

The bioavailability of psilocybin is estimated to be 50%.[20] According to Hasler et al, the bioavailability for psilocin following oral administration of 10 to 20 mg of psilocybin was 52.7 ± 20%.[21]

Distribution

Psilocybin is uniformly distributed throughout the body and is detectable in plasma within 20 to 40 minutes of administration in significant concentrations.[12] Psilocin is also uniformly distributed throughout the body—including the brain, as it readily passes through the blood-brain barrier.[15] Psychological effects may be perceptible once psilocybin has reached plasma levels of 4 to 6 μg/mL and tend to peak within 60 to 90 minutes of ingestion.[20]

Metabolism

As noted earlier, the primary metabolite of psilocybin is psilocin. Within 5 hours, up to 80% of psilocin undergoes glucuronidation via glucuronosyltransferase enzymes UGT1A9 and UGT1A10 to form psilocin O-glucuronide, which is then excreted through urine.[22] Psilocin is also metabolized by demethylation and oxidative deamination through liver monoamine oxidase (MAO) or aldehyde dehydrogenase to yield 4-hydroxyindole-3-acetaldehyde and then 4-hydroxytryptophol and 4-hydroxyindole-3-acetic acid.[15] A third metabolic pathway occurs in the liver and converts psilocin into psilocin iminoquinone.[22]

Elimination and Excretion

Psilocybin's elimination half-life is 160 minutes, while psilocin's is only 50 minutes.[15] It is estimated that 3% to 10% of psilocybin is eliminated through the kidneys unaltered.[20] However, in rat studies, that figure is notably higher, with 25% of the unaltered dose being excreted.[15] Rat studies also showed that psilocin is excreted primarily through urine (65%), as well as bile and feces (15%-20%) within 8 hours and psilocin excretion being complete within 24 hours.[12] Rat studies suggest that some psilocin metabolites may be detectable in urine for up to 7 days.[15]

Pharmacodynamics

Mechanism of Action

The molecular structures of psilocybin and psilocin are similar to tryptamine (see Figure 9.1), which is converted into serotonin. However, psilocybin does not cross the blood-brain barrier, whereas psilocin does, acting as a partial agonist at multiple serotonin receptors, most notably 5-HT$_{2A}$ (see Table 9.1).[23] Psilocin has greater than 40% activation efficacy at 5-HT$_{2A}$ and is also a ligand at 5-HT$_{2C}$, 5-HT$_{1A}$, and 5-HT$_{1B}$ receptors. As is the case with all classic psychedelics, alterations in perception are primarily mediated via 5-HT$_{2A}$ receptors, which modulate glutamatergic signaling across a range of subcortical and cortical afferents.[13]

The stimulation of postsynaptic 5-HT$_{2A}$ receptors found in pyramidal neurons located in the deepest layers of the cortex leads to increased levels of extracellular glutamate in the prefrontal cortex. This release of glutamate activates α-amino-3-hydroxy-5-methyl-4-isoxazole propionic acid (AMPA) and *N*-methyl-D-aspartate (NMDA) receptors. The activation of these three receptors (5-HT$_{2A}$, AMPA, and NMDA) is believed to then cause an increase in brain-derived neurotrophic factor (BDNF).[24] High levels of BDNF are positively correlated with neuroplasticity, as well

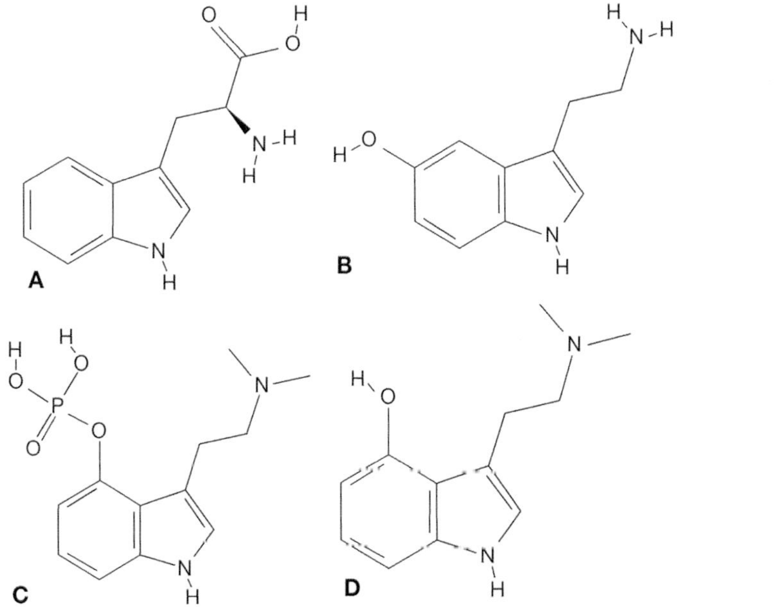

Figure 9.1 From left to right: chemical structures of tryptophan (A), serotonin (B), psilocybin (C), and psilocin (D).

TABLE 9.1 Binding Affinity of Psilocin at Select Receptor Sites

Receptor	K_i Value (nM)
5-HT$_{1A}$	62.6
5-HT$_{1B}$	305
5-HT$_{1D}$	18.6
5-HT$_{1E}$	44.3
5-HT$_{2A}$	339.6
5-HT$_{2B}$	4.7
5-HT$_{2C}$	141.2
5-HT$_{5A}$	69.9
5-HT$_6$	71.7
5-HT$_7$	71.6
D$_1$	19.9
D$_2$	>10,000
D$_3$	101.2
D$_4$	>10,000
D$_5$	>10,000
α_{1A}	>10,000
α_{1B}	>10,000
α_{2A}	2,044
α_{2B}	1,271
α_{2C}	4,404
SERT	851.6

5-HT, serotonin receptor; α, alpha-adrenergic receptor; D, Dopamine receptor; nM, nanomoles; SERT, serotonin transporter.

Ray TS. Psychedelics and the human receptorome. *PLoS One*. 2010;5(2):e9019. doi:10.1371/journal.pone.0009019. Erratum in: *PLoS One*. 2010;5(3). doi:10.1371/annotation/e580a864-cf13-40c2-9bd9-b9687a6f0fe4. PMID: 20126400; PMCID: PMC2814854.

as neurogenesis and, conversely, negatively associated with depression and neuroinflammation.[25]

Moliner and colleagues also demonstrated that psilocin has a high affinity for tropomyosin receptor kinase B (TrkB) and allosterically potentiates the signaling of BDNF.[26] Of note, antidepressants such as fluoxetine and imipramine, as well as ketamine, also bind to TrkB, but with affinities that are several magnitudes lower than either psilocin or LSD.[26]

Like other tryptamine psychedelics, psilocin induces alterations in brain dynamics and functional connectivity between areas of the brain, resulting in disruption of normal communication between connected pathways such as the default-mode network and the task-positive network.[27] The default-mode network is believed to be central in the formation and retention of the concept of self or ego, and disruptions in its normal activity may serve as the neural correlates of the subjective feeling of ego dissolution or oceanic boundlessness, which are frequently described in psychedelic literature.[28] Psilocybin also reduces hyperactivity within the medial prefrontal cortex, as well as the interaction between the medial prefrontal cortex and posterior cingulate cortex, which may disrupt the normal neural hierarchy of top-down information transfer.[29] These disruptions can then result in difficulties with attention and impaired associative learning, episodic recall, and working memory.[13] Additionally, disruptions in functional connectivity of the claustrum and other brain regions may be associated with perceived changes in executive function.[13]

Administration of psilocybin is associated with increases in extracellular dopamine.[30] Unlike many other psychedelics, psilocin's activity at dopamine D_2 receptors is minimal, but administration of haloperidol (a D_2 antagonist) has reportedly attenuated psilocybin-induced euphoria, depersonalization, and derealization.[30] In addition, serotonergic activity at 5-HT_{1A} and 5-HT_{2A} may be indirectly responsible for increases in dopamine levels via the striatum.

Therapeutic Index

Psilocybin has the most favorable safety profile of any known psychedelics.[31] It has an especially wide therapeutic index, with an average lethal dose (LD_{50}) of approximately 280 mg/kg in rodents.[20] This would translate into the consumption of approximately 17 kg of mushrooms, which would be unrealistic for either rats or humans.[32]

Tolerance, Dependence, and Withdrawal

Though tolerance to psilocybin is established, it dissipates quickly. Cross-tolerance to other classical psychedelics has also been observed since tolerance is mediated through the downregulation of 5-HT$_{2A}$ receptors.[6] However, physical dependence and withdrawal symptoms are extremely rare.

Other Psychotropic Compounds in Mushrooms

Psilocybin and psilocin are not the only psychotropic tryptamines found in the fungi kingdom. The active metabolites aeruginascin, baeocystin, and norbaeocystin, which are oftentimes found alongside psilocybin, may play a role in the therapeutic effects of psilocybin or they may affect the subjective experience following ingestion of psychedelic mushrooms.

Aeruginascin

Aeruginascin is the *N*-trimethyl analogue of psilocybin. Its active metabolite, 4-hydroxy-*N*,*N*,*N*-trimethyltryptamine (4-HO-TMT), has a relatively high affinity at human serotonin receptors 5-HT$_{1A}$, 5-HT$_{2A}$, and 5-HT$_{2B}$ (K_i = 4,400, 670, and 120 nM, respectively). Although these findings suggest that the compound has psychotropic effects due to serotoninergic activity in vitro, quaternary trimethylammonium compounds like 4-HO-TMT typically do not cross the blood-brain barrier, though there have been reports of quaternary trimethylammonium salts passing the blood-brain barrier through transporters.[33]

Research into the pharmacology of aeruginascin and the metabolite 4-HO-TMT is preliminary. Although it seems unlikely that 4-HO-TMT can cause significant psychotropic effects on its own or to enhance the effects of psilocin, it remains a possibility.

Baeocystin and Norbaeocystin

Baeocystin and norbaeocystin were isolated in 1968 and are both derivatives and analogues of psilocybin.[34] At this time, very little is known about the therapeutic applications of either compound, and there is some debate about whether or not they possess psychedelic properties.

Somatic Effects

Those who ingest psilocybin will frequently feel a wave of nausea before the psychotropic effects of the drug take effect. Nausea may persist during the onset of these effects, though it typically passes well before the peak experience is attained. Autonomic effects typically include mydriasis, accelerated heart rate, and hypertension. A review by Vargas and colleagues examining three studies and 92 patients found systolic blood pressure, diastolic blood pressure, and heart rate all increased following the administration of psilocybin. Their findings indicate that systolic blood pressure is at its highest during the second and fourth hours and that it stays elevated for up to 6 hours. Diastolic blood pressure is highest between the first and third hours and remains elevated for 5 hours. Heart rate increases were highest at the third and fourth hours following administration and stabilized after 6 hours.[35]

Subjective Effects

The subjective effects of psilocybin are akin to other classic psychedelics. These effects involve alterations in perception; synesthesia; euphoria; and an increased fondness for music, art, and nature. Visual imagery may involve intricate geometric patterns or visions that borrow from memory, especially when the individual's eyes are closed. One is typically aware that these images are not real. They may also lose their subjective self-identity (ego dissolution), which may be accompanied by the feeling that they have died, and then reborn as the ego reconstructs itself. This may be terrifying for some people, but others find the act of surrender to be liberating.

Mystical-Type Experiences

Mystical-type experiences are also common with psilocybin, and some of the most well-known studies involving psilocybin have focused on the drug's ability to occasion these kinds of states. These include Pahnke's Good Friday Experiment of 1962 and the 2006 paper by Griffiths and colleagues that is often regarded as the catalyst for the launch of the recent psychedelic renaissance. Although the Good Friday Experiment has been critiqued for methodological flaws, particularly in Rick Doblin's 1991 paper, "Pahnke's 'Good Friday Experiment': a long-term follow-up and methodological critique," the Griffiths paper is highly valued.[36] Aspects of the experiment have also been replicated several times, oftentimes in groups of individuals who are experiencing existential duress on account of a terminal diagnosis.[37]

While Pahnke's experiment is historically important, Griffith's paper was groundbreaking because it took place in a clinical setting and shed light on the psychological effects of psychedelics in healthy adults. It also laid the foundation for a standardized procedure to some extent when administering psychedelics. Each participant in the study became familiar with the primary monitor over the course of four 2-hour meetings before the first session and then spoke with the primary monitor in four 1-hour meetings following each session. A total of 36 volunteers were randomly assigned to participate in two 8-hour sessions ($n = 30$) or three 8-hour sessions ($n = 6$), which were spaced

2 months apart. During the first session, among the group of 30, half were randomly assigned to receive psilocybin (30 mg/70 kg), while the other half received methylphenidate hydrochloride (40 mg/70 kg), and the alternative drug was administered during the second session. The three-session group received active placebo during the first two sessions, followed by an unblinded dose of psilocybin during their third session 2 months later.[38] For each session, participants completed questionnaires assessing the level of mystical experience attained 7 hours after dose, and questionnaires were completed again 2 months later.

The questionnaires completed by the participants included the hallucinogen rating scale, APZ (*abnormale Geisteszustände* [German to English: Abnormal Mental States], which contains questions designed to assess oceanic boundlessness, dread of ego dissolution, and visionary restructuralization), addiction research center inventory, states of consciousness questionnaire, and Mysticism Scale. At 2-month follow-up, participants also completed the Persisting Effects Questionnaire, Mysticism Scale-Lifetime, Spiritual Transcendence Scale, NEO Personality Inventory, and Positive and Negative Affect Schedule (PANAS) Expanded Form. Three individuals who had close contact with each participant were also interviewed to assess observational changes in behavior.[38] Overall, it was an exceptionally thorough study.

Of the 36 participants, 22 (61%) had what qualified as a "complete" mystical experience, and 24 (67%) participants described it as either the single most meaningful experience or among the top five most meaningful experiences of their lives. According to the authors, "the volunteers judged the meaningfulness of the experience to be similar, for example, to the birth of a first child or death of a parent."[38] Participants also reported elevations in mood, sociability, and positive attitudes following their psilocybin sessions that far exceeded controls.[38]

At 14-month follow-up, these results had barely changed. No participant said that the experience had decreased their sense of well-being or satisfaction with life, while 64% said that it had increased their sense of well-being and satisfaction with life moderately or very much. Additionally, 58% and 67% of participants rated the experience as being among the five most personally meaningful experiences and the five most spiritually significant experiences of their lives, respectively. Additionally, 17% felt it was the single most spiritually significant experience in their lifetime, while for 11% it was the single most meaningful experience of their lives.[39]

The authors concluded that "When administered to volunteers under supportive conditions, psilocybin occasioned experiences similar to spontaneously occurring mystical experiences."[38] Moreover, these experiences were felt to be personally meaningful and to have spiritual significance.

Potential Uses

As of this writing, the FDA has not approved psilocybin use for any condition, and it remains a Schedule I drug. However, three breakthrough therapy designations have been issued by the FDA for the use of psilocybin or an analogue in treating depressive disorders. The first designation was issued in 2018 following publication of a study that relied on Compass Pathways' psilocybin formulation, COMP360, and showed efficacy of psilocybin therapy coupled with psychological support in the treatment of treatment-resistant depression.[40] The Usona Institute then received breakthrough therapy designation in 2019 for the use of psilocybin in the treatment of major depressive disorder.[41]

Most recently, in March 2024, FDA awarded breakthrough therapy designation to Cybin for the use of CYB003, a deuterated psilocybin analogue, for the treatment of major depressive disorder. Enrollment of phase 3 trials for CYB003 is set to begin in the summer of 2024.[42]

In addition to the work of the above-mentioned commercial entities, there has been an enormous amount of noncommercial research into the potential uses of psilocybin, with dozens of studies examining the potential use of psilocybin within the context of psychedelic-assisted psychotherapy. The strongest evidence in favor of psilocybin's efficacy is in mood disorders, as well as anxiety and depression associated with terminal illnesses. Though less convincing, there is some evidence for psilocybin's use in the treatment of substance use disorders, OCD, anorexia nervosa, body dysmorphic disorder, migraines, and cluster headaches.

Primary Depression

Numerous studies have examined the effects of psilocybin on treatment-resistant depression, major depressive disorder, and depression associated with terminal illness. The first two subsets of depressive disorders will be examined in this section. A discussion of the literature on depression associated with a terminal illness will be described in "Anxiety and Depression in a Palliative Context" section.

In addition to the work conducted by commercial enterprises, research work done at Johns Hopkins Medicine (Davis et al) and the Heffter Research Institute (von Rotz et al) will be discussed. More importantly, unless mentioned specifically, all studies included a washout period, had multiple sessions where the participant had the opportunity to become acquainted with therapists, and engaged in integrative psychotherapy sessions following the administration of psilocybin.

Early Research

Before delving into the phase 2 trials described earlier, it's important to note Robin Carhart-Harris's study published in *The Lancet* in 2016 describing an open-label feasibility trial in 12 patients with moderate-to-severe, unipolar, treatment-resistant depression.[43] Participants received two oral doses of psilocybin 7 days apart. The first was 10 mg, with a second dose of 25 mg. Follow-ups were conducted 1 day after treatment with the 25-mg dose, then again at week 1, week 2, week 3, week 5, and month 3 posttreatment. Mean clinical rating at baseline for Quick Inventory of Depressive Symptoms (QIDS), which served as the primary efficacy outcome, was 19.2, and then declined to 7.4, 6.3, 6.4, 8.2, and 10.0 at week 1, week 2, week 3, week 5, and month 3, respectively. Secondary outcomes were measured using the Montgomery-Åsberg Depression Rating Scale (MADRS), Global Assessment of Functioning, Beck Depression Inventory (BDI), Spielberger's State-Trait Anxiety Inventory (STAI), but just the trait version [STAI-T]), and the Snaith-Hamilton Pleasure Scale. Most notably, the response rate to psilocybin at 1 week after treatment was 67% (8) according to Hamilton Depression Scale (HAM-D) and BDI scores, and 58% (7) maintained response until assessment at 3 months posttreatment. According to the same scales, 58% (7) of patients achieved remission 1 week after treatment and 42% (5) remained in remission at 3 months. No serious adverse events were reported, though several participants experienced headache in the wake of dosing.[43]

Extended data on the 12 participants, plus an additional 8 participants (though only 7 completed the full trial), showed similar effects at 6 months. Mean scores declined from baseline to month 3 and then remained significantly lower than baseline through month 6.[44] Though there was no control arm in the study, the results appear promising and suggest potential for future research in a larger cohort in a double-blind fashion.

Usona Institute Studies

In 2023, Raison and colleagues published the results of their phase 2 trial examining the efficacy of single-dose psilocybin treatment in 104 participants who had been diagnosed with major depressive disorder. The randomized, two-group trial was conducted between December 2019 and June 2022 across 11 sites within the United States. Participants received either a 25-mg dose of synthetic psilocybin ($n = 50$) or a 100-mg dose of niacin ($n = 54$). The primary outcome measure was a comparison of MADRS scores at baseline to 43 days posttreatment, while secondary outcomes measured the MADRS scores at baseline and 8 days posttreatment while the Sheehan Disability Scale (SDS) score was assessed at baseline and 43 days posttreatment. Eligible participants completed baseline assessments before undergoing 6 to 8 hours of preparatory sessions. Of note, no later than 7 days after the assessment, participants received either psilocybin or active placebo psilocybin, while postdosing assessments were conducted at 5 points (days 2, 8, 15, 29, and 43) with day 43 being the endpoint of the study.

The primary results of the trial showed greater efficacy of psilocybin than placebo, with MADRS scores declining from baseline to day 43 by 19.1 (range: 22.7-15.5) for the psilocybin group, while in the placebo group, it was 6.8 (range: 10.5-3.1), resulting in a mean difference of 12.3 between the two groups. Similar disparities were reported on days 8, 15, 29, and 43, but not day 2, when both groups reported a mean decline in MADRS scores of 2.7. For the psilocybin group, SDS scores declined by 4.07 between baseline and day 43, while the placebo group saw a decline over the same period of only 1.76. Similar declines for both groups were observed on day 8 and remained largely constant through the posttreatment period.

Of the 50 individuals in the psilocybin group, 4 (8%) experienced a severe adverse event, including 1 migraine, 1 headache, 1 illusion, and 1 episode of paranoia combined with a panic attack. There were no serious treatment-emergent adverse events (TEAEs).[45]

Of note, phase 3 trials are currently underway (ClinicalTrials.gov Identifier: NCT06308653).

Compass Pathways Studies

There are three relevant Compass Pathways studies that highlight the use of the COMP360 treatment, which is a synthetic form of psilocybin. The first study published, in November 2022, was a phase 2 double-blind trial for individuals with treatment-resistant depression. Participants were given one of the three following doses of psilocybin: a moderate dose (25 mg; $n = 79$), a low dose (10 mg; $n = 75$), and a subperceptual dose (1 mg; $n = 79$) that served as a control. The primary end point was 3 weeks following dosing and utilized MADRS to assess the severity of depressive symptom, while the secondary endpoint was 12 weeks posttreatment. This trial is notable for the diversity of sites involved, with 22 across 10 countries (Canada, the Czech Republic, Denmark, Germany, Ireland, the Netherlands, Portugal, Spain, the United Kingdom, and the United States).

At baseline, mean MADRS scores for the 25-, 10-, and 1-mg groups were 31.9 (±5.4), 33 (±6.3), and 32.7 (±6.2), respectively. The mean overall MADRS score was 32.5 (±6.0). Thirty percent of participants had moderate symptoms (MADRS score 20-30), while 68% had a score that constituted severe depression (MADRS scores ≥31).

The least-squares mean change from baseline to week 3 in the MADRS scores of the 25-, 10-, and 1-mg groups were −12.0, −7.9, and −5.4, respectively. Response rates (≥50% decrease in MADRS scores between baseline and week 3) for the 25-, 10-, and 1-mg groups were 37%, 19%, and 18%, respectively. Remission rates (MADRS score ≤10 at week 3) for the 25-, 10-, and 1-mg groups were 29%, 9%, and 8%, respectively. Sustained responses (week 3 response sustained until week 12) for the 25-, 10-, and 1-mg groups were 18%, 8%, and 10%, respectively.

According to the authors, adverse events occurred in 84% of the 25-mg group, 75% of the 10-mg group, and 72% of the 1-mg group. Within the 25-mg group, the most common adverse events included headache, nausea, dizziness, and fatigue, which occurred on the day of dosing. Although there were no serious adverse events, 4% of participants in the 25-mg group reported severe adverse events (compared to 8% in the 10-mg group and 1% in the 1-mg group). Of note, following the day of dosing and week 3, severe events were reported by members of the 25-, 10-, and 1-mg groups at a rate of 9%, 7%, and 1%, respectively. Serious events in the 25-mg group during this period included suicidal ideation (two participants) and nonsuicidal self-injurious behavior (two participants). The 10-mg group saw similar serious events, with two participants reporting suicidal ideation, one participant reporting intentional self-injury, and one participant needing hospitalization for severe depression. No serious events were reported for the 1-mg group. Between week 3 and week 12, severe adverse events were reported by 3% of the 25-mg group, 4% of the 10-mg group, and 0 in the 1-mg group.

What's important to note is that, in many cases, the trial with psilocybin represented a third-, fourth-, or fifth-line treatment, which may indicate why MADRS scores were lower than in the Usona Institute trial. It may also help explain the relatively high rate of adverse events. Similarly, it should be taken into consideration that suicidality was not part of the study's exclusion criteria and that suicidal ideation was reported by 21 participants (27%) in the 25-mg group, 27 (36%) in the 10-mg group, and 19 (24%) in the 1-mg group. Despite the adverse events, the authors concluded that psilocybin was effective at reducing depressive symptoms in some patients.[46]

A second paper expanding upon the initial study reported on multiple exploratory endpoints that are outlined in Table 9.2. Some of the highlights include the decline in SDS scores from baseline to week 12 between the 25-and 1-mg groups (−8.8 and −2.3, respectively), as well as in the Work and Social Adjustment Scale scores between the 25-and 1-mg

TABLE 9.2 Clinical Characteristics of Psilocybin Treatment in Patients With Treatment-Resistant Depression, From Baseline to 12 Weeks Following Dose

Measure	25 mg (n = 79) Baseline (SD)	25 mg (n = 79) Change Week 12 (SE)	10 mg (n = 75) Baseline (SD)	10 mg (n = 75) Change Week 12 (SE)	1 mg (n = 79) Baseline (SD)	1 mg (n = 79) Change Week 12 (SE)
QIDS-SR-16; range: 0-27	16.1 (4.14)	−6.3 (0.66)	16.3 (4.16)	−5.2 (0.68)	15.8 (3.96)	−3.6 (0.67)
PANAS positive affect; range: 10-50	19.5 (5.69)	5.9 (0.96)	19.5 (7.19)	1.3 (1.02)	19.6 (6.41)	−0.3 (0.99)
PANAS negative affect; range: 10-50	24.6 (8.37)	−6.7 (0.87)	24.7 (8.08)	−5.1 (0.92)	24.0 (7.54)	−3.5 (0.89)
GAD-7; range: 0-21	11.6 (5.21)	−5.1 (0.57)	13.2 (4.92)	−3.8 (0.6)	12.8 (4.97)	−3.3 (0.59)
SDS; range: 0-30	21.7 (5.21)	−8.8 (1.05)	21.6 (4.47)	−6.3 (1.12)	21.7 (5.44)	−2.3 (1.19)
SDS days lost[a]	2.9 (2.79)	−1.5 (0.26)	2.7 (2.71)	−0.5 (0.28)	2.8 (2.77)	−0.3 (0.27)
SDS days unproductive[a]	5.7 (1.91)	−2.7 (0.30)	5.7 (1.59)	−1.9 (0.32)	5.4 (2.22)	−1.1 (0.31)
WSAS; range: 0-40	28.9 (6.83)	−9.2 (1.2)	30.2 (5.56)	−7.2 (1.28)	29.6 (6.21)	−4.1 (1.24)
EQ-5D-3L; range: −0.594 to 1.0	0.49 (0.236)	0.20 (0.033)	0.46 (0.236)	0.14 (0.035)	0.43 (0.267)	0.14 (0.034)
EQ-VAS; range: 0-100	51.2 (20.50)	11.1 (2.58)	46.9 (20.17)	8.7 (2.74)	45.8 (19.09)	4.4 (2.66)
DSST; range: 0-100	30.8 (10.07)	6.4 (0.84)	32.1 (10.08)	5.4 (0.87)	34.1 (9.61)	4.8 (0.84)

DSST, Digit Symbol Substitution Test; EQ-5D-3L, EuroQol-5 Dimensions-3 Levels; EQ-VAS, EuroQol-Visual Analog Scale; GAD-7, Generalized Anxiety Disorder-7 item; n, number of participants; PANAS, Positive and Negative Affect Schedule; QIDS-SR-16, Quick Inventory of Depressive Symptomatology-16 item; SD, standard deviation; SDS, Sheehan Disability Scale; WSAS, Work and Social Adjustment Scale.

[a]The analysis of SDS days lost and SDS days unproductive was post hoc and not a prespecified exploratory efficacy endpoint.

Goodwin GM, Aaronson ST, Alvarez O, et al. Single-dose psilocybin for a treatment-resistant episode of major depression: impact on patient-reported depression severity, anxiety, function, and quality of life. *J Affect Disord*. 2023;327:120-127. doi:10.1016/j.jad.2023.01.108. PMID: 36740140.

groups (−9.2 and −4.1, respectively). Improvements from baseline to week 12 in PANAS scores were reported between the 25-and 1-mg groups for negative total scores (−6.7 and −3.5, respectively) and positive total scores (5.9 and −0.3, respectively). These results suggest that the efficacy of psilocybin extends beyond depressive symptoms among patients with treatment-resistant depression and can also positively impact their quality of life and ability to function on a daily basis.[47]

The third paper from Compass Pathways involves a significantly smaller cohort of patients ($n = 19$) with treatment-resistant depression who were allowed to continue taking selective serotonin reuptake inhibitors (SSRIs) during the phase 2 exploratory trial. SSRI medications included:

- Sertraline (Zoloft)—six participants
- Escitalopram (Lexapro)—six participants
- Fluoxetine (Prozac)—three participants
- Vilazodone (Viibryd)—two participants
- Paroxetine (Paxil)—one participant
- Citalopram (Celexa)—one participant

The open-label study involved a single dosing session with 25 mg of psilocybin with psychological support. Like the first Compass Pathways study, the primary endpoint was 3 weeks posttreatment. MADRS total score was taken at baseline and week 3. The study also reported responders and remitters at week 3, TEAEs, and changes in Clinical Global Impression-Severity (CGI-S) scores between baseline and week 3.

At baseline, the mean MADRS score was 31.7. At week 3, the mean MADRS score had fallen to 16.8, representing a decline of 14.9. Of the 19 participants, response and remission were evident in 8 for each category. The mean CGI-S score at baseline was 4.3 (moderately ill) and fell to 2.0 (borderline mentally ill) by week 3.

Of the 19 participants, 12 (63.2%) reported a total of 17 TEAEs. Of the 17 TEAEs, 11 occurred on the day of psilocybin administration and 8 resolved the same day. The six remaining TEAEs occurred in four participants, and all but two resolved within 1 day. The most commonly reported TEAEs were headache (6) and increased blood pressure (3), though increased blood pressure was only reported on the day of psilocybin administration. In two cases, the blood pressure increases were considered severe and treated with clonidine. There were no serious adverse events and, moreover, no participants reported suicidal ideation at baseline or at week 3 assessment.[48]

Cybin

As of spring 2024, only topline results have been released regarding the phase 2 trial of CYB003 for the treatment of major depressive disorder. According to a press release issued by Cybin, the trial involved a dosage of 12 or 16 mg of CYB003. In both cohorts, mean MADRS scores declined 22 points from baseline to the primary endpoint of the study (4 months). Response and remission rates are outlined in Table 9.3. Moreover, all adverse events were reportedly mild or moderate in intensity.[49]

Johns Hopkins Medicine

The Center of Psychedelic and Consciousness Research at Johns Hopkins Bayview Medical Center in Baltimore conducted a randomized, waiting list–controlled clinical trial with 27 participants who had been diagnosed with major depressive disorder but were not using antidepressant medications. Exclusion criteria included a history of psychotic disorder, serious suicide attempt, or previous hospitalization for a psychiatric disorder. The trial included two psilocybin sessions (20 mg/70 kg in session 1 and 30 mg/70 kg in session 2) that were administered to both the immediate ($n = 15$) and the delayed treatment arm ($n = 12$). Of the 27 participants, 24 completed the trial.

For the immediate treatment arm, preparation meetings were held during weeks 1 and 2 of the trial, and psilocybin dosing sessions occurred in weeks 3 and 4 while depression assessments were conducted in weeks 5 and 8. In the delayed treatment arm, there was inactivity between baseline and week 4, and the group was then assessed in week 5 and again during week 8. Preparation meetings for the psilocybin sessions

TABLE 9.3 Response and Remission Rates to CYB003 in Phase 2 Trials

	Responders		Remitters	
Time	12 mg ($n = 15$) (%)	16 mg ($n = 8$) (%)	12 mg ($n = 15$) (%)	16 mg ($n = 8$) (%)
Day 21	53	44	20	22
Day 42	7	75	79	50
Day 126	73	75	60	75

Business Wire. Cybin receives FDA breakthrough therapy designation for its novel psychedelic molecule CYB003 and announces positive four-month durability data in major depressive disorder. Published March 13, 2024. Accessed April 19, 2024. https://www.businesswire.com/news/home/20240313731043/en/Cybin-Receives-FDA-Breakthrough-Therapy-Designation-for-its-Novel-Psychedelic-Molecule-CYB003-and-Announces-Positive-Four-Month-Durability-Data-in-Major-Depressive-Disorder then began, lasting through week 10 while psilocybin sessions occurred in weeks 11 and 12. Further assessments were taken only for the delayed treatment arm in weeks 13 and 16.

The mean GRID-Hamilton Depression Rating Scale (GRID-HAMD) score across both groups was 22.8 at baseline. The differences between the two groups' responses were expectedly dramatic at week 5. In the immediate group, the mean baseline GRID-HAMD score was 22.9, but dropped to 8.0, before rising slightly to 8.5 in week 8. For the delayed treatment arm, GRID-HAMD scores in weeks 5 and 8 were 23.8 and 23.5. To clarify, the delayed treatment arm did not receive psilocybin until week 11.

At the end of the study, 17 of the 24 participants (71%) who completed the study had a clinically significant response in the week following their second psilocybin treatment (defined as a 50% or greater decrease in GRID-HAMD score). The same number of participants had a clinically significant response 4 weeks after their second psilocybin dose. Posttreatment remission criteria were met in 14 participants (58%) at week 1 and 13 participants (54%) at week 4.[50]

The 24 participants who completed the initial trial attended all follow-up visits through the 12-month timepoint, and both response and remission rates remained surprisingly steady, as measured by GRID-HAMD scores. Response rates were 67%, 79%, and 75% at 3, 6, and 12 months, respectively. Remission rates were 54%, 71%, and 58% at 3, 6, and 12 months, respectively. The same trends were observed for QIDS and BDI-II scores over the same period.[51]

There were no serious adverse events during the trial. Mild to moderate transient headaches were reported in 16 (33%) of the total psilocybin sessions and in 14 (29%) instances during follow-up sessions. Additional adverse events during sessions included four heartrate events and two blood pressure events though both resolved quickly and without intervention. In addition, the following adverse events were reported within 2 weeks of the sessions:

- Headache (14)
- Physical discomfort (1)
- Mild controllable muscle motion (1)
- Visual distortion (3)
- Tenseness/soreness (2)
- Chest tightness (1)
- Vivid dreams (1)
- Altered body sensation (1)

Heffter Research Institute—Zurich

A double-blind, randomized clinical trial involving 52 participants with major depressive disorder at the Psychiatric University Hospital Zurich has also reported promising results. Participants received either placebo or a moderate dose of psilocybin (0.215 mg/kg) in conjunction with psychological support. MADRS and BDI scores were utilized to gauge efficacy over the course of 14 days from baseline. A clinically relevant response was defined as a decline in MADRS score of 50% or more from baseline or a prospectively determined threshold of less than 10 points or both. Remission was defined as a score of less than 10. Of note, BDI is analogous to MADRS.

Two weeks posttreatment, the psilocybin group's mean MADRS score had fallen from a baseline of 24.3 to 11.3 (a change of -13.0), while BDI had fallen from a baseline of 26.9 to 13.7 (a change of -13.2). This trial demonstrated that psilocybin clearly outperformed placebo, which produced only minor declines in MADRS and BDI scores. Two weeks posttreatment, the between-group differences for MADRS and BDI were 13.0 and 10.5, respectively. Fifty-eight percent of participants in the psilocybin group experienced significant declines in MADRS scores so as to meet criteria for treatment response compared to only 16% in placebo group. For BDI scores, those figures were 54% and 12% for the psilocybin group and placebo group, respectively.

A total of 11 adverse events were reported that persisted longer than the acute effects of the psilocybin, including headache and dizziness, though all side effects were described as mild.[52]

Psilocybin Versus Escitalopram

In 2021, Carhart-Harris and colleagues published a phase 2, double-blind, randomized, controlled trial that compared the efficacy of psilocybin to escitalopram. Fifty-nine participants were enrolled who had been diagnosed with moderate-to-severe major depressive disorder. Of the 59, 30 were assigned to the psilocybin group and 29 to the escitalopram group. Those within the psilocybin group received two 25-mg doses 3 weeks apart.

The primary clinical outcome measured the change in the 16-item Quick Inventory of Depressive Symptomatology-Self Report (QIDS-SR-16) at 6 weeks following the final doses. The secondary outcomes assessed response and remission at 6 weeks, as measured by QIDS-SR-16. Adverse events were similar in the two groups (87% in the psilocybin group and 83% in the escitalopram group), with the most common complaint within the psilocybin group being headache. No serious events were reported in either group.

The mean change in QIDS-SR-16 was −8.0 (±1.0) for the psilocybin group and −6.0 (±1.0) for the escitalopram group, indicating no significant difference. However, secondary outcomes favored psilocybin over escitalopram. Furthermore, at 6 weeks, the psilocybin group reported a response rate of 70% (21) and a remission rate of 57% (17), while the escitalopram group reported a 48% (14) response rate and a remission rate of 28% (8).

Considering the results of this trial, a follow-up study with a larger cohort will help better define how psilocybin compares to more conventional treatments.

Treatment-Resistant Major Depressive Disorder and Bipolar II Disorder

Another study recently published in 2024 by Rosenblat and colleagues deserves special mention, largely due to the diagnostic complexity of the population enrolled in the trial. Many who were allowed to participate would have been excluded from other trials due to psychiatric comorbidities (particularly borderline personality disorder), severity of depressive symptoms, number of treatment failures, or suicidality. However, this trial accepted participants with either major depressive disorder ($n = 26$) or bipolar II disorder ($n = 4$). Most studies exclude individuals if they so much as have a family history of the latter. Of the enrollees, 40% had received intensive interventions like electroconvulsive therapy or ketamine therapy without response, and the mean number of failed medication trials was 11.27.

Participants were randomized to receive immediate treatment ($n = 16$) or delayed treatment ($n = 14$). Of the 30 individuals, 29 remained until the end of the 2-week study meeting the primary endpoint. The mean baseline MADRS score for the immediate treatment arm (33.0) was higher than the delayed treatment arm (27.6) but was lower at the endpoint, as the former declined by 9.6 (to 23.4), while the latter declined only by 3 (to 24.6).

Another unique aspect of this open-label feasibility study was that it allowed greater flexibility in dosing over the 6-month follow-up period, with some participants receiving two or three doses of psilocybin over the course of the trial. Consequently, 17 participants received a second dose, while 5 participants received a third dose, which led to further declines in MADRS scores with each subsequent dose.

During the course of the study, there were no serious adverse events; only two participants reported transient worsening of suicidality within 24 to 48 hours of dosing but did not require additional intervention, and only one TEAE persisted for more than 48 hours. However, one adverse event that has never been documented in a trial involving psilocybin before was persistent genital arousal that lasted through the entire duration of the 6-month follow-up.[53]

Bipolar Disorders

A nonrandomized open-label study involving 15 individuals (6 males and 9 females) with bipolar II disorder experiencing a major depressive episode during the trial was published in 2023. Participants received a single 25-mg dose of synthetic psilocybin in conjunction with psychotherapy. Prior to the 8-h dosing session, participants met with therapists 3 times and then for three integration sessions. The study represents the first prospective and systematic report of the clinical experience of individuals with bipolar disorder II experiencing a major depressive episode during the study who received a treatment involving psilocybin and psychotherapy.

The primary outcome measure was a comparison of MADRS scores at baseline and 3 weeks posttreatment. All 15 participants reported lower MADRS scores at end point with a mean decrease of 24, while 12 met response criterion (50% decrease in MADRS) and 11 met the criterion for remission (MADRS score of ≤10). More importantly, at 12-week follow-up, 12 patients met both response and remission criteria. Participants also reported notable improvements in QIDS and Quality of Life Enjoyment and Satisfaction Questionnaire-Short Form scores. The authors also noted, "Despite the high remission rate, there was an association between general intensity of the psychedelic experience and clinical benefit." Perhaps just as important, psilocybin administration did not lead to any significant adverse events.[54]

The most notable limitations of the trial were its short duration (12 weeks), small sample size, and lack of control.

Anxiety and Depression in a Palliative Context

Psychedelic-assisted therapy with psilocybin has been especially helpful for patients with terminal illnesses like cancer. Griffiths and colleagues published a paper in 2016 reporting that patients ($n = 51$) with life-threatening cancer diagnoses who experienced anxiety and depression had significant improvements in mood and attitude after treatment with psilocybin. Community observer ratings also indicated improvement. Of note, during the follow-up 6 months later, these results were largely unchanged. The authors reported, "For the clinician-rated measures of depression and anxiety, respectively, the overall rate of clinical response at 6 months was 78% and 83% and the overall rate of symptom remission was 65% and 57%."[55] Clinician-rated measures included GRID-HAM-D-17 and the Hamilton Anxiety Rating Scale (HAM-A). Similar results were reported by Grob and colleagues in their 2011 paper after performing a randomized clinical trial involving 12 patients with advanced-stage cancer.[56]

A 2016 paper by Ross and colleagues ($n = 29$) found that a single dose of psilocybin, in conjunction with psychotherapy, was effective in reducing existential distress, and these effects were sustained for as long as 26 weeks.[57] The majority of patients reported anxiolytic and antidepressant effects, improved attitudes toward death, and increases in overall quality of life. A long-term follow-up from Ross' 2016 study ($n = 14$) was published in 2020 and included participants who were still alive since the last trial. The first and second follow-ups were completed on average 3.2 years (range: 2.3-4.5 years) and 4.5 years (range: 3.5-5.5 years) following the participants' dosing date, respectively. Primary outcomes showed clinically significant anxiolytic and antidepressant responses via the STAI, BDI, and Hospital Anxiety and Depression Scale (HADS).[i] At the second follow-up, 57% of participants showed a clinically significant decline in HADS-A scores, 71% reported clinically significant declines in HADS-T scores, while clinical responses for depression on HADS-D and BDI ranged from 57% to 79%. Additionally, remission rates for depressive symptoms ranged from 50% to 79%. Secondary outcomes measuring hopelessness, demoralization, and death anxiety showed improvement over baseline.[58]

Substance Use Disorders

Since the 1960s, psilocybin has shown promise as a treatment for substance use disorder, especially alcohol use disorder.[59] Though those initial studies are relevant, this section will focus exclusively on more recent studies.

Alcohol Use Disorder

In 2015, Bogenschutz and colleagues conducted a proof-of-concept study by administering psilocybin to 10 volunteers with alcohol dependency. Although the psilocybin treatment did not result in widespread abstinence, all participants reported decreases in alcohol use.[60]

---

[i] The HADS includes a total score (HAD-T), a subscale for only depression (HADS-D) and a subscale for only anxiety (HADS-A).

A more recent double-blind, randomized clinical trial conducted by Bogenschutz and colleagues included 95 participants diagnosed with alcohol use disorder. The trial was conducted over the course of 36 weeks with assessments at weeks 0 (baseline), 4, 5, 8, 9, 12, 24, and 36. Participants were randomly assigned in a 1:1 ratio to receive either psilocybin (25 mg/70 kg first dosing session, 25-40 mg/70 kg second dosing session) or diphenhydramine (50 mg first dosing session, 50-100 mg second dosing session) at weeks 4 and 8. All participants were offered a total of 12 psychotherapy sessions—4 prior to the first dosing session, 4 between the first and second dosing sessions, and 4 following the second dosing session. Of the 49 participants in the psilocybin arm, 48 participated in the first dosing session and 43 received a second dose. Of the 46 participants in the diphenhydramine group, 45 participated in the first dosing session, while only 35 received a second dose.

In the 12 weeks prior to screening, the participants' mean percentage of drinking days (PDD) was 74.9%. The percentage of heavy drinking days (PHDD) (defined as five or more drinks in a day for a man and four or more drinks in a day for a woman) was 52.7%. Participants consumed an average of 7.1 standard drinks per drinking day (DPD). Between screening and week 4 (prior to drug administration), PHDD, PDD, and DPD declined in both groups. In the group that would subsequently receive psilocybin, PHDD declined by a mean of 32.37, whereas it dropped by a mean of 27.26 in the diphenhydramine group. For PDD, the mean declines for the psilocybin group and diphenhydramine groups were 25.05 and 25.69, respectively. For DPD, the mean declines for the psilocybin group and diphenhydramine groups were 2.43 and 2.19, respectively. At the follow-up period 32 weeks later, these three metrics were notably better in the psilocybin group. Mean PHDD (SD) was 9.71 (26.21) for the psilocybin group compared to 23.57 (26.21) for the diphenhydramine group, representing a difference in mean of 13.86. At week 32, mean PDD and DPD continued to decline for the psilocybin group, but actually began to drift upward for the diphenhydramine group (though they remained far below where they had been at baseline for both groups). Additionally, the authors report that "participants who were treated with psilocybin were more likely than those receiving diphenhydramine to have no heavy drinking days."

The treatment was well tolerated, though there were 204 adverse events reported (119 in the psilocybin group and 85 in the diphenhydramine group). Headaches, anxiety, and nausea were commonly reported following the administration of psilocybin. Three serious adverse events were reported in the diphenhydramine group, while none were reported in the psilocybin group.[61]

Tobacco Use Disorder

Johnson and colleagues published a paper in 2017 involving 15 cigarette smokers who were enrolled in a 15-week open-label pilot study that included cognitive behavioral therapy (CBT), as well as psilocybin administration at weeks 5, 7, and 13. During the initial 4 weeks, patients participated in CBT while still being allowed to smoke. However, during week 5, subjects had to quit smoking, which coincided with the first dose of psilocybin which was administered as either 20 mg/70 kg or 30 mg/70 kg.

Of the 15 subjects in the study, 12 (80%) participants were smoke free at 6-month follow-up and 10 (67%) were smoke free at 12-month follow-up. Only 12 of the 15 participants returned for a long-term follow-up (mean: 30 months after target quit date; range: 16-57 months). Of those 12, 9 participants had effectively quit, while 7 of the 9 had been abstinent since the target quit date. Of note, these results are significantly better than those produced by CBT alone.[62]

According to the authors, "In controlled studies, the most effective smoking cessation medications typically demonstrate less than 31% abstinence at 12 months post-treatment."[62]

Obsessive-Compulsive Disorder

One of the earliest studies involving the use of psilocybin in the second wave of psychedelic research was published by Moreno and colleagues in 2006. The study was conducted between November 2001 and November 2004. Although this trial only involved nine participants with OCD, the multidose, partially blinded crossover study heeded notable improvements in symptom severity as measured by the Yale-Brown Obsessive Compulsive Disorder Scale (YBOCS). Doses were semirandomized and differed considerably—25 µg/kg (very low), 100 µg/kg (low), 200 µg/kg (medium), and 300 µg/kg (high)—and each dose was administered in a controlled environment over the course of 8 hours. Scale measurement was done 24 hours after psilocybin administration with decreases in YBOCS that ranged from 23% to 100%. Of the nine patients, eight showed a greater than or equal to 25% decline in symptoms as per YBOCS 24 hours after ingesting psilocybin. Additionally, six of the nine saw a decrease of 50% 24 hours after the session. Of note, symptom improvement lasted well over 24 hours though these effects did not appear to have any correlation to dosage.[63]

Unfortunately, since the publication of that study, there have only been a handful of case studies on the use of psilocybin in the treatment of OCD. It is noteworthy to mention one such patient who is currently part of a double-blind, randomized placebo-controlled trial of single-dose psilocybin in treatment-resistant OCD that is being conducted at Yale University (NCT03356483) and is expected to be completed in late 2024.

According to the case study, a participant identified by the pseudonym Daniel had a profound experience while under the influence of psilocybin when he experienced a moment of nothingness or death, followed by rebirth. He reported going from nothingness to becoming a sapling, then a mature tree, and thereafter living through several seasons. Daniel was then reborn as a human being and relived memories from his youth, all the while realizing that suppressing his emotions had led to many of the difficulties he faced later in life. According to the study's authors, "He realized that he had been living as if 'chasing perfection was the answer' to 'being happy' or 'living a life.' At one point during the dosing session, Daniel stated aloud, 'This is giving me my life back.'" In terms of scale measurement, Daniel's YBOCS was 21 at baseline. One week after psilocybin administration, it was 4; it then declined to 1 at 4 weeks, remained at 1 at 8 weeks, and then fell to 0 at 12 weeks.[64]

Anorexia Nervosa

A phase 1, open-label feasibility study involving 10 adult females diagnosed with anorexia nervosa who received a single 25-mg dose of synthetic psilocybin in conjunction with psychological support was recently conducted at the University of California, San Diego. At 3-month follow-up, 9 of 10 participants felt more positive about life endeavors, 8 of 10 said the experience was one of the top five most meaningful events of their lives, while 7 of 10 felt a positive shift in personal identity and overall quality of life.[65]

More pertinently, 4 of the 10 participants demonstrated a clinically significant reduction in eating disorder pathology at 3-month follow-up, though there was no significant effect on body mass index (though this may be due to the short duration between administration and follow-up). Adverse events were mild and transient at 3-month follow-up with the exception of one participant's report of increased heart rate due to orthostasis. These findings suggest that psilocybin is well tolerated and may be effective in treating anorexia nervosa.[65]

Results from a phase 1 trial conducted at Johns Hopkins (NCT04052568) have yet to be published.

Body Dysmorphic Disorder

In a small pilot study, eight women and four men with moderate-to-severe nondelusional body dysmorphic disorder were given a single oral dose of psilocybin (25 mg) with psychological support before, during, and after the dosing session. At 12-week follow-up, all 12 involved in the study reported decreases in Yale-Brown Obsessive Compulsive Disorder Scale Modified for Body Dysmorphic Disorder (BDD-YBOCS). At the end of the trial (12 weeks following psilocybin dose), 7 of the 12 participants (58%) reported a decrease of 30% or greater in BDD-YBOCS scores, and no serious adverse events were reported.[66]

Migraines

An exploratory, double-blind, placebo-controlled, crossover study in adults with migraines ($n = 10$) reported some efficacy when treated with moderate doses of psilocybin (0.143 mg/kg) compared to placebo. The trial included two dosing sessions 2 weeks apart. The psilocybin group reported a reduction in mean weekly migraine days of −1.65 (−2.53 to −0.77) compared to a mean reduction of 0.15 days (−1.13 to 0.83). To clarify, the placebo group experienced an increase in mean weekly migraine days, whereas the psilocybin group did not. Within the psilocybin group, 80% had a 25% reduction in weekly migraine days; 50% had a 50% reduction in weekly migraine days; and 30% had a 75% reduction in weekly migraine days. Within the placebo group, 20% had a 25% reduction in weekly migraine days; 20% had a 50% reduction in weekly migraine days; and 0% had a 75% reduction in weekly migraine days.

As psilocybin may induce headaches, the study's authors measured both the time to first attack and the time to second attack following dosing. The time to the first attack was similar in both groups, though greater in the psilocybin group. The number of days until the second attack was significantly greater in the psilocybin group (10.30 [1.61] days) when compared to placebo (5.00 [1.13] days).

All adverse events were transient, self-limiting, and mild to moderate, and there were no serious adverse events.[67]

Cluster Headaches

Anecdotal evidence of classic psychedelics helping with cluster headaches has existed for a very long time, but there is limited clinical evidence to support the use of psilocybin in the treatment of cluster headaches. The ongoing research of Emmanuelle Schindler from Yale University who is also the medical director of the Headache Center of Excellence has pioneered several preliminary studies into the utility of classic psychedelics like psilocybin in the treatment of cluster headaches.[67-69]

Precautions and Adverse Events

Psilocybin and psychedelic-assisted therapy in general are typically contraindicated for people with a family history of severe and persistent mental illnesses or existing psychiatric comorbidities that make them more susceptible to psychosis. Even those who view psychedelics in a positive light may experience adverse psychological effects during the acute phase of the treatment, including confusion, fear, paranoia, and unpleasant hallucinations.

Other common adverse effects include headache, tachycardia, nausea, and increased blood pressure. Headaches are also frequently reported in the 24 to 36 hours following the use of moderate or large doses of psilocybin. Additional adverse events that have been reported include fatigue, dizziness, and paranoia.

Drug Interactions

Serotonin receptors are the targets of many antidepressants and some antipsychotic medications (see Table 9.4). Consequently, patients will

TABLE 9.4 Drug-Drug Interactions Between Antidepressants and Classic Psychedelics

Drug Type	Examples
Monoamine oxidase inhibitors	Isocarboxazid, moclobemide, phenelzine, selegiline, tranylcypromine
Noradrenergic and specific serotonergic antidepressants	Mianserin, mirtazapine, setiptiline
Selective serotonin reuptake inhibitors	Citalopram, escitalopram, fluvoxamine, fluoxetine,[a] paroxetine, sertraline
Serotonin modulators	Nefazodone, trazodone, vilazodone, vortioxetine
Serotonin-norepinephrine reuptake inhibitors	Desvenlafaxine, duloxetine, levomilnacipran, venlafaxine
Serotonin partial agonist reuptake inhibitors	Vilazodone, vortioxetine
Tricyclic antidepressants	Amitriptyline, chlorpheniramine, clomipramine, desipramine, imipramine, nortriptyline
Other	Buspirone

Listed drugs should be tapered and discontinued at least 2 weeks prior to acute psychedelic therapy.
[a]Fluoxetine should be tapered and discontinued at least 6 weeks prior to acute psychedelic therapy.

likely be asked to taper and discontinue any medications that affect serotonin levels at least 2 weeks prior to the administration of psilocybin. Due to its long half-life, fluoxetine should be tapered and discontinued at least 6 weeks prior to psychedelic therapy. There is some risk of patients developing serotonin syndrome if psilocybin is taken with another drug capable of increasing serotonin levels (see Table 9.5). There is also some evidence to suggest that the coadministration of classic psychedelics with lithium may increase the risk of seizure.[70]

Other drug interactions have not been identified at this time.

Special Populations

Pregnant and Nursing Women

Pregnant and nursing women should not ingest psilocybin.

TABLE 9.5 Drugs Associated With Elevated Serotonin Levels and Serotonin Syndrome

Drug Type	Examples
Analgesics	Fentanyl, meperidine, pentazocine, tramadol
Antibiotics	Linezolid, ritonavir
Anticonvulsants	Valproate
Antidepressants	Buspirone, clomipramine, nefazodone, trazodone, venlafaxine
Antiemetics	Granisetron, metoclopramide, ondansetron
Antimigraine medications	Sumatriptan
Bariatric drugs	Sibutramine
Monoamine oxidase inhibitors	Clorgiline, isocarboxazid, moclobemide, phenelzine
Over-the-counter drugs	Dextromethorphan
Selective serotonin reuptake inhibitors	Citalopram, fluoxetine, fluvoxamine, paroxetine, sertraline, and others

Individuals With Cardiovascular Disease

Psilocybin may increase blood pressure and heart rate. Consequently, individuals with severe cardiovascular disease may not be optimal candidates for trials or treatments involving this drug.

Dosage and Administration

There are no guidelines on administering psilocybin at this time. In most cases, patients receive one to three doses of psilocybin while under the supervision of one or two clinicians. Standard doses tend to fall within the 20- to 35-mg range. Prior to dosing sessions, patients are typically screened for personal or family history of psychotic disorders or suicidality, though emerging evidence seems to suggest that psilocybin may be beneficial in contexts where patients are expressing suicidal ideation. However, this remains a controversial matter at this point in time.

Following sessions with psilocybin, patients will meet with clinicians to help process the experience.

Conclusion

The strongest evidence in favor of the use of psilocybin in psychiatry comes from the numerous trials involving patients with depressive disorders. However, given the evidence of its efficacy in treating other disorders and in palliative care settings, it seems as though psilocybin addresses transdiagnostic processes that are associated with depression, addiction, and anxiety and cannot be fully addressed solely with conventional pharmacotherapies.

As noted throughout the book, there is strong evidence indicating that psilocybin's efficacy is not due to activity at 5-HT_{2A} receptors or any constellation of receptors alone. Although there is no doubt that the drug's pharmacology is instrumental in explaining some of its clinical utility in treating numerous disorders, a purely biological receptor-mediated explanation seems insufficient. Instead, the efficacy of psilocybin and other psychedelics appears to be linked to the psychedelic experience itself. In some cases, these qualify as mystical-type experiences, while in others the patient is afforded a new perspective, and this new perspective often allows them to make psychological breakthroughs that, through therapy alone, may have only been contrived after several years of difficult work.

Although these revelatory experiences can occur without guidance, current research and centuries of anecdotal evidence indicate that the psychedelic experience is most beneficial when the patient is prepared, meaning that they are in the correct mindset (set) and surroundings (settings), but also in the presence of a person (or persons) who can help them process the experience while under the influence of the drug and during subsequent sessions. Mental health practitioners are in a unique position to fill that role.

REFERENCES

1. Shao LX, Liao C, Gregg I, et al. Psilocybin induces rapid and persistent growth of dendritic spines in frontal cortex in vivo. *Neuron.* 2021;109(16):2535-2544.e4. doi:10.1016/j.neuron.2021.06.008. PMID: 34228959; PMCID: PMC8376772.
2. Froese T, Guzmán G, Guzmán-Dávalos L. On the origin of the genus Psilocybe and its potential ritual use in ancient Africa and Europe. *Econ Bot.* 2016;70(2):103-114.
3. Nichols DE. Psilocybin: from ancient magic to modern medicine. *J Antibiot (Tokyo).* 2020;73(10):679-686. doi:10.1038/s41429-020-0311-8. PMID: 32398764.
4. Pollan M. *How to Change Your Mind: What the New Science of Psychedelics Teaches Us About Consciousness, Dying, Addiction, Depression, and Transcendence*. Penguin Books; 2019:104-114.
5. Wasson RG. Seeking the magic mushroom. *Life.* 1957;42(19):100-120.
6. Lowe H, Toyang N, Steele B, et al. The therapeutic potential of psilocybin. *Molecules.* 2021;26(10):2948. doi:10.3390/molecules26102948. PMID: 34063505; PMCID: PMC8156539.
7. Reiff CM, Richman EE, Nemeroff CB, et al. Psychedelics and psychedelic-assisted psychotherapy. *Am J Psychiatry.* 2020;177(5):391-410. doi:10.1176/appi.ajp.2019.19010035. PMID: 32098487.
8. Hoffman A. *LSD: My Problem Child*. Multidisciplinary Association for Psychedelic Studies; 2005:85-87.
9. Rucker JJH, Iliff J, Nutt DJ. Psychiatry & the psychedelic drugs. Past, present & future. *Neuropharmacology.* 2018;142:200-218. doi:10.1016/j.neuropharm.2017.12.040
10. Richards WA. *Sacred Knowledge: Psychedelics and Religious Experience*. Columbia University Press; 2015:4.
11. Strauss D, Ghosh S, Murray Z, Gryzenhout M. An overview of the taxonomy, phylogenetics and ecology of the psychedelic genera *Psilocybe, Panaeolus, Pluteus* and *Gymnopilus*. *Front for Glob Change.* 2022;5:813998. doi:10.3389/ffgc.2022.813998
12. MacCallum CA, Lo LA, Pistawka CA, Deol JK. Therapeutic use of psilocybin: practical considerations for dosing and administration. *Front Psychiatry.* 2022;13:1040217. doi:10.3389/fpsyt.2022.1040217. PMID: 36532184; PMCID: PMC9751063.
13. Barrett FS, Krimmel SR, Griffiths RR, Seminowicz DA, Mathur BN. Psilocybin acutely alters the functional connectivity of the claustrum with brain networks that support perception, memory, and attention. *Neuroimage.* 2020;218:116980. doi:10.1016/j.neuroimage.2020.116980. PMID: 32454209; PMCID: PMC10792549.
14. Lenz C, Wick J, Braga D, García-Altares M, Lackner G, Hertweck C, Gressler M, Hoffmeister D. Injury-triggered blueing reactions of *Psilocybe* "Magic" mushrooms. *Angew Chem Int Ed Engl.* 2020;59(4):1450-1454. doi:10.1002/anie.201910175. PMID: 31725937; PMCID: PMC7004109.
15. Coppola M, Bevione F, Mondola R. Psilocybin for treating psychiatric disorders: a psychonaut legend or a promising therapeutic perspective? *J Xenobiot.* 2022;12(1):41-52. doi:10.3390/jox12010004. PMID: 35225956; PMCID: PMC8883979.
16. Serreau R, Amirouche A, Benyamina A, Berteina-Raboin S. A review of synthetic access to therapeutic compounds extracted from *Psilocybe. Pharmaceuticals (Basel).* 2022;16(1):40. doi:10.3390/ph16010040. PMID: 36678537; PMCID: PMC9867295.

17. Nicholas CR, Henriquez KM, Gassman MC, et al. High dose psilocybin is associated with positive subjective effects in healthy volunteers. *J Psychopharmacol.* 2018;32(7):770-778. doi:10.1177/0269881118780713. PMID: 29945469; PMCID: PMC7751062.
18. Garcia-Romeu A, Barrett FS, Carbonaro TM, Johnson MW, Griffiths RR. Optimal dosing for psilocybin pharmacotherapy: considering weight-adjusted and fixed dosing approaches. *J Psychopharmacol.* 2021;35(4):353-361. doi:10.1177/0269881121991822. PMID: 33611977; PMCID: PMC8056712.
19. Ley L, Holze F, Arikci D, et al. Comparative acute effects of mescaline, lysergic acid diethylamide, and psilocybin in a randomized, double-blind, placebo-controlled cross-over study in healthy participants. *Neuropsychopharmacology.* 2023;48(11): 1659-1667. doi:10.1038/s41386-023-01607-2
20. Passie T, Seifert J, Schneider U, Emrich HM. The pharmacology of psilocybin. *Addict Biol.* 2002;7(4):357-364. doi:10.1080/1355621021000005937. PMID: 14578010.
21. Hasler F, Bourquin D, Brenneisen R, Bär T, Vollenweider FX. Determination of psilocin and 4-hydroxyindole-3-acetic acid in plasma by HPLC-ECD and pharmacokinetic profiles of oral and intravenous psilocybin in man. *Pharm Acta Helv.* 1997;72(3):175-184. doi:10.1016/s0031-6865(97)00014-9. PMID: 9204776.
22. Dinis-Oliveira RJ. Metabolism of psilocybin and psilocin: clinical and forensic toxicological relevance. *Drug Metab Rev.* 2017;49(1):84-91. doi:10.1080/03602532.2016 .1278228. PMID: 28074670.
23. Ray TS. Psychedelics and the human receptorome. *PLoS One.* 2010;5(2):e9019. doi:10.1371/journal.pone.0009019. Erratum in: *PLoS One.* 2010;5(3). doi:10.1371/annotation/e580a864-cf13-40c2-9bd9-b9687a6f0fe4. PMID: 20126400; PMCID: PMC2814854.
24. Smausz R, Neill J, Gigg J. Neural mechanisms underlying psilocybin's therapeutic potential—the need for preclinical in vivo electrophysiology. *J Psychopharmacol.* 2022;36(7):781-793. doi:10.1177/02698811221092508. PMID: 35638159; PMCID: PMC9247433.
25. Calabrese F, Rossetti AC, Racagni G, Gass P, Riva MA, Molteni R. Brain-derived neurotrophic factor: a bridge between inflammation and neuroplasticity. *Front Cell Neurosci.* 2014;8:430. doi:10.3389/fncel.2014.00430. PMID: 25565964; PMCID: PMC4273623.
26. Moliner R, Girych M, Brunello CA, et al. Psychedelics promote plasticity by directly binding to BDNF receptor TrkB. *Nat Neurosci.* 2023;26:1032-1041. doi:10.1038/s41593-023-01316-5
27. Carhart-Harris RL, Leech R, Erritzoe D, et al. Functional connectivity measures after psilocybin inform a novel hypothesis of early psychosis. *Schizophr Bull.* 2013;39(6):1343-1351. doi:10.1093/schbul/sbs117. PMID: 23044373; PMCID: PMC3796071.
28. Gattuso JJ, Perkins D, Ruffell S, et al. Default mode network modulation by psychedelics: a systematic review. *Int J Neuropsychopharmacol.* 2023;26(3):155-188. doi:10.1093/ijnp/pyac074. PMID: 36272145; PMCID: PMC10032309.
29. Carhart-Harris RL, Erritzoe D, Williams T, et al. Neural correlates of the psychedelic state as determined by fMRI studies with psilocybin. *Proc Natl Acad Sci U S A.* 2012;109(6):2138-2143. doi:10.1073/pnas.1119598109. PMID: 22308440; PMCID: PMC3277566.
30. Vollenweider FX, Vontobel P, Hell D, Leenders KL. 5-HT modulation of dopamine release in basal ganglia in psilocybin-induced psychosis in man—a PET study with [11C]raclopride. *Neuropsychopharmacology.* 1999;20(5):424-433. doi:10.1016/S0893-133X(98)00108-0. PMID: 10192823.
31. Hendricks PS, Johnson MW, Griffiths RR. Psilocybin, psychological distress, and suicidality. *J Psychopharmacol.* 2015;29(9):1041-1043. doi:10.1177/0269881115598338. PMID: 26395582; PMCID: PMC4721603.
32. Daniel J, Haberman M. Clinical potential of psilocybin as a treatment for mental health conditions. *Ment Health Clin.* 2018;7(1):24-28. doi:10.9740/mhc.2017.01.024. PMID: 29955494; PMCID: PMC6007659.

33. Chadeayne AR, Pham DNK, Reid BG, Golen JA, Manke DR. Active metabolite of Aeruginascin (4-hydroxy-N,N,N-trimethyltryptamine): synthesis, structure, and serotonergic binding affinity. *ACS Omega*. 2020;5(27):16940-16943. doi:10.1021/acsomega.0c02208. PMID: 32685863; PMCID: PMC7365549.
34. Leung AY, Paul AG. Baeocystin and norbaeocystin: new analogs of psilocybin from *Psilocybe baeocystis*. *J Pharm Sci*. 1968;57(10):1667-1671. doi:10.1002/jps.2600571007. PMID: 5684732.
35. Vargas AS, Luís Â, Barroso M, Gallardo E, Pereira L. Psilocybin as a new approach to treat depression and anxiety in the context of life-threatening diseases-a systematic review and meta-analysis of clinical trials. *Biomedicines*. 2020;8(9):331. doi:10.3390/biomedicines8090331. PMID: 32899469; PMCID: PMC7554922.
36. Doblin R. Pahnke's "Good Friday Experiment": a long-term follow-up and methodological critique. *J Transpers Psychol*. 1991;23(1):1-28. Accessed on April 20, 2024. https://www.atpweb.org/jtparchive/trps-23-91-01-001.pdf
37. Barrett FS, Griffiths RR. Classic hallucinogens and mystical experiences: phenomenology and neural correlates. *Curr Top Behav Neurosci*. 2018;36:393-430. doi:10.1007/7854_2017_474. PMID: 28401522; PMCID: PMC6707356.
38. Griffiths RR, Richards WA, McCann U, Jesse R. Psilocybin can occasion mystical-type experiences having substantial and sustained personal meaning and spiritual significance. *Psychopharmacology (Berl)*. 2006;187(3):268-283; discussion 284-292. doi:10.1007/s00213-006-0457-5. PMID: 16826400.
39. Griffiths R, Richards W, Johnson M, McCann U, Jesse R. Mystical-type experiences occasioned by psilocybin mediate the attribution of personal meaning and spiritual significance 14 months later. *J Psychopharmacol*. 2008;22(6):621-632. doi:10.1177/0269881108094300. PMID: 18593735; PMCID: PMC3050654.
40. Compass Pathways. Compass Pathways receives FDA breakthrough therapy designation for psilocybin therapy for treatment-resistant depression. Published October 23, 2018. Accessed April 17, 2024. https://ir.compasspathways.com/News--Events-/news/news-details/2018/COMPASS-Pathways-receives-FDA-Breakthrough-Therapy-designation-for-psilocybin-therapy-for-treatment-resistant-depression/default.aspx
41. Usona Institute. FDA grants breakthrough therapy designation to Usona Institute's psilocybin program for major depressive disorder. Published November 22, 2019. Accessed April 17, 2024. https://www.usonainstitute.org/updates/fda-grants-breakthrough-therapy-designation-to-usona-institutes-psilocybin-program-for-major-depressive-disorder
42. Cybin. Cybin announces positive end-of-phase 2 meeting with FDA for CYB003 in major depressive disorder and phase 3 program design. Published March 14, 2024. Accessed April 16, 2024. https://ir.cybin.com/investors/news/news-details/2024/Cybin-Announces-Positive-End-of-Phase-2-Meeting-with-FDA-for-CYB003-in-Major-Depressive-Disorder-and-Phase-3-Program-Design/default.aspx
43. Carhart-Harris RL, Bolstridge M, Rucker J, et al. Psilocybin with psychological support for treatment-resistant depression: an open-label feasibility study. *Lancet Psychiatry*. 2016;3(7):619-627. doi:10.1016/S2215-0366(16)30065-7. PMID: 27210031.
44. Carhart-Harris RL, Bolstridge M, Day CMJ, et al. Psilocybin with psychological support for treatment-resistant depression: six-month follow-up. *Psychopharmacology (Berl)*. 2018;235(2):399-408. doi:10.1007/s00213-017-4771-x. PMID: 29119317; PMCID: PMC5813086.
45. Raison CL, Sanacora G, Woolley J, et al. Single-dose psilocybin treatment for major depressive disorder: a randomized clinical trial. *JAMA*. 2023;330(9):843-853. doi:10.1001/jama.2023.14530. Erratum in: *JAMA*. 2024;331(8):710. PMID: 37651119; PMCID: PMC10472268.
46. Goodwin GM, Aaronson ST, Alvarez O, et al. Single-dose psilocybin for a treatment-resistant episode of major depression. *N Engl J Med*. 2022;387(18):1637-1648. doi:10.1056/NEJMoa2206443. PMID: 36322843.

47. Goodwin GM, Aaronson ST, Alvarez O, et al. Single-dose psilocybin for a treatment-resistant episode of major depression: impact on patient-reported depression severity, anxiety, function, and quality of life. *J Affect Disord*. 2023;327:120-127. doi:10.1016/j.jad.2023.01.108. PMID: 36740140.
48. Goodwin GM, Croal M, Feifel D, et al. Psilocybin for treatment resistant depression in patients taking a concomitant SSRI medication. *Neuropsychopharmacology*. 2023;48(10):1492-1499. doi:10.1038/s41386-023-01648-7. PMID: 37443386; PMCID: PMC10425429.
49. Business Wire. Cybin receives FDA breakthrough therapy designation for its novel psychedelic molecule CYB003 and announces positive four-month durability data in major depressive disorder. Published March 13, 2024. Accessed April 19, 2024. https://www.businesswire.com/news/home/20240313731043/en/Cybin-Receives-FDA-Breakthrough-Therapy-Designation-for-its-Novel-Psychedelic-Molecule-CYB003-and-Announces-Positive-Four-Month-Durability-Data-in-Major-Depressive-Disorder
50. Davis AK, Barrett FS, May DG, et al. Effects of psilocybin-assisted therapy on major depressive disorder: a randomized clinical trial. *JAMA Psychiatry*. 2021;78(5):481-489. doi:10.1001/jamapsychiatry.2020.3285. Erratum in: *JAMA Psychiatry*. 2021. PMID: 33146667; PMCID: PMC7643046.
51. Gukasyan N, Davis AK, Barrett FS, et al. Efficacy and safety of psilocybin-assisted treatment for major depressive disorder: Prospective 12-month follow-up. *J Psychopharmacol*. 2022;36(2):151-158. doi:10.1177/02698811211073759. PMID: 35166158; PMCID: PMC8864328.
52. von Rotz R, Schindowski EM, Jungwirth J, et al. Single-dose psilocybin-assisted therapy in major depressive disorder: a placebo-controlled, double-blind, randomised clinical trial. *EClinicalMedicine*. 2022;56:101809. doi:10.1016/j.eclinm.2022.101809. Erratum in: *EClinicalMedicine*. 2023;56:101841. PMID: 36636296; PMCID: PMC9830149.
53. Rosenblat JD, Meshkat S, Doyle Z, et al. Psilocybin-assisted psychotherapy for treatment resistant depression: a randomized clinical trial evaluating repeated doses of psilocybin. *Med*. 2024;5(3):190-200.e5. doi:10.1016/j.medj.2024.01.005. PMID: 38359838.
54. Aaronson ST, van der Vaart A, Miller T, et al. Single-dose synthetic psilocybin with psychotherapy for treatment-resistant bipolar type II major depressive episodes: a nonrandomized open-label trial. *JAMA Psychiatry*. 2024;81(6):555-562. doi:10.1001/jamapsychiatry.2023.4685. Erratum in: *JAMA Psychiatry*. 2024. PMID: 38055270; PMCID: PMC10701666.
55. Griffiths RR, Johnson MW, Carducci MA, et al. Psilocybin produces substantial and sustained decreases in depression and anxiety in patients with life-threatening cancer: a randomized double-blind trial. *J Psychopharmacol*. 2016;30(12):1181-1197. doi:10.1177/0269881116675513. PMID: 27909165; PMCID: PMC5367557.
56. Grob CS, Danforth AL, Chopra GS, et al. Pilot study of psilocybin treatment for anxiety in patients with advanced-stage cancer. *Arch Gen Psychiatry*. 2011;68(1):71-78. doi:10.1001/archgenpsychiatry.2010.116. PMID: 20819978.
57. Ross S, Bossis A, Guss J, et al. Rapid and sustained symptom reduction following psilocybin treatment for anxiety and depression in patients with life-threatening cancer: a randomized controlled trial. *J Psychopharmacol*. 2016;30(12):1165-1180. doi:10.1177/0269881116675512. PMID: 27909164; PMCID: PMC5367551.
58. Agin-Liebes GI, Malone T, Yalch MM, et al. Long-term follow-up of psilocybin-assisted psychotherapy for psychiatric and existential distress in patients with life-threatening cancer. *J Psychopharmacol*. 2020;34(2):155-166. doi:10.1177/0269881119897615. PMID: 31916890.
59. Ziff S, Stern B, Lewis G, Majeed M, Gorantla VR. Analysis of psilocybin-assisted therapy in medicine: a narrative review. *Cureus*. 2022;14(2):e21944. doi:10.7759/cureus.21944. PMID: 35273885; PMCID: PMC8901083.

60. Bogenschutz MP, Forcehimes AA, Pommy JA, Wilcox CE, Barbosa PC, Strassman RJ. Psilocybin-assisted treatment for alcohol dependence: a proof-of-concept study. *J Psychopharmacol*. 2015;29(3):289-299. doi:10.1177/0269881114565144. PMID: 25586396.
61. Bogenschutz MP, Ross S, Bhatt S, et al. Percentage of heavy drinking days following psilocybin-assisted psychotherapy vs placebo in the treatment of adult patients with alcohol use disorder: a randomized clinical trial. *JAMA Psychiatry*. 2022;79(10):953-962. doi:10.1001/jamapsychiatry.2022.2096. Erratum in: *JAMA Psychiatry*. 2022. PMID: 36001306; PMCID: PMC9403854.
62. Johnson MW, Garcia-Romeu A, Griffiths RR. Long-term follow-up of psilocybin-facilitated smoking cessation. *Am J Drug Alcohol Abuse*. 2017;43(1):55-60. doi:10.3109/00952990.2016.1170135. Erratum in: *Am J Drug Alcohol Abuse*. 2017;43(1):127. PMID: 27441452; PMCID: PMC5641975.
63. Moreno FA, Wiegand CB, Taitano EK, Delgado PL. Safety, tolerability, and efficacy of psilocybin in 9 patients with obsessive-compulsive disorder. *J Clin Psychiatry*. 2006;67(11):1735-1740. doi:10.4088/jcp.v67n1110. PMID: 17196053.
64. Kelmendi B, Kichuk SA, DePalmer G, et al. Single-dose psilocybin for treatment-resistant obsessive-compulsive disorder: a case report. *Heliyon*. 2022;8(12):e12135. doi:10.1016/j.heliyon.2022.e12135. PMID: 36536916; PMCID: PMC9758406.
65. Peck SK, Shao S, Gruen T, et al. Psilocybin therapy for females with anorexia nervosa: a phase 1, open-label feasibility study. *Nat Med*. 2023;29(8):1947-1953. doi:10.1038/s41591-023-02455-9. PMID: 37488291; PMCID: PMC10427429.
66. Schneier FR, Feusner J, Wheaton MG, et al. Pilot study of single-dose psilocybin for serotonin reuptake inhibitor-resistant body dysmorphic disorder. *J Psychiatr Res*. 2023;161:364-370. doi:10.1016/j.jpsychires.2023.03.031. PMID: 37004409; PMCID: PMC10967229.
67. Schindler EAD, Sewell RA, Gottschalk CH, et al. Exploratory controlled study of the migraine-suppressing effects of psilocybin. *Neurotherapeutics*. 2021;18(1):534-543. doi:10.1007/s13311-020-00962-y. PMID: 33184743; PMCID: PMC8116458.
68. Schindler EAD, Sewell RA, Gottschalk CH, et al. Exploratory investigation of a patient-informed low-dose psilocybin pulse regimen in the suppression of cluster headache: results from a randomized, double-blind, placebo-controlled trial. *Headache*. 2022;62(10):1383-1394. doi:10.1111/head.14420. PMID: 36416492.
69. Schindler EAD, Sewell RA, Gottschalk CH, et al. Psilocybin pulse regimen reduces cluster headache attack frequency in the blinded extension phase of a randomized controlled trial. *J Neurol Sci*. 2024;460:122993. doi:10.1016/j.jns.2024.122993. PMID: 38581739.
70. Nayak SM, Gukasyan N, Barrett FS, Erowid E, Erowid F, Griffiths RR. Classic psychedelic coadministration with lithium, but not lamotrigine, is associated with seizures: an analysis of online psychedelic experience reports. *Pharmacopsychiatry*. 2021;54(5):240-245. doi:10.1055/a-1524-2794. PMID: 34348413.

10

Lysergic Acid Diethylamide

Lysergic acid diethylamide 25 (known as LSD-25 or just LSD) is an ergoline derivative that was first synthesized in 1938 and is known to cause changes in consciousness and alterations in perception even at very small doses (>100 μg). It is a partial agonist at serotonin 2A receptors (5-HT_{2A}), which is believed to be the site through which its subjective effects are mediated. Particularly in the United States and the Global North, LSD has been the protagonist in the story of psychedelics, with drugs such as psilocybin, mescaline, and 3,4-methylenedioxymethamphetamine (MDMA) playing secondary, albeit vital, roles. Throughout this time, LSD has been referred to in a variety of ways, including hallucinogen, psychomimetic, psychedelic, and entheogen. It has also been characterized as a great corrupter of youth as well as a means of unlocking the full potential of the human spirit. One thing that everyone seems to agree on is that perhaps no other drug is as polarizing as LSD with the possible exception of cannabis.

One of the reasons why LSD has been so controversial is that it can result in mystical-type experiences, and these can leave an ever-lasting impression on people. Without a doubt, there is no other class of drugs that can induce such a phenomenological experience. Particularly, first-time users recount the experience as though they were struck by a bolt of lightning, with revelations that are considered being one of the most important events in their lives. Consequently, it is understandable why a drug such as LSD had such an enormous impact on American culture of the 1960s and particularly among the millions of young people who experimented with it, especially during the Vietnam War. These experiences led them to reexamine their lives and challenge the moral and spiritual authorities of organized religions, as well as the ethical authority of the government that they believed was engaging in an unjust war. A drug such as LSD also provided them with a unifying experience at a time when they felt the world was coming apart.

Many clinicians who came of age following the passage of the Controlled Substances Act of 1970 view classic psychedelics such as LSD as either relics of the 1960s counterculture or drugs of misuse devoid of therapeutic value, befitting their status as Schedule I substances. However, LSD and other classic psychedelics have experienced a major resurgence in recent years, and interest in LSD-assisted psychotherapy has been coupled with a thawing in research. There is now some evidence to suggest that LSD, when used in a clinical setting, may help alleviate symptoms of anxiety, depression, substance use disorders, and existential distress among terminally ill patients. A formulation of LSD pioneered by one of the psychedelic companies has even received breakthrough designation from the U.S. Food and Drug Administration (FDA) for the treatment of generalized anxiety disorder.

History

Lysergic acid diethylamide (LSD) was first synthesized from ergoline alkaloids in 1938 by Swiss chemist Albert Hofmann while working at the Sandoz pharmaceutic research laboratory in Basel, Switzerland. Hofmann was attempting to develop novel medicines by combining lysergic acid with more than two dozen amines. Nothing seemed particularly special about the 25th substance within this series (lysergic acid diethylamide 25 or LSD-25) until 5 years later, on April 16, 1943, when Hofmann resynthesized the compound and accidentally absorbed a small portion of it. He felt a bit strange, but the effects quickly wore off.[1(pp35-47)]

On April 19, 1943, Hofmann took a dose of 0.25 mg LSD tartrate, becoming the first human to experience the full effects of the drug. While the initial experience was frightening for Hofmann, he noted the following day being greeted by "a sensation of well-being and renewed life," which seemed to flow through him.[1(p50)] He informed his superiors, Professor Arthur Stoll, and the director of the pharmacologic department, Professor Ernst Rothlin, of his discovery. Both read Hofmann's report incredulously, and Rothlin and two of his assistants repeated Hofmann's experiment with one-third the dose. They stopped being incredulous after that experiment.[1(p52)]

The first systematic investigation of LSD in humans was conducted in the psychiatry clinic at the University of Zurich by Werner A. Stoll. Doses ranged from 0.02 to 0.13 mg of LSD tartrate and the results were published in 1947. While Stoll documented the effects of LSD, which were compared to mescaline, the active agent in peyote, he left the question of therapeutic applications unanswered. However, he felt that the drug held immense promise for research in psychiatry.[1(pp63-78)]

Within the same year, Sandoz began marketing LSD under the name Delysid for use in analytic psychotherapy and experimental studies. Early research on LSD suggested that its effects mimicked a type of "model psychosis," and many believed that it could be used to better understand the mechanisms behind schizophrenia.[1(pp63-78)] In fact, there was a widespread belief in the 1940s and 1950s that an endogenous hallucinogen or "substance-M" existed and that it was potentially responsible for the development of schizophrenia.[2] There is no doubt that there are parallels between schizophrenia and the effects of LSD. Even relatively recent studies have suggested that individuals with premorbid schizoid and paranoid traits, as well as individuals with a family history of schizophrenia, are more likely to exhibit psychotic symptoms while experiencing the acute effects of LSD compared to healthy controls.[3] However, the theory that dysregulation of a single endogenous substance leads to schizophrenia has been abandoned.

As recounted in Chapter 3, psychoanalysts recognized that LSD could enhance some patients' experiences, and clinical use became more popular during the 1950s and into the early 1960s. Clinical work during this time revealed that LSD could be used effectively to treat substance use disorder (particularly alcoholism) and to help terminally ill patients with existential anxiety and distress. Of note, many researchers also self-experimented with the drug.[4]

Recreational use of LSD became more prevalent as the 1960s progressed, particularly among various countercultural movements. The surge in nonmedicinal use and experimentation led Sandoz to cease production and distribution of the drug in 1965,[1(pp85-87)] before becoming illegal in 1968.[3] Following that, it was placed on the list of Schedule I drugs according to the Controlled Substances Act of 1970. By this point in time, the cultural shift that had come as a result of a confluence of factors (but seemed to be somewhat catalyzed by LSD and psychedelics) had made research into these drugs highly stigmatized within academia. Those who had once championed psychedelics became less vocal about their promise or publicly dismissed their value in psychiatry, medicine, and the study of consciousness.

With very few exceptions, what ensued was a deep freeze on psychedelic research that lasted over 30 years (from 1970 until the early 2000s). Over time, the research conducted during the 1940s, 1950s, and 1960s was forgotten, and many younger scientists and researchers came to know of LSD and other psychedelics solely as drugs of misuse. Outside of academic discourse, LSD became synonymous with tie-dye clothing, rose-hued glasses, bands like the Grateful Dead, and the Summer of Love. To talk about LSD as being a tool to study consciousness or to change one's perception was to brand oneself a relic, a kook, or a drug pusher.

Though this perception of LSD persists in many circles, it is once again being recognized as a powerful tool that can help us better understand the inner workings of the brain, as well as a therapeutic agent that, when coupled with psychotherapy, may be capable of helping patients with several very difficult to treat conditions that include not only substance use disorders and end-of-life anxiety but also anxiety disorders, depressive disorders, attention-deficit/hyperactivity disorder (ADHD), and other conditions to be explored in this chapter.

Pharmacology

Description

LSD is a semisynthetic product of lysergic acid, which is produced by the rye fungus ergot (*Claviceps purpurea*). The D-LSD isomer of LSD is the sole isomer with psychoactive properties.[5] It is a water-soluble, white crystalline substance that is typically found in a solution. Its molar mass is 323.42 g/mol.[5] The molecular structure of LSD is shown in Figure 10.1.

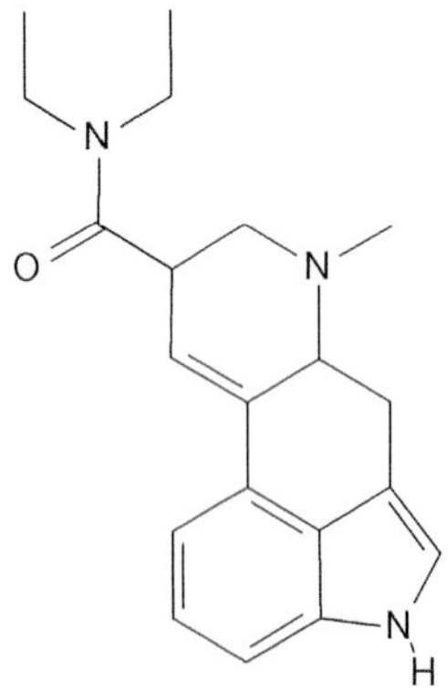

Figure 10.1 The chemical structure of lysergic acid diethylamide (LSD).

Route of Administration

LSD is extremely potent. Whereas a typical dose of orally administered mescaline falls within the range of a few hundred milligrams (200-500 mg) and a typical dose of orally administered psilocybin falls within the range of 10 to 25 mg, oral doses of LSD are typically administered within the range of 0.10 to 0.25 mg (100-250 μg). In other words, a typical dose of psilocybin is two orders of magnitude larger than a typical dose of LSD and a typical dose of mescaline is three orders of magnitude larger than a typical dose of LSD.

As a consequence of its potency, LSD is almost always encountered in solution. It can be injected, but it is far more commonly administered orally. In some cases, it is administered sublingually or buccally with an eyedropper. One may also use an eyedropper to first put a dose on mediums such as blotter paper, gelatin sheets, or food items (eg, sugar cubes).

Pharmacokinetics

Onset of action occurs within 1 minute with intraspinal injection, 3 to 5 minutes with intravenous (IV) injection, 15 to 20 minutes with intramuscular injection, and 30 to 45 minutes when taken orally. Peak effects typically occur in approximately 1 hour when injected or 1 to 2.5 hours following oral administration, and effects may persist for 9 to 12 hours following any type of administration.[5]

Absorption and Bioavailability

Following oral administration, LSD is completely absorbed in the digestive tract and has an estimated bioavailability of 71%.[6] Absorption typically occurs within 1 hour but may be slowed if administration is preceded by a meal.[5] Dolder and colleagues found average C_{max} for 100-μg (n = 24) and 200-μg (n = 16) doses to be 1.3 ng/mL (range: 0.3-3.7 ng/mL) and 3.1 ng/mL (range: 1.9-7.1 ng/mL), respectively.[6] Ley and colleagues found C_{max} for a 100-μg dose (n = 32) to be 2.1 ng/mL (range: 1.1-3.6 ng/mL).[7] T_{max} was similar for Ley (1.4 hours; range: 0.5-3.5 hours) and both the 100-μg and the 200-μg doses in the Dolder study—1.4 hours (1.3-2.1 hours) and 1.5 hours (1.3-2.4 hours), respectively.

Distribution

LSD is rapidly distributed throughout the body, but a full understanding of how it is distributed across organ systems has yet to be quantified. In mice, LSD was found in nearly all organs within 10 minutes of iv administration, and the highest concentration was found to occur in the liver.[5]

LSD crosses the blood-brain barrier, but it is unclear how readily it does so. Following administration, the areas with the highest concentrations of LSD within the central nervous system are the hippocampus, the basal ganglia, periventricular gray matter, and the frontoparietal cortex.[5]

Metabolism

LSD undergoes extensive first-pass metabolism in humans and is almost fully metabolized into inactive metabolites. The major human metabolite of LSD is 2-oxo-3-hydroxy LSD. Other metabolites include lysergic acid ethylamide (LAE), lysergic acid ethyl-2-hydroxyethylamide (LEO), nor-LSD, 2-oxo-LSD, and 13- or 14-hydroxy-LSD glucuronide. CYP1A2, CYP2C19, CYP2D6, CYP2E1, and CYP3A4 each play a role in the metabolism of LSD.[8] Less than 1% of LSD is excreted unchanged.[5]

Elimination and Excretion

LSD appears to follow linear dose and elimination kinetics for up to 12 hours after administration.[6] Its half-life is estimated to be approximately 2.3 to 4.8 hours.[7] It is excreted primarily through urine within 8 hours and may be detectable in urine for 96 hours following administration, with the rate of excretion reaching a maximum rate of 4 to 6 hours after administration.[5]

Pharmacodynamics

LSD can produce a wide variety of effects ranging from euphoria and minor sensory distortions in small doses (<100 μg po) to mystical-like experiences in larger doses. As is the case with most if not all psychedelics, the intensity of one's subjective experience is dose dependent and can be influenced by experience with psychedelics, as well as mental outlook and environmental factors (ie, "set and setting").

Mechanism of Action

LSD is a partial agonist of 5-HT_{2A} receptors. Its most acute effects can be eliminated via the administration of the 5-HT_{2A} antagonist ketanserin. Repeated doses of psychedelics such as LSD have also been linked with the downregulation of 5-HT_{2A} receptors.[9]

LSD's activity at thalamic 5-HT_{2A} receptors alters communication between the thalamus and the cerebral cortex, thereby disrupting the brain's ability to filter sensory stimuli and convert experienced reality into a familiar narrative, thereby accounting for patients' increasingly disorganized thoughts while experiencing the acute effects of the drug.[10] Disruptions to typical cerebral cortex functioning via LSD's activity at

5-HT$_{2A}$ receptors may also contribute to its acute effects on mood, social behavior, personality expression, and executive functioning, as explored in Chapter 7.

In addition to 5-HT$_{2A}$ receptors, LSD has been shown to have an affinity for several 5-HT subtypes and other receptors (see Table 10.1),

TABLE 10.1 Lysergic Acid Diethylamide Affinity at Select Receptor Sites

Receptor	K$_i$ Value (nM)
5-HT$_{1A}$	7.3
5-HT$_{1B}$	3.9
5-HT$_{1D}$	7.8
5-HT$_{1E}$	92.8
5-HT$_{2A}$	11.3
5-HT$_{2B}$	30
5-HT$_{2C}$	30.6
5-HT$_{5A}$	9
5-HT$_6$	6.9
5-HT$_7$	6.6
D1	177
D2	110.1
D3	27
D4	158.4
D5	344.4
α_{1A}	1,127.7
α_{1B}	8,677
α_{2A}	45.8
$\beta 1$	1,600.7
$\beta 2$	3,460.9

5-HT, serotonin receptor; α, alpha-adrenergic receptor; β, beta-adrenergic receptor; D, dopamine receptor.
From Ray TS. Psychedelics and the human receptorome [published correction appears in *PLoS One*. 2010;5(3). doi:10.1371/annotation/e580a864-cf13-40c2-9bd9-b9687a6f0fe4]. *PLoS One*. 2010;5(2):e9019. doi:10.1371/journal.pone.0009019. PMID: 20126400; PMCID: PMC2814854.

though a full understanding of the relationship between the activation of these receptors and the subjective effects of the drug are still poorly understood. It has a particularly high affinity for 5-HT$_{1A}$ receptors, where it is a partial agonist.[5] Downstream effects on dopaminergic pathways and the glutamate system may also be partially responsible for LSD's effects on mood and the phenomenon of ego dissolution.[11] Similarly, evidence has indicated that LSD and other psychedelics increase levels of brain-derived neurotrophic factor (BDNF), but these indirect effects have not been fully elucidated.[9] Ley and colleagues report that LSD is associated with increases in plasma oxytocin levels.[7]

Therapeutic Index

The average lethal dose (LD$_{50}$) of LSD is 16.5 mg/kg (IV) for rats and 50 to 60 mg/kg (IV) for mice. An effective dose in a human is estimated to be 0.0003 to 0.001 mg/kg.[1(p55)] Assuming similar toxicity in humans as in mice, a fatal dose would have to be in the range of 50,000 to 100,000 times greater than an effective dose.

Despite the chasm between effective and lethal doses, numerous deaths have been linked to LSD, largely because of accidents that have occurred while under the influence of the drug. There have been reports of suicide and self-inflicted harm by healthy participants while under the influence of LSD, too.[12] Ostensibly, these occurrences are rare but represent one of the many reasons why individuals should not use psychedelics outside of a clinical or ceremonial setting—or at the very least without a responsible chaperone.

Tolerance, Dependence, and Withdrawal

Tolerance to LSD is rapidly established but dissipates quickly, typically within 3 to 4 days.[5] Cross-tolerance with other classical psychedelics including mescaline and psilocybin has also been observed.[5] Physical dependence and symptoms of withdrawal are extremely rare.

Subjective Effects

In addition to elevations in mood (euphoria), as well as increased capacity for introspection and creativity whether real or imagined, LSD can induce non-ordinary states of consciousness. Changes in perception can be extreme, as those feeling the acute effects of LSD may experience illusions, visions, pseudohallucinations (with eyes open or with eyes closed), changes to how they experience time, and synesthesia (eg, seeing music as color). Mystical-type experiences have also been recorded, especially at higher doses. These experiences are often profound and ineffable. Individuals who have more experience with psychedelics tend to be capable of delving deeper into the experience and have reported states of spiritual awareness that resemble *baqá wa faná* in Islam, *sekhel mufla* in Judaism, *samadhi* in Hinduism, *nirvana* or *satori* in Buddhism, the *beatific vision* in Christianity, or *wu wei* in Taoism.[13] Alterations in ego function and body image may also occur and may be of clinical utility in some settings.

Most individuals find the LSD experience to be transforming, enlightening, or at the very least rewarding. However, in some cases, the experience can be traumatic and hellish (ie, a "bad trip"). Literature suggests that these kinds of experiences are more common in uncontrolled settings and that supportive conditions with proper guidance from a clinician or individual well versed in the administration of psychedelics can ensure that the experience remains positive.

Somatic Effects

LSD increases diastolic and systolic blood pressure, heart rate, and body temperature (hyperthermia).[6] Additional autonomic changes include diaphoresis, flushing of the face, hyperglycemia, hypersialosis, hypertonia, mydriasis, and tachypnea. LSD may also cause nausea, though vomiting or diarrhea is rare. Appetite is frequently diminished while under the influence of LSD.

Therapeutic Indications

LSD is a Schedule I drug. At present, it does not have any accepted uses in medicine.

Potential Uses

Literature from the 1950s suggests that LSD is well suited for use in psychiatry. It was found to be particularly good at treating alcoholism, as well as end-of-life anxiety.[1] More recent research has corroborated these findings and proposed several other uses for LSD. Moreover, in March 2024, one psychedelic company received breakthrough designation from the FDA for its LSD treatment (known as MM-120 [lysergic D-tartrate]).[14]

Generalized Anxiety Disorder

A 5-arm, phase 2 clinical trial ($n = 198$) involving the administration of placebo or a single dose of MM-120 (25 µg, 50 µg, 100 µg, or 200 µg) showed clinically meaningful improvements on the Hamilton Anxiety rating scale (HAM-A) at both primary and secondary end points. The primary end point was 4 weeks after administration, while the secondary end point was 12 weeks after administration. The 100-μg dose was identified as the optimal dose, as patients in this group experienced the most significant response. Participants in this group showed a 7.7-point improvement in HAM-A scores over placebo at secondary end point (−21.9 MM-120 vs −14.2 placebo). The clinical response rate was 65% and 48% of participants experienced remission of anxiety symptoms.[14] As of this writing, the paper documenting these findings has not been peer reviewed.

Substance Use Disorders

As noted in the previous chapter, classic psychedelics such as LSD, psilocybin, mescaline, and *N,N*-dimethyltryptamine (DMT, often in the form of ayahuasca) have all demonstrated efficacy in the treatment of substance use disorders. Studies from the 1950s and 1960s using LSD for the treatment of alcohol use disorder appeared to be particularly promising in terms of improving quality of life and general health.[15]

Unfortunately, recent studies using LSD to treat substance use disorders are currently lacking. Most trials have instead used psilocybin (see Chapter 9). One exception is a phase 2 trial that is currently underway in Switzerland (NCT05474989) and is expected to be completed in 2028.

Palliative Care

In their double-blind, placebo-controlled, randomized phase 2 trial, Holze and colleagues administered LSD during two treatment sessions. The number of randomized patients was 44, with 21 being assigned to the group who received LSD in the first session and 23 who received placebo in the first session. There were seven dropouts. The authors found that LSD "induced rapid and lasting reductions in anxiety, depression, and general psychiatric symptomology for up to 16 weeks."[16]

Another phase 2 trial is currently studying LSD's efficacy in helping patients in a palliative care setting (NCT05883540). The estimated study completion is in 2027.

Depression

There has been significant anecdotal evidence about the ability of psychedelics such as LSD to boost mood. However, it is unclear if these effects are transient or if they can be sustained over the long term with a single dose. Unfortunately, clinical trials on the participants are lacking, though a randomized, double-blind, active-placebo-controlled trial using moderate to high doses of LSD does appear to have produced promising results. The results of this trial (NCT03866252) have yet to be made public.

A double-blind, placebo-controlled, crossover study investigating the use of microdosed LSD (26 µg) found that patients with moderate depressive symptoms (as identified by scoring 17 or above on the Beck Depression-II Inventory [BDI]) reported greater improvements in mood 48 h after sessions than individuals with BDI scores below 17.[17]

Cluster Headaches

There has long been anecdotal evidence about the efficacy of classic psychedelics in treating cluster headaches. Additionally, Shirane and colleagues note, "Several medications routinely used in headache management share chemical or pharmacologic properties with psychedelic drugs. For example, triptans, dihydroergotamine (DHE), and methysergide are all serotonergic compounds that share an indolamine structure with psilocybin, LSD, and DMT."[18]

Unfortunately, solid clinical evidence establishing the efficacy of psychedelics in the treatment of cluster headaches is still lacking, but two clinical trials are in the process of examining the effects of LSD on cluster headaches. As of this writing, NCT03781128 is underway and NCT05477459 is in preparation.

Adult Attention-Deficit/Hyperactivity Disorder

At present, the evidence to support the use of LSD to treat ADHD in adults is not particularly strong. A naturalistic, prospective study that examined the effects of microdosing on ADHD symptoms showed promising results, but the study lacked a placebo arm and there were several participant biases that favored positive findings.[19] As of this writing, a proof-of-concept trial by one company is underway investigating the use of MM-120 (20 µg) in treating ADHD (NCT05200936).

Alzheimer Disease

There is some speculation that psychedelics such as LSD may be of use in treating Alzheimer disease, largely because they have been shown to increase neuroplasticity, stimulate neurogenesis, and reduce inflammation. Each of these factors is relevant to the pathology of

Alzheimer disease, but there is currently no clinical evidence to support the use of LSD in the treatment of the disease.[20]

Precautions and Adverse Effects

LSD and psychedelic-assisted psychotherapy in general are typically contraindicated for people with a personal or family history of severe and persistent mental illnesses or existing psychiatric comorbidities that make them more susceptible to psychosis. It is also not recommended for patients who express significant fear about psychedelics, as they are prone to negative experiences that are both frightening and not therapeutically useful.

Even those who view psychedelics in a positive light may experience adverse psychological effects during the acute phase of the treatment, including confusion, fear, paranoia, and unpleasant hallucinations. Other common adverse effects include headache, pupil dilation, tachycardia, nausea, and increased blood pressure. Consequently, patients with cardiovascular disease may not be suitable candidates for psychedelic-assisted therapy.

A paper published in 1967 suggested that LSD causes chromosomal damage, but that theory was disproven in 1971.[21]

Risk of Overdose

Given the LD_{50} of LSD, there is minimal risk of fatal overdose in humans, especially in a clinical setting. Within a controlled setting, there also appears to be very low risk of long-term psychosis following the use of LSD, especially among patients who are otherwise healthy adults.

In a trio of case reports, Haden and Woods describe a woman who ingested the equivalent of 550 recreational doses of LSD and reported positive effects on pain levels and voluntary cessation of morphine for 5 days. Though she resumed morphine use, it was at a lower level. The woman continued to microdose LSD every 3 days. After 2 years, she stopped using both morphine and LSD.[22] Haden and Woods also note that a patient experienced reductions in mania and psychotic features following accidental ingestion of LSD that have been sustained for two decades.[22]

Drug Interactions

LSD targets serotonin receptors, which are also the targets of many antidepressants as well as atypical antipsychotic medications. Acute administration of selective serotonin reuptake inhibitors (SSRIs) potentiates the effects of psilocybin and LSD, whereas chronic administration downregulates serotonin receptors, thereby attenuating the effects of these drugs. Most medicines that alter the effects of psychedelics should be tapered and discontinued at least 2 weeks prior to initiating psychedelic therapy. Considering the long half-life of fluoxetine, it should be tapered and discontinued at least 6 weeks prior to beginning psychedelic therapy. For a more robust list of drug-drug interactions, see Table 10.2.

There is a mild-to-moderate risk of patients developing serotonin syndrome if psilocybin and LSD are taken concurrently with another drug that increases serotonin levels (see Table 10.3). There is also some evidence to suggest that coadministration of classic psychedelics with lithium may increase the risk of seizure.[23]

TABLE 10.2 Drug-Drug Interactions Between Antidepressants and Classic Psychedelics

Drug Type	Examples
Monoamine oxidase inhibitors	Isocarboxazid, moclobemide, phenelzine, selegiline, tranylcypromine
Noradrenergic and specific serotonergic antidepressants	Mianserin, mirtazapine, setiptiline
Selective serotonin reuptake inhibitors	Citalopram, escitalopram, fluvoxamine, fluoxetine,[a] paroxetine, sertraline
Serotonin modulators	Nefazodone, trazodone, vilazodone, vortioxetine
Serotonin norepinephrine reuptake inhibitors	Desvenlafaxine, duloxetine, levomilnacipran, venlafaxine
Serotonin partial agonist reuptake inhibitors	Vilazodone, vortioxetine
Tricyclic antidepressants	Amitriptyline, chlorpheniramine, clomipramine, desipramine, imipramine, nortriptyline
Other	Buspirone

Listed drugs should be tapered and discontinued at least 2 weeks prior to acute psychedelic therapy.
[a]Fluoxetine should be tapered and discontinued at least 6 weeks prior to acute psychedelic therapy.

TABLE 10.3 Drugs Associated With Elevated Serotonin Levels and Serotonin Syndrome

Drug Type	Examples
Analgesics	Fentanyl, meperidine, pentazocine, tramadol
Antibiotics	Linezolid, ritonavir
Anticonvulsants	Valproate
Antidepressants	Buspirone, clomipramine, nefazodone, trazodone, venlafaxine
Antiemetics	Granisetron, metoclopramide, ondansetron
Antimigraine medications	Sumatriptan
Bariatric drugs	Sibutramine
Monoamine oxidase inhibitors	Clorgiline, isocarboxazid, moclobemide, phenelzine
Over-the-counter drugs	Dextromethorphan
Selective serotonin reuptake inhibitors	Citalopram, fluoxetine, fluvoxamine, paroxetine, sertraline

Use in Pregnancy and Lactation

Though some small studies have suggested that LSD use during pregnancy does not lead to an increase in birth defects and no direct correlation has been established between birth defects and LSD, its use is not advised while pregnant. As LSD levels in human breast milk have not been established, its use while nursing is not advised.

Dosage and Administration

Research is ongoing to establish proper dosing guidelines, though a rough protocol has taken shape. In most cases, patients receive one to three doses of LSD while under the supervision of one or two clinicians. Prior to sessions with LSD, patients are screened for personal or family history of mental illness. If no conflicts arise during screening, patients will undergo one or more preparational sessions with clinicians. Following sessions with LSD, patients will meet with clinicians to help process the experience. Historically, oral doses have tended to range from 100 to 250 μg.

Guidelines for microdosing have not been established.

Conclusions

As mentioned, numerous times in this book, there is reason for optimism in terms of the potential applications of psychedelics. LSD in particular appears to hold a lot of promise for the treatment of several psychiatric disorders, especially substance use disorders and generalized anxiety disorder. However, this optimism should be tempered with recognition that psychedelics are not panaceas and that far more clinical evidence is needed to establish best practices in the administration of even familiar psychedelics such as LSD.

REFERENCES

1. Hofmann A. *LSD: My Problem Child*. Multidisciplinary Association for Psychedelic Studies (MAPS); 2009.
2. Friesen P. Psychosis and psychedelics: historical entanglements and contemporary contrasts. *Transcult Psychiatry*. 2022;59(5):592-609. doi:10.1177/13634615221129116. PMID: 36300247; PMCID: PMC9660273.
3. Reiff CM, Richman EE, Nemeroff CB, et al. Psychedelics and psychedelic-assisted psychotherapy. *Am J Psychiatry*. 2020;177(5):391-410. doi:10.1176/appi.ajp.2019.19010035. PMID: 32098487.
4. Grof S. Foreword. In: Hofmann A, ed. *LSD: My Problem Child*. Multidisciplinary Association for Psychedelic Studies (MAPS); 2009:5-21.
5. Passie T, Halpern JH, Stichtenoth DO, Emrich HM, Hintzen A. The pharmacology of lysergic acid diethylamide: a review. *CNS Neurosci Ther*. 2008;14(4):295-314. doi:10.1111/j.1755-5949.2008.00059.x. PMID: 19040555; PMCID: PMC6494066.
6. Dolder PC, Schmid Y, Steuer AE, et al. Pharmacokinetics and pharmacodynamics of lysergic acid diethylamide in healthy subjects. *Clin Pharmacokinet*. 2017;56(10):1219-1230. doi:10.1007/s40262-017-0513-9. PMID: 28197931; PMCID: PMC5591798.
7. Ley L, Holze F, Arikci D, et al. Comparative acute effects of mescaline, lysergic acid diethylamide, and psilocybin in a randomized, double-blind, placebo-controlled cross-over study in healthy participants. *Neuropsychopharmacology*. 2023;48(11):1659-1667. doi:10.1038/s41386-023-01607-2
8. Luethi D, Hoener MC, Krähenbühl S, Liechti ME, Duthaler U. Cytochrome P450 enzymes contribute to the metabolism of LSD to nor-LSD and 2-oxo-3-hydroxy-LSD: Implications for clinical LSD use. *Biochem Pharmacol*. 2019;164:129-138. doi:10.1016/j.bcp.2019.04.013. PMID: 30981875.
9. Murnane KS. Serotonin 2A receptors are a stress response system: implications for post-traumatic stress disorder. *Behav Pharmacol*. 2019;30(2 and 3):151-162. doi:10.1097/FBP.0000000000000459. PMID: 30632995; PMCID: PMC6422730.
10. Delli Pizzi S, Chiacchiaretta P, Sestieri C, et al. LSD-induced changes in the functional connectivity of distinct thalamic nuclei. *Neuroimage*. 2023;283:120414. doi:10.1016/j.neuroimage.2023.120414. PMID: 37858906.

11. Gattuso JJ, Perkins D, Ruffell S, et al. Default mode network modulation by psychedelics: a systematic review. *Int J Neuropsychopharmacol*. 2023;26(3):155-188. doi:10.1093/ijnp/pyac074. PMID: 36272145; PMCID: PMC10032309.
12. Le Daré B, Gicquel T, Baert A, Morel I, Bouvet R. Self-inflicted neck wounds under influence of lysergic acid diethylamide: a case report and literature review. *Medicine*. 2020;99(27):e20868. doi:10.1097/MD.0000000000020868
13. Bache CM. *LSD and the Mind of the Universe: Diamonds from Heaven*. Park Street Press; 2019.
14. Kuntz L. FDA grants breakthrough designation to MM-120 for generalized anxiety disorder. *Psychiatric Times*. Published March 7, 2024. Accessed April 9, 2024. https://www.psychiatrictimes.com/view/fda-grants-breakthrough-designation-to-mm-120-for-generalized-anxiety-disorder
15. Fuentes JJ, Fonseca F, Elices M, Farré M, Torrens M. Therapeutic use of LSD in psychiatry: a systematic review of randomized-controlled clinical trials. *Front Psychiatry*. 2020;10:943. doi:10.3389/fpsyt.2019.00943. PMID: 32038315; PMCID: PMC6985449.
16. Holze F, Gasser P, Müller F, Dolder PC, Liechti ME. Lysergic acid diethylamide-assisted therapy in patients with anxiety with and without a life-threatening illness: a randomized, double-blind, placebo-controlled phase II study. *Biol Psychiatry*. 2023;93(3):215-223. doi:10.1016/j.biopsych.2022.08.025. PMID: 36266118.
17. Molla H, Lee R, Tare I, et al. Greater subjective effects of a low dose of LSD in participants with depressed mood. *Neuropsychopharmacology*. 2024;49:774–781. doi:10.1038/s41386-023-01772-4
18. Shirane RA, Gottschalk CH, Schindler EAD. Headache horizons: the study and use of psychedelics in cluster headache. Practical Neurology. Published August 2023. Accessed April 9, 2024. https://practicalneurology.com/articles/2023-aug/headache-horizons-the-study-and-use-of-psychedelics-in-cluster-headache
19. Haijen ECHM, Hurks PPM, Kuypers KPC. Microdosing with psychedelics to self-medicate for ADHD symptoms in adults: a prospective naturalistic study. *Neurosci Appl*. 2022;1:101012. doi:10.1016/j.nsa.2022.101012
20. Vann Jones SA, O'Kelly A. Psychedelics as a treatment for Alzheimer's disease dementia. *Front Synaptic Neurosci*. 2020;12:34. doi:10.3389/fnsyn.2020.00034
21. Bower B. In 1967, LSD was briefly labeled a breaker of chromosomes. *ScienceNews*. Published March 23, 2017. Accessed April 10, 2024. https://www.sciencenews.org/article/1967-lsd-was-briefly-labeled-breaker-chromosomes
22. Haden M, Woods B. LSD overdoses: three case reports. *J Stud Alcohol Drugs*. 2020;81(1):115-118. PMID: 32048609.
23. Nayak SM, Gukasyan N, Barrett FS, Erowid E, Erowid F, Griffiths RR. Classic psychedelic coadministration with lithium, but not lamotrigine, is associated with seizures: an analysis of online psychedelic experience reports. *Pharmacopsychiatry*. 2021;54(5):240-245. doi:10.1055/a-1524-2794. PMID: 34348413.

11
N, N-Dimethyltryptamine (DMT) and Ayahuasca

N, N-Dimethyltryptamine (DMT) is an indole alkaloid and derivative of tryptamine found in plants and animals, including humans. It is also the principal psychedelic/entheogenic compound in ayahuasca, yagé, and several other decoctions that are used for ceremonial or medicinal purposes throughout the Amazon Basin. Both endogenous and exogenous DMT are partial agonists at a variety of serotonergic receptors (like all serotonergic psychedelics, this includes 5-HT$_{2A}$), but it also appears to be a ligand at trace amine-associated receptors (TAAR1s). It also binds to sigma-1 (σ-1) receptors, showing agonist-like effects at low micromolar levels (EC50 = 14 μM).[1] Emerging evidence suggests that activity at σ-1 receptors could be responsible for the neuroprotective, antidepressant, and anxiolytic effects of DMT and ayahuasca, as well as other psychedelics.

Historically, clinicians have paid significantly less attention to DMT than other psychedelics. This is largely due to its brief duration of action, which some have speculated could limit its utility in psychiatry.[2] Rapid onset is achieved when DMT is smoked, insufflated, or administered parenterally as a bolus. Peak effects may last only a few minutes, with the entire experience lasting approximately 30 minutes. Of note, the effects of DMT can be extended when it is coadministered with a monoamine oxidase inhibitor (MAOI) since DMT is quickly degraded by monoamine oxidase (MAO). Therefore, orally administered decoctions that have DMT (eg, ayahuasca) must contain MAOIs to be psychoactive. The effects of preparations like ayahuasca may not be felt for as long as 30 minutes and may persist for several hours, but they are far less intense than preparations that have a more rapid onset and shorter duration of action.

The subjective effects of high doses of nonoral preparations of DMT are some of the most unique within the world of psychedelics. In addition to seeing vivid geometric patterns, individuals often feel as though they have traveled through a tunnel or transitionary space and then had a "breakthrough" to an alternate reality or realm that is inhabited by intelligent or even superintelligent beings. These creatures are often described as godlike or alien, and these experiences are often accompanied by a sense of oceanic boundlessness.[3] Moreover, according to individuals who have experienced both, they are phenomenologically similar to near-death experiences (NDEs).[4]

Although short in duration, the intensity of the DMT experience is also similar to NDEs because it may lead to significant changes in cosmologic and spiritual beliefs, while also serving as a catalyst for greater introspection.[4] Consequently, some researchers have asserted that DMT could be a useful adjunct in talk therapy and that it may have applications in the treatment of multiple psychiatric disorders.

History

As described in Chapter 2, archaeological evidence indicates that individuals throughout the Western Hemisphere for centuries, if not millennia, have been ingesting plants that contain DMT or close relatives of DMT (eg, bufotenin, 5-methoxy-*N*, *N*-dimethyltryptamine [5-MeO-DMT]). Routes of administration vary from culture to culture, but two of the most common were via insufflation (snuffs) and oral ingestion of decoctions. Traditionally, snuffs were administered using hollowed-out reeds or bird bones, and paraphernalia associated with the practice (including these snuffing instruments and snuff trays) have been recovered from archaeological sites that are over 3,000 years old (dated to 1200 BCE).[5] Evidence of using smoking pipes that contain trace amounts of these compounds goes back even further (2130 BCE).[5] The oral traditions of these cultures often place "teacher plants" that contain these compounds at the center of their cosmology.

As for the historical record, this begins with Friar Ramón Pané, who accompanied Christopher Columbus on his second voyage to the Western Hemisphere in 1494. He remained on Hispaniola (modern-day Haiti and the Dominican Republic) for several years. Though seen through a Eurocentric lens, Pané's chronicle provides a firsthand look at the indigenous people of the island and their culture. His accounts suggest that *cohoba*, a snuff comprised of the ground seeds of *Anadenanthera peregrina*, was used to induce nonordinary states of consciousness for a variety of reasons (eg, healing, prophecy, discerning the disposition of local deities [zemi'no]), though its use seemed to be restricted to men of higher social status.[6] In addition to containing DMT, *A. peregrina* contains the psychedelic compounds bufotenin and 5-MeO-DMT, which will both be covered in Chapter 16.

Snuffs containing these compounds also have a long history of use among many shamanistic cultures within the Amazon Basin, and they have been used in concert with psychoactive and sacramental decoctions made from a variety of plant-based ingredients. The two plants most commonly used in these decoctions are *Psychotria viridis* and *Banisteriopsis caapi*. *P. viridis* is a shrubby flowering plant that belongs to the coffee family, and its leaves are a source of DMT, while *Diplopterys cabrerana* may also be used as a source of DMT.[7] Meanwhile, *B. caapi* is a liana and a source of the alkaloids harmine, harmaline, and tetrahydroharmine, which serve as MAOIs.

More than simply delaying the onset and prolonging the effects of DMT, MAOIs are necessary to make orally ingested DMT psychoactive. Though DMT may be considered the active ingredient in these decoctions, the most well-known being ayahuasca, it is the harmala alkaloids found in the bank of *B. caapi* which are the potentiators. In fact, the translation of "ayahuasca" from the original Quechua is "the vine of the dead" or "the vine of the soul" in reference to *B. caapi*.[4]

Though the term ayahuasca refers to a specific decoction created by a specific culture, it has become a catchall for all DMT-containing decoctions from the Amazon. Although this chapter does not delve enough into specifics to warrant the abandonment of this convention, readers should be aware that there may be innumerable variations of ayahuasca (yagé, hoasca, caapi, mihi, dapa, natema, pinde, damine, and vegetal, to name a few) within the Amazon Basin that contain DMT. These include *P. viridis* or *D. cabrerana*, β-carboline alkaloids from *B. caapi*, and an assortment of secondary ingredients capable of modulating the subjective or therapeutic effects of the brew. There may also be other plant-based sources of DMT and MAOIs that are more readily available in various cultures depending on the flora of their immediate landscape.

DMT Spreads Outside of the Amazon

DMT was first synthesized in 1931 by the Canadian chemist Richard Manske, though its pharmacology was not assessed at that time. In 1946,

Oswaldo Gonçalves de Lima, a microbiologist, discovered its presence in plants such as *Mimosa hostilis*. Ten years later, in 1956, Stephen Szára tested intramuscular doses of DMT and determined that its effects were similar in nature to lysergic acid diethylamide (LSD), even though the tryptamine structure of the DMT molecule bears more of a resemblance to psilocin, the active metabolite of psilocybin.[8] There was early interest in DMT's potential role in schizophrenia, and it was even suggested that DMT may be a schizotoxin—a compound capable of inducing schizophrenia and theoretically similar to a psychotomimetic.[9] Current models of schizophrenia have discredited the notion of such a substance, though it is still possible that endogenous DMT may play a role in psychosis.

Clinical work with DMT was largely pioneered by Rick Strassman in the 1990s, who was the first person to conduct human research with drugs classified as hallucinogens since the last administration of psilocybin in 1977 at the Maryland Psychiatric Research Center. Strassman's work focused on the physiologic effects and self-reports of individuals who had received DMT in controlled settings. His 2001 book, *DMT: The Spirit Molecule*, helped to bring awareness of the compound to a wider audience. Despite Strassman's work and its historical use within a shamanistic context, the clinical applications of DMT and ayahuasca remain understudied by practitioners of conventional medicine.

There are several churches in Brazil that have been granted the right to use ayahuasca (or *hoasca*, as it is known in Portuguese) as a sacrament. This includes the O Centro Espirita Beneficiente União Do Vegetal (UDV) and the Santo Damie, which were founded in 1961 and 1940, respectively.[10] In 2006, the US Supreme Court determined that ayahuasca use by the New Mexico branch of the UDV was legal even though DMT is a Schedule I drug.[10]

Recreational or illicit use of DMT has been documented in the United States at least since the 1960s, though it's unclear how widespread the practice currently is.[11] Similarly, it is unclear how common is the use of concoctions comprised of freebase DMT and an MAOI like Syrian rue or synthetic harmaline (known as *pharmahuasca*). Neither DMT nor ayahuasca seems well suited for casual use, and ayahuasca's purgative effects make it an especially poor choice in a club or festival setting.

That said, throughout the Americas, there has been a rise in ayahuasca use for spiritual purposes or within wellness-oriented settings that rely on psychedelic therapies.[12] In parallel with ibogaine (see Chapter 13), there has been some concern recently that *B. caapi*, *P. viridis*, and other plants that form the constituents of ayahuasca may be under threat from overharvesting.[13]

Endogenous *N, N*-dimethyltryptamine

Unlike other compounds described in this book, DMT is not only found in plants, but it is also an endogenous substance found within animals, including humans. There has been speculation about its function, including claims that it may be a neurotransmitter or neurohormone, though no specific role for DMT has been established at this time. It is speculated that DMT plays a role in psychosis, dreams, imagination, religious ecstasy, NDEs, and even during death itself. There is also some evidence suggesting that endogenous DMT is released in the central nervous system (CNS) when the body is under extreme stress (eg, cardiac arrest) and plays a role in preserving neurons when the brain is in a state of hypoxia.[14] It is also entirely possible that the role of endogenous DMT is entirely distinct from the effects observed following the administration of exogenous DMT.

What is clear is that both endogenous and exogenous DMT are active at multiple sites outside of the serotonergic system, including TAAR1s, as well as σ-1 receptors, and that DMT can be locally sequestered in neurotransmitter storage vesicles before being released.[1] DMT has also been demonstrated to be neuroprotective, and it may activate pathways that result in increased expression of brain-derived neurotrophic factor (BDNF) and possibly glial-derived neurotrophic factor (GDNF).[15,16] Curiously, some studies have contradicted the relationship between exogenous DMT administration and increased levels of plasma BDNF.[17] Clearly, more studies are required to better understand this complex relationship.

Biosynthesis

Synthesis of DMT begins with tryptophan, an essential amino acid that is a regular part of most human diets. It is found in animal sources (beef, poultry, lamb, dairy), as well as in legumes, whole grains, nuts, and seeds. Once ingested, tryptophan is then decarboxylated to form tryptamine. Tryptamine is transmethylated by aromatic-L-amino acid decarboxylase (AADC), and indolethylamine-*N*-methyltransferase (INMT), which also methylates another amine, histamine.[14] Catalyzation of INMT with additional methyl groups results in *N*-methyltryptamine (NMT) and DMT.[1] A visualization of this process is shown in Figure 11.1.

INMT is expressed throughout peripheral tissue, with the highest levels found in the adrenal gland, thyroid, and lungs. Intermediate concentrations are observed in the stomach, small intestine, pancreas,

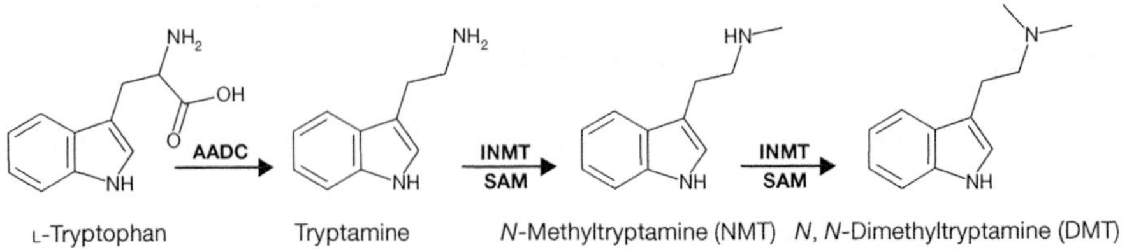

Figure 11.1 The synthesis of DMT from tryptophan. AADC, aromatic-L-amino acid decarboxylase; DMT, N, N-dimethyltryptamine; INMT, indolethylamine-N-methyltransferase; SAM, S-adenosyl-methionine.

heart, skeletal muscle, retina, placenta, and lymph nodes.[1] Within the CNS, the highest concentrations of INMT have been observed in the spinal cord, pineal gland, medulla, uncus, amygdala, frontal cortex, fronto-parietal, and temporal lobes.[1] Carbonaro and Gatch note that high concentrations in the CNS are relatively important, because "the wide distribution of INMT implies a wide distribution of DMT."[1]

Prevalence

Strassman once hypothesized that DMT production occurred primarily in the pineal gland, but this appears to be incorrect. Research by Dean and colleagues has convincingly shown that the cortex is the major source of DMT in the brain, while the pineal gland's role is more ancillary—if it plays a role at all. In unstressed rodent models, concentrations of DMT measured in cortical microdialysates ranged from 0.25 to 2.2 nM (average 1.02 nM), which is similar in range to serotonin (0.12-3.4 nM; average: 0.87 nM), dopamine (0.07-4.9 nM; average: 1.5 nM), and norepinephrine (0.19-4.4 nM; average: 1.77 nM). Dean and colleagues also found that DMT concentrations in the CNS increase dramatically following induced cardiac arrest in rodent models.[14] *This gives credence to the notion that DMT may be released as a neuroprotectant during times of extreme stress and hypoxia, which could possibly account for the parallels between NDEs and the subjective effects of exogenous DMT.*

Although there is no doubt that DMT is present in the CNS, it appears to be synthesized in peripheral organs, particularly the lungs. It is then transported to the CNS and stored within neurons via a three-step process articulated by Frecska and colleagues.[18] Only a small fraction of DMT that is synthesized or stored intracellularly is released into the blood.[1] This has made detecting endogenous DMT difficult.

Pharmacology

The pharmacology described below refers to exogenous DMT, which is found in a variety of plant sources of the genera *Acacia, Delosperma, Desmodium, Diplopterys Mimosa, Phalaris, Psychotria,* and *Virola,* among others.[1] Although it is also found throughout the animal kingdom, there is no evidence to suggest that any culture has harvested DMT from sources outside of the plant kingdom.

It's also important to note that this section focuses on the pharmacology of just DMT and will not go into depth describing the pharmacology of the various β-carbolines found in *B. caapi*, such as harmine, harmaline, and tetrahydroharmine. Though these are common constituents of ayahuasca and potentiate DMT, their clinical use is not pertinent to this discussion.

Description

In its purified form, DMT is a white or colorless crystalline powder with a molar mass of 188.27 g/mol and a melting point of 46 °C.[19] Less pure forms of DMT may appear slightly orange and waxy.[11] DMT powder may be smoked or vaporized. The structure of DMT is shown in Figure 11.2.

DMT may also be administered parenterally as a bolus, either intramuscularly or intravenously.[20] DMT fumarate, which contains two molecules of DMT and one molecule of fumaric acid, was patented as SPL026 by Small Pharma, which was later acquired by Cybin. It is more water soluble and shelf stable than freebase DMT, making it an attractive option for researchers.

The small size and hydrophobic nature of DMT allow it to easily cross the blood-brain barrier, but it is also rapidly metabolized by MAO.[8] Consequently, MAOIs are frequently administered in conjunction with

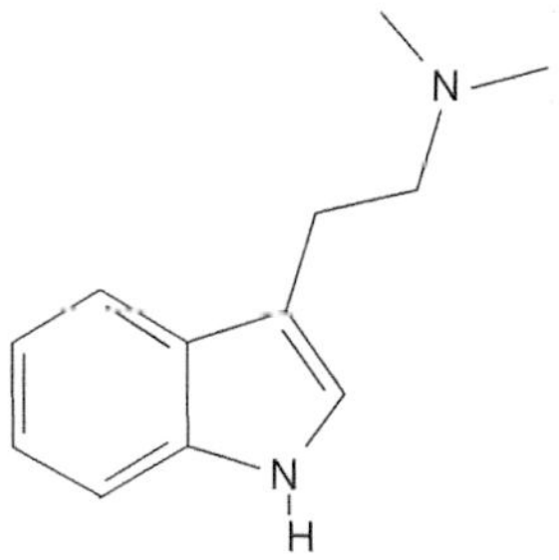

Figure 11.2 The molecular structure of DMT. DMT, *N, N*-dimethyltryptamine.

DMT, as is the case with decoctions such as ayahuasca or yagé. In these preparations, plant matter is gathered and boiled for several hours before being decanted. The resultant liquid is brown, oily, and thick, with a notably bitter taste.[10]

Doses of DMT in different samples of ayahuasca were found to range from 8.8 mg to 42 mg, which is similar to the disparity in caffeine content between a cup of green tea and a cup of drip coffee.[10] The exogenous DMT found in ayahuasca typically comes from the leaves of *P. viridis*, which may contain as little as 0.1% DMT by dry weight or as much as 0.66%, while concentrations of β-carboline alkaloids found in *B. caapi* range from 0.05% to 1.95% by dry weight.[10]

Route of Administration

When taken orally in conjunction with an MAOI, DMT's onset of action is arrested. The subjective effects may not be felt for upward of 30 minutes, with peak effects occurring 90 minutes after administration. These effects may persist for several hours, and individuals may not feel totally normal for a few days.[21]

When smoked or administered via intravenous injection, the onset of action is instantaneous, as DMT can access cerebral circulation in a matter of seconds.[8] Peak effects are reached within approximately 3 minutes and, depending on dose, begin to resolve within 10 minutes. The effects are far more intense than when administered as ayahuasca, though an individual may return to a normal state and not experience any lingering subjective effects 30 minutes after the dose. Meanwhile, intramuscular administration has a slightly slower onset of a few minutes and may last between 30 and 60 minutes.[1]

Pharmacokinetics

DMT is rapidly absorbed into the bloodstream when insufflated or smoked, while intravenous administration of DMT reaches peak blood concentrations approximately within 2 minutes.[8,1]

Plasma concentrations must reach the level of 12 to 90 μg/L with an apparent volume of distribution of 36 to 55 L/kg for the psychedelic effects of DMT to become discernible.[1] Peak plasma concentrations (C_{max}) and area under the curve at the last time point (AUC_{last}) appear to be dose dependent, though to what extent is difficult to determine since there is also a great deal of interpersonal variability.[22] DMT has poor permeability and plasma protein binding,[22] and the plasma half-life is estimated to be 10 to 12 minutes following intravenous infusion.[22]

DMT is primarily metabolized by peripheral MAO, with common metabolites being NMT, DMT-N-oxide (DMT-NO), 6-hydroxy-DMT (6-OH-DMT), 6-OH-DMT-NO, and indole-3-acetic acid (IAA).[1] However, the major metabolite of DMT is IAA.[22] Neither IAA nor any of the other noted metabolites are believed to be pharmacologically active.

When administered in conjunction with an MAOI, DMT may also be metabolized by cytochrome P450 isoenzyme CYP2D6 and to a lesser extent CYP2C19.[22]

According to Good and colleagues, who published a study on the effects of DMT in vitro using human hepatocyte and liver mitochondrial fractions with and without MAOIs, the intrinsic clearance of DMT (0.62 µM, $n = 2$) was 175.0 µL/min/mg protein (half-life, 7.9 minutes).[22] They noted that higher concentrations (3.1 µM) had a notable impact on the intrinsic clearance of DMT. The clearance "was reduced by >90% (approximately 11-fold) by the MAO-A inhibitor compared to vehicle control (<3.9 vs 42.9 µL/min/mg protein) with an accompanying increase in half-life (>373.7 vs 33.7 minutes)."[22] The team found intrinsic hepatocyte clearance at 0.62 µM was 19.4 ± 0.8 µL/min/million cells with a mean half-life of 98.9 (± 3.9 SD) and was minimally affected by MAOIs.[22] Good and colleagues also performed in vivo studies using a variety of intravenous doses, finding that DMT is largely cleared before it reaches the human liver, meaning that CYP enzymes likely play a minor role in DMT metabolism except when it is administered orally in conjunction with an MAOI.[22]

Less than 1% of the parent compound is excreted unchanged in urine. Approximately 8.3% of an intravenous DMT dose is detected as IAA in urine in human volunteers.[1] However, following administration of ayahuasca, 50% of the DMT dose is recovered as IAA and 10% as DMT-NO.[23]

Pharmacodynamics

The pharmacodynamics and mechanism of action of DMT are similar to other classic psychedelics. It is recommended that readers review Chapter 7 to gain an understanding of these drugs' mechanism of action and how these drugs affect the CNS. Like other psychedelics, DMT appears to decrease alpha power and increase entropy, delta and gamma power, and global functional connectivity.[24] The entropic modality that is common following the administration of classic psychedelics, including but not limited to DMT, may account for the distinct phenomenology of these drugs, though it does not account for subtle variations in the subjective effects of LSD, psilocybin, DMT, and other drugs covered in this book.

Mechanism of Action

DMT is a partial agonist at multiple serotonin receptors (see Table 11.1), especially serotonin 2A (5-HT$_{2A}$), as well as at σ-1 receptors and TAAR1s. The acute psychedelic effects are believed to be mediated primarily via 5-HT$_{2A}$ receptors, though this seems unsatisfactory as a complete explanation, given the unique visionary states caused by DMT. As is the

TABLE 11.1 DMT Receptor Interactions and Effects of Receptor Activation

Receptor	Affinity: K_i (nM)	DMT Action	Signaling Pathway(s)	Downstream Effects
5-HT$_{1D}$	39	Agonist	G$_i$/G$_0$	Inhibits neurotransmission
5-HT$_{2A}$	127	Agonist	G$_q$	Increases phosphoinositide hydrolysis, increases mechanistic target of rapamycin (mTOR)-dependent structural plasticity, neurite growth, and spinogenesis
5-HT$_{1B}$	129	Agonist	G$_i$/G$_0$	Inhibits neurotransmission
5-HT$_{1A}$	183	Agonist	G$_i$/G$_0$	Acute inhibition of dorsal raphe firing, anxiolytic, and antidepressant
5-HT$_{2B}$	184	Agonist	G$_q$ and β-arrestin 2	Transport and regulation of serotonin plasma levels, vasoconstriction and platelet morphology, maintains cardiac valve leaflets
5-HT$_7$	206	Partial agonist	Adenyl cyclase; CDK, and GTPase Cdc42	Serotonergic system-related neuropsychiatric disorders, prolonged activation of dendritic spine formation and synaptogenesis in cortical and striatal neurons, acute activation of neurite elongation in striatal and cortical neurons, establishment of correct neuronal cytoarchitecture during development and remodeling of neuronal circuits in the mature brain

TABLE 11.1 DMT Receptor Interactions and Effects of Receptor Activation (*continued*)

Receptor	Affinity: K_i (nM)	DMT Action	Signaling Pathway(s)	Downstream Effects
5-HT$_{2C}$	360	Agonist	G$_q$	Desensitizes over time, unlike 5-HT$_{2A}$
5-HT$_6$	464	Partial agonist	G$_S$, Erk1/2, Jun, mTOR	Modulation of cognitive processes, mood regulation, and motivated behaviors
5-HT$_{1E}$	517	Agonist	G$_i$/G$_0$	Inhibits neurotransmission
5-HT$_{5A}$	213	Partial agonist	G$_i$ and G$_0$	Control of circadian rhythms, mood, and cognitive function, and implicated in schizophrenia
Sigma-1	K_d ~15 μM	Agonist	BDNF and EGF	Neural plasticity, protection from oxidative stress, and antidepressant
TAAR1	Unknown	Agonist	G$_S$	Dopamine efflux via dopamine transporter internalization

5-HT, serotonin; BDNF, brain-derived neurotrophic factor; CDK, cyclic-dependent kinases; DMT, N, N-dimethyltryptamine; EGF, epidermal growth factor; GTP, guanosine triphosphate; TAAR1, trace amine-associated receptor.
Adapted from Colosimo FA, Borsellino P, Krider RI, Marquez RE, Vida TA. The clinical potential of dimethyltryptamine: breakthroughs into the other side of mental illness, neurodegeneration, and consciousness. *Psychoactives*. 2024;3(1):93-122. doi:10.3390/psychoactives3010007

case with other psychedelics, the mechanisms behind these effects are not totally understood.

Similarly, the therapeutic effects of DMT are difficult to explain. On the one hand, activity at serotonin and σ receptors is associated with reductions in inflammation, which may account for some of the anxiolytic and antidepressant effects of psychedelics, including DMT. Szabo has even suggested that DMT could potentially be used to treat chronic inflammatory conditions and autoimmune disorders because σ-1 agonists increase levels of GDNF, thereby promoting neuronal cell survival and differentiation.[16]

Classic psychedelics like DMT have also been shown to promote neuroplasticity, synapse formation, and dendritic spine growth by increasing BDNF via tropomyosin receptor kinase B (TrkB)- and mTOR-dependent mechanisms, though the exact mechanisms of these interactions are not fully understood.[15] Conversely, Vogt and colleagues found that DMT does not appear to have any effect on BDNF levels.[17] In fact, it is possible that synaptogenesis is promoted through other routes like 5-HT$_6$ and HT$_7$ receptors, where DMT is an agonist.[8]

Therapeutic Index

The median lethal dose (LD$_{50}$) for DMT in a murine model was measured to be 47 mg/kg when administered intraperitoneally and 32 mg/kg when administered intravenously.[10] Good and colleagues found that intravenous doses of 17 mg DMT (well under 1 mg/kg in adult humans) are sufficient to produce a "breakthrough" psychedelic experience and, more importantly, that DMT is minimally toxic when administered responsibly in a clinical setting.[22]

The LD$_{50}$ of the principal β-carboline alkaloids in ayahuasca is estimated to be in the range of 2 g/kg, indicating that the primary source of concern for acute lethality is DMT. Based on the extremely conservative calculations by Gable, the safety margin for ayahuasca is extremely wide, with a potentially toxic dose needing to be 20 times greater than a median dose (presuming LD$_{50}$ of oral DMT to be 8 mg/kg [560 mg for a 70 kg individual] and an average ceremonial dose of 27 mg).[10]

Tolerance, Dependence, and Withdrawal

Early studies of DMT indicate that it does not produce tolerance or cross-tolerance with other classic psychedelics. However, tolerance to DMT and cross-tolerance with other 5-HT$_{2A}$ agonists can occur with frequent administration at higher doses (eg, 3.2-10 mg/kg every 2 hours for 21 days).[1] One caveat is that the tolerance is more applicable to the somatic effects of DMT and less so to the subjective/psychotropic experiences of an individual.

Like most other psychedelics, the risk of abuse or dependence is considered to be very low. There appear to be no studies reporting withdrawal symptoms following DMT use.

Subjective Effects

Intravenous injection or inhalation of DMT avoids the immediate clearance by MAO, resulting in a very intense albeit brief psychedelic experience. There is extensive literature on the subject, especially on the internet, describing these mystical-like experiences that are more immersive than other tryptamine psychedelics as well as more visually intricate than other psychedelics.

Those who take a dose sufficient to experience a breakthrough may feel as though they have visited another realm possessed with hyperrealistic qualities that are at the same time characterized by a profound sense of otherness. Additionally, they may report time distortion (individuals oftentimes claim to have experienced "eternity"), oceanic boundlessness, and a sense of unity with the universe.[10] In some instances, individuals have claimed to have encountered sentient life-forms that have been described as deities (eg, angels, demons, gods) or extraterrestrial beings.[25] Many people feel convinced that these life-forms possess an independent existence and are not figments of their imagination even after the effects of DMT have dissipated. These experiences are also commonly associated with descriptions of religious ecstasy within Christianity (*beatific vision*), Hinduism (*samadhi*), and Zen Buddhism (*satori*). It is unclear if there is any clinical utility to these experiences that are distinct from the mystical-like experiences while using ayahuasca or other drugs mentioned throughout this book.

The subjective effects of ayahuasca are distinct, but similar to other tryptamine psychedelics like psilocybin or LSD. While one is experiencing these effects, they may observe rapidly moving patterns and scenes with eyes open or closed, as well as changes to visible objects (they may appear to vibrate or pulsate as if breathing, increase in brightness, or change in size [become more diminutive or elongated]).[10]

DMT and Near-Death Experiences

Common experiences for those who have gone through an NDE include out-of-body experiences, feelings of inner peace, travel through a void or tunnel, bright lights, and interactions with sentient beings. Curiously, these experiences are frequently reported by individuals who take large doses of DMT. Timmermann and colleagues note that "the near-death experience has been associated with long-term positive changes in psychological well-being and related outcomes," including reductions in anxiety or distress about one's mortality, increases in concern for others, a greater appreciation of nature, and improvements in self-esteem.[4]

The phenomenological similarities between DMT and NDEs were measured by Timmermann and colleagues. In their placebo-controlled, single-blind study, various doses of intravenous DMT were administered to 13 healthy individuals (six females and seven males). Results were compared to a gender and age-matched sample of 13 individuals who had reported NDEs. The two groups each completed the Near-Death Experience scale (NDE scale), the Ego Dissolution Inventory (EDI), and the Mystical Experiences Questionnaire (MEQ).

There were significant overlaps in scores, though a notable disparity was that the NDE group was more likely to feel as though type had encountered a "point of no return," most likely because of antecedent illness or injury. Scores were slightly lower on the NDE scale for the DMT group, but scores were nearly identical with respect to the experience of unity with the universe and a sense of joy. The authors of the paper note, "The so-called 'unitive experience' was originally identified as the core component of the mystical experience by its most influential scholar, Walter Stace."[26]

One important thing to note is that baseline delusional thinking was strongly associated with NDE scores.[26] Rather than discrediting these experiences as being delusions, this can be interpreted to mean that individuals who have higher-than-average delusional thinking are more receptive to the idea of paranormal phenomena and may view something like an NDE as being within reason.

Somatic Effects

When injected or smoked, individuals may not be aware of their surroundings for several minutes even though they are awake. When consumed as ayahuasca, individuals will maintain the ability to speak and navigate through space with greater ease. Like many other psychedelics, nausea and oftentimes violent purging are common following the administration of ayahuasca or other decoctions containing DMT. During the initial stages of the ayahuasca experience, vomiting and diarrhea are very common but tend to pass well before the subjective effects of the drug have worn off.

The somatic effects of injected, smoked, or insufflated DMT primarily concern increases in heart rate and both systolic and diastolic blood pressure. Within 2 minutes of an intravenous dose of 0.4 mg/kg, Strassman and Qualls reported an increase in heart rate of 26 beats per minute, as well as raised blood pressure (35 mm Hg systolic; 30 mm Hg diastolic). With ayahuasca, cardiac stress has also been observed, but at a rate of one-third that of intravenous DMT. For comparison, a study involving 77 individuals who were asked to give a 3-minute speech found an average increase in heart rate of 30 beats per minute and an average increase in systolic and diastolic blood pressures of 28 mm Hg and 21 mm Hg, respectively.[10]

Therapeutic Indications

DMT is a Schedule I drug. There are no accepted indications for its use.

Potential Uses

At present, the most likely uses for DMT within a clinical setting appear to be for major depressive disorder and substance use disorders. DMT, rather than ayahuasca, has been recognized as a desirable alternative to other psychedelics because of the minimal duration of its effects, its short half-life, and its rapid onset, especially when administered parenterally. Anecdotal reports have suggested that ayahuasca may be used to treat any number of psychiatric conditions, but the evidence to support these claims has not been corroborated by clinical evidence. Future studies may find that ayahuasca and DMT are effective treatments for many of the conditions described in Chapter 8.

Major Depressive Disorder

Ayahuasca has demonstrated rapid antidepressant effects similar to other psychedelics, and open-label studies have shown promising results for up to 21 days among healthy individuals and individuals with mood disorders.[8] Similarly, Timmermann and colleagues found that intravenous DMT improved depression scores in healthy individuals 1 to 2 weeks following administration.[26] They also noted, "a significant relationship was found between acute experiences of 'Oceanic Boundlessness' induced by DMT and post-DMT improvements in depression and anxiety."[26] However, long-term efficacy has yet to be established.

Substance Use Disorders

Ayahuasca has shown some efficacy in treating alcohol use disorder, cocaine use disorder, tobacco use disorder, and polysubstance use disorder, according to multiple studies. Unfortunately, there are significant limitations in these studies, as they were largely retrospective and without controls.[27]

Potential Dangers

The acute effects of DMT can increase heart rate and blood pressure, potentially resulting in adverse cardiac events. Individuals with heart conditions may not be suitable candidates for treatment with DMT. Additionally, DMT and ayahuasca may not be suitable for individuals with severe and persistent mental illnesses, as the experience can be psychologically demanding and difficult.

Like all psychedelics, set and setting are integral to the productive use of DMT and ayahuasca. If an individual is not psychologically prepared, they will derive limited therapeutic value from the experience.

Adverse Effects

A study involving 32 participants (placebo group = 8; drug groups = 24) conducted by Good and colleagues reported that 13 subjects experienced drug-related treatment-emergent adverse events, all of which were mild or moderate and transient in nature. The most common adverse events were pain at the administration site, sleep disorders, euphoria, tachycardia, pallor, and headache. No serious adverse events were reported.[22]

Any toxic effects of long-term DMT use are unknown at this writing.

Risk of Overdose

Although the toxicity of DMT and ayahuasca is low, it is common to feel as though one has taken an overdose because of excessive vomiting and diarrhea, fever, and intense visions.

Pregnant and Nursing Women

There is not enough information to establish the safety of DMT or ayahuasca in pregnant and nursing individuals. Consequently, use of DMT or ayahuasca is not advised in these populations.

Drug Interactions

There is very little clinical evidence about drug-drug interactions with DMT or ayahuasca. As DMT targets serotonin receptors, individuals who are on antidepressant drugs that affect serotonin (see Table 11.2) may be at risk of developing serotonin syndrome if DMT is taken concurrently. Similarly, individuals taking MAOIs may experience prolonged effects of DMT or ayahuasca, so a washout period of at least 2 weeks is recommended.

There is also some evidence to suggest that the coadministration of classic psychedelics with lithium may increase the risk of seizure.[28]

TABLE 11.2 Drugs Associated With Elevated Serotonin Levels and Serotonin Syndrome

Drug Type	Examples
Analgesics	Fentanyl, meperidine, pentazocine, tramadol
Antibiotics	Linezolid, ritonavir
Anticonvulsants	Valproate
Antidepressants	Buspirone, clomipramine, nefazodone, trazodone, venlafaxine
Antiemetics	Granisetron, metoclopramide, ondansetron
Antimigraine medications	Sumatriptan
Bariatric drugs	Sibutramine
Monoamine oxidase inhibitors	Clorgiline, isocarboxazid, moclobemide, phenelzine
Over-the-counter drugs	Dextromethorphan
Selective serotonin reuptake inhibitors	Citalopram, fluoxetine, fluvoxamine, paroxetine, sertraline

Dosage and Administration

There are currently no standard clinical guidelines for administering DMT. A typical dose of smoked or inhaled freebase DMT has been estimated to be 40 to 50 mg, with exceptionally high doses being near 100 mg. When individuals have too large a dose of DMT, they may lose consciousness or experience amnesia. According to Szára, who first experimented with DMT in the 1950s, intramuscular injections of 50 to 60 mg were capable of producing profound visions, but doses larger than 125 mg would induce catatonia or loss of consciousness.[11] DMT content in ayahuasca varies, though Gable estimated 24 mg for 100 mL of brew.[10]

Studies involving the intravenous administration of DMT have bolus doses of 20 mg with limited adverse effects.[24] Continuous intravenous infusions of up to 18 mg administered at 1.9 mg/min were well tolerated in healthy individuals.[20]

Conclusion

Clinical research into DMT and ayahuasca is just beginning. The latter has been used ceremonially and medicinally since before the historical record began, indicating that it can be used safely. Like other psychedelics, it may prove to be an effective therapeutic instrument, particularly when treating patients with complex and multilayered pathologies resulting in multiple psychiatric disorders and symptoms. Meanwhile, the former remains one of the most unique compounds in this book due to its near instantaneous onset and the tendency to produce breakthrough experiences. These experiences are associated with DMT's rapid antidepressant effects, as well as profound changes to one's outlook on life and spirituality. What remains to be seen is whether or not these experiences lead to lasting behavioral changes or sustained improvements in mood.

REFERENCES

1. Carbonaro TM, Gatch MB. Neuropharmacology of N,N-dimethyltryptamine. *Brain Res Bull.* 2016;126(pt 1):74-88. doi:10.1016/j.brainresbull.2016.04.016. PMID: 27126737; PMCID: PMC5048497.
2. Nardou R, Sawyer E, Song YJ, et al. Psychedelics reopen the social reward learning critical period. *Nature.* 2023;618:790-798. doi:10.1038/s41586-023-06204-3
3. Lawrence DW, Carhart-Harris R, Griffiths R, et al. Phenomenology and content of the inhaled N, N-dimethyltryptamine (N, N-DMT) experience. *Sci Rep.* 2022;12(1):8562. doi:10.1038/s41598-022-11999-8
4. Timmermann C, Roseman L, Williams L, et al. DMT models the near-death experience. *Front Psychol.* 2018;9:1424. doi:10.3389/fpsyg.2018.01424
5. Samorini G. The oldest archeological data evidencing the relationship of Homo sapiens with psychoactive plants: a worldwide overview. *J Psychedelic Stud.* 2019;3(2):63-80. doi:10.1556/2054.2019.008
6. Wassen SH. Anthropological survey of the use of South American snuffs. In: Efron DH, ed. *Ethnopharmacologic Search for Psychoactive Drugs: Proceedings of a Symposium Held in San Francisco, California January 28-30, 1967.* Vol I. Synergetic Press; 2018:233-289.
7. Luna LE. Ayahuasca: a powerful epistemological wildcard in a complex, fascinating and dangerous world. In: Prance GT, ed. *Ethnopharmacologic Search for Psychoactive Drugs: 50th Anniversary Symposium, June 6-8, 2017.* Vol II. Synergetic Press; 2018:24-35.
8. Colosimo FA, Borsellino P, Krider RI, Marquez RE, Vida TA. The clinical potential of dimethyltryptamine: breakthroughs into the other side of mental illness, neurodegeneration, and consciousness. *Psychoactives.* 2024;3(1):93-122. doi:10.3390/psychoactives3010007
9. Gillin JC, Kaplan J, Stillman R, Wyatt RJ. The psychedelic model of schizophrenia: the case of N,N-dimethyltryptamine. *Am J Psychiatry.* 1976;133(2):203-208. doi:10.1176/ajp.133.2.203. PMID: 1062171.
10. Gable RS. Risk assessment of ritual use of oral dimethyltryptamine (DMT) and harmala alkaloids. *Addiction.* 2007;102(1):24-34. doi:10.1111/j.1360-0443.2006.01652.x. PMID: 17207120.

11. Meyer P. Apparent communication with discarnate entities induced by dimethyltryptamine (DMT). *Psychedelic Monogr Essays*. 1993;6:29-67.
12. Kamin D. The rise of psychedelic retreats. *New York Times*. Published November 25, 2021. Accessed April 3, 2024. https://www.nytimes.com/2021/11/25/travel/psychedelic-retreat-ayahuasca.html
13. Brooks K. Ancient medicine in today's world. Omnia. Published April 25, 2023. Accessed April 3, 2024. https://omnia.sas.upenn.edu/story/doctoral-student-Taylor-Dysart-studies-ancient-medicine-today
14. Dean JG, Liu T, Huff S, et al. Biosynthesis and extracellular concentrations of N,N-dimethyltryptamine (DMT) in mammalian brain. *Sci Rep*. 2019;9:9333. doi:10.1038/s41598-019-45812-w
15. Ly C, Greb AC, Cameron LP, et al. Psychedelics promote structural and functional neural plasticity. *Cell Rep*. 2018;23(11):3170-3182. doi:10.1016/j.celrep.2018.05.022. PMID: 29898390; PMCID: PMC6082376.
16. Szabo A, Frecska E. Dimethyltryptamine (DMT): a biochemical Swiss Army knife in neuroinflammation and neuroprotection? *Neural Regen Res*. 2016;11(3):396-397. doi:10.4103/1673-5374.179041. PMID: 27127466; PMCID: PMC4828992.
17. Vogt SB, Ley L, Erne L, et al. Acute effects of intravenous DMT in a randomized placebo-controlled study in healthy participants. *Transl Psychiatry*. 2023;13(1):172. doi:10.1038/s41398-023-02477-4. PMID: 37221177; PMCID: PMC10206108.
18. Frecska E, Szabo A, Winkelman MJ, Luna LE, McKenna DJ. A possibly sigma-1 receptor mediated role of dimethyltryptamine in tissue protection, regeneration, and immunity. *J Neural Transm (Vienna)*. 2013;120(9):1295-1303. doi:10.1007/s00702-013-1024-y. PMID: 23619992.
19. American Chemical Society. Molecule of the week archive: N,N-dimethyltryptamine. Published September 17, 2018. Accessed March 26, 2024. https://www.acs.org/molecule-of-the-week/archive/d/dimethyltryptamine.html
20. Luan LX, Eckernäs E, Ashton M, et al. Psychological and physiological effects of extended DMT. *J Psychopharmacol*. 2024;38(1):56-67. doi:10.1177/02698811231196877
21. Barker SA. N, N-dimethyltryptamine (DMT), an endogenous hallucinogen: past, present, and future research to determine its role and function. *Front Neurosci*. 2018;12:536. doi:10.3389/fnins.2018.00536. PMID: 30127713; PMCID: PMC6088236.
22. Good M, Joel Z, Benway T, et al. Pharmacokinetics of N,N-dimethyltryptamine in humans. *Eur J Drug Metab Pharmacokinet*. 2023;48(3):311-327. doi:10.1007/s13318-023-00822-y. PMID: 37086340; PMCID: PMC10122081.
23. Riba J, McIlhenny EH, Valle M, Bouso JC, Barker SA. Metabolism and disposition of N,N-dimethyltryptamine and harmala alkaloids after oral administration of ayahuasca. *Drug Test Anal*. 2012;4(7-8):610-616. doi:10.1002/dta.1344. PMID: 22514127.
24. Timmermann C, Roseman L, Haridas S, et al. Human brain effects of DMT assessed via EEG-fMRI. *Proc Natl Acad Sci U S A*. 2023;120(13):e2218949120. doi:10.1073/pnas.2218949120. PMID: 36940333; PMCID: PMC10068756.
25. Michael P, Luke D, Robinson O. An encounter with the other: a thematic and content analysis of DMT experiences from a naturalistic field study. *Front Psychol*. 2021;12:720717. doi:10.3389/fpsyg.2021.720717. PMID: 34975614; PMCID: PMC8716686.
26. Timmermann C, Zeifman RJ, Erritzoe D, Nutt DJ, Carhart-Harris RL. Effects of DMT on mental health outcomes in healthy volunteers. *Sci Rep*. 2024;14:3097. doi:10.1038/s41598-024-53363-y
27. Zafar R, Siegel J, Harding R, et al. Psychedelic therapy in the treatment of addiction: the past, present and future. *Front Psychiatry*. 2023;14:1183740. doi:10.3389/fpsyt.2023.1183740. PMID: 37377473; PMCID: PMC10291338.
28. Nayak SM, Gukasyan N, Barrett FS, Erowid E, Erowid F, Griffiths RR. Classic psychedelic coadministration with lithium, but not lamotrigine, is associated with seizures: an analysis of online psychedelic experience reports. *Pharmacopsychiatry*. 2021;54(5):240-245. doi:10.1055/a-1524-2794. PMID: 34348413.

12

Mescaline

Mescaline was described as "the forgotten psychedelic" by Vamvakopoulou and colleagues in their 2022 paper published in *Neuropharmacology*.[1] This continues to be an accurate, though unfortunate, distinction. Although the use of peyote (a cactus that contains high concentrations of mescaline) continues to be central to the practices of the Native American Church (NAC), there has been little interest in its clinical use during the so-called psychedelic renaissance in recent years. Despite being the first psychedelic to receive significant attention during the first half of the 20th century, far fewer studies have been dedicated to the potential benefits of mescaline in psychiatry than other classic psychedelics like psilocybin and lysergic acid diethylamide (LSD). This is surprising considering the fact that it played an instrumental role in instigating clinical research into psychedelics during the 1950s and early 1960s (topics explored in previous chapters of this book).

A PubMed search of articles with "mescaline" or "peyote" in the title reveals a modest number of publications through the 1950s and 1960s, with a small surge in the 1970s, an enormous decline during the 1980s through the early 2010s, and a ripple of renewed interest only in recent years (see Figure 12.1A). When the search is filtered to include only clinical trials, the number of publications drops precipitously (see Figure 12.2A). There are a total of eight results—one from each of the

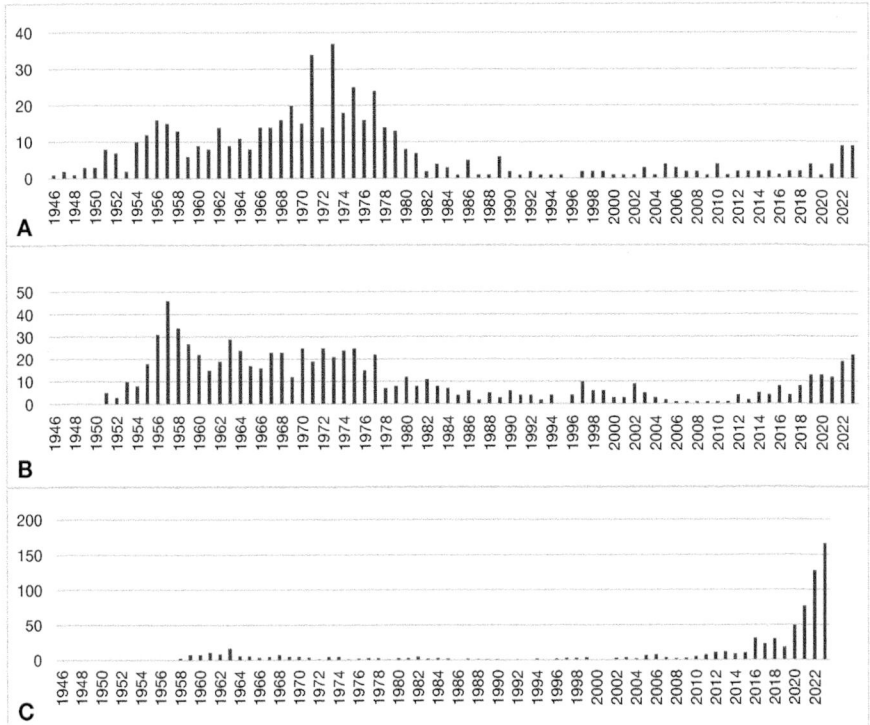

Figure 12.1 The above graphs show the frequency of appearance of classic psychedelics mescaline (A), LSD (B), and psilocybin (C) in the titles of all journal articles from 1946 through 2023. LSD, lysergic acid diethylamide.

following years: 1966, 1967, 1968, 1970, 1971, 1975, 2005, and 2023. Of all, only the 2023 publication qualifies as a randomized controlled trial.[2] By comparison, interest in LSD and psilocybin has been far more pronounced (see Figures 12.1B,C and 12.2B,C), considering that just in 2022 there were 11 randomized controlled trials of psilocybin.

It is possible that even if studies about mescaline have lagged behind other psychedelics, new research will lead to greater interest in the coming years. Consequently, clinicians should have some background information about its pharmacology and potential uses in clinical practice. Mescaline's use within the NAC and the history of its nonceremonial use in the United States have already been described, so this text will provide only a brief overview of the history of mescaline before moving on to its pharmacology and potential therapeutic uses. For information on the relationship between classic psychedelics like mescaline and consciousness, see Chapter 7.

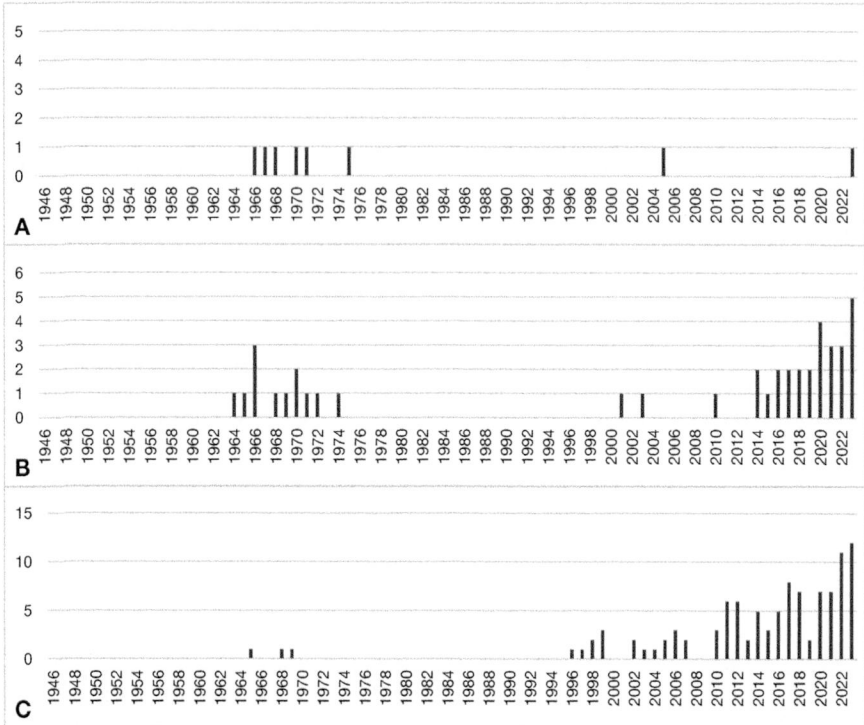

Figure 12.2 The above graphs show the frequency of appearance of classic psychedelics mescaline (A), LSD (B), and psilocybin (C) in the titles of articles about clinical trials from 1946 through 2023. LSD, lysergic acid diethylamide.

History

Like many other psychotropic substances discussed in this book, mescaline is a naturally occurring alkaloid. It is found in several species of cacti throughout the Americas, with the highest concentrations occurring in the North American peyote cactus (*Lophophora williamsii*) and the South American San Pedro cactus (*Echinopsis pachanoi*). Mescaline is also found in lower concentrations among other members of the genus *Echinopsis*—namely *E. peruviana* (the Peruvian torch cactus) and *E. lageniformis* (the Bolivian torch cactus)—with trace amounts having been detected in *Acacia berlandieri*, *Vachellia rigidula*, as well as other members within the Fabaceae family.[3,4] In addition, mescaline is found in small quantities in the leaves of Barbados gooseberry (*Pereskia aculeata*).[5]

The psychotropic properties of peyote and San Pedro cacti have long been recognized by the indigenous peoples of the Americas, who have used them for ceremonial, spiritual, and medicinal purposes. Unlike Western medicine, where health concerns are typically viewed as physiologic problems that have biological solutions, the line between spirituality and medicine is considerably more blurred among many cultures indigenous to the Americas. Even today, many indigenous individuals view illnesses not solely as physical problems but consider them to be potentially spiritual ones as well. Accordingly, practitioners believe that one must engage with these problems on a spiritual or metaphysical level if they are to resolve them and restore patients' health. This approach grants not only the patient or the healer, but both, access to the metaphysical realm, though this also depends on how the psychedelic compounds like mescaline are administered.

Archaeological records indicate that the use of peyote and San Pedro cacti predate the most well-known pre-Columbian civilizations of Central and South Americans by thousands of years. The earliest evidence of San Pedro consumption dates back to 8600 BCE.[6] Ceremonial use of the San Pedro has been evinced by carvings at the site Chavín de Huántar, which sits 270 miles to the north of Lima at over 10,000 feet above sea level. Radiocarbon dating indicates that these carvings were etched into rock around 1200 BCE.[7(p15)] The earliest evidence of peyote's use was found in Texas and dates back to 5,700 years ago.[8]

The colonization of the Americas by Europeans led to the prohibition of shamanistic forms of healing and the use of psychedelic medicines, as noted in Chapter 2. Throughout New Spain, the Catholic Church proved to be especially proscriptive in their view of mescaline, and countless individuals were prosecuted for using either the San Pedro in South America or peyote (*raiz diabólica* [devilish root]) in territories that have since become present-day Mexico and Texas. As a result, the use of mescaline became more surreptitious in areas where colonial rule was firmly established. In the rugged deserts of parts of Mexico, Spanish (and then Mexican) authorities struggled to assert their control, and peyote ceremonies among cultures like the Huichol—who reside primarily in the mountainous regions of Nayarit, Jalisco, Zacatecas, and Durango—continued virtually unabated.[7(pp33-49)]

Among Europeans, Charles Lemaire and Prince Joseph de Salm-Dyck were the first to describe peyote in 1840.[7(p65)] The first account of the effects of peyote was written 17 years later in the *New Orleans Picayune*, where it was referred to as "whiskey root" and said to produce an effect "precisely the same as alcoholic drinks."[7(p65)] The ignorance would not stop there, and in the 1880s, some confusion arose about mescaline and mescal bean due to the similarity of the two words. The former refers to *L. williamsii*, whereas the latter refers to *Dermatophyllum secundiflorum* or *Sophora secundiflora*, which contain cytisine (an alkaloid with a high affinity for the $α_4β_2$ subtype of nicotinic acetylcholine receptor) and are quite toxic.[9] Even among scholars, there was some confusion in the classification of peyote, but in 1894, it was placed in the genus *Lophophora* by American botanist John Merle Coulter.[10]

The next year, Daniel Webster Prentiss and Francis Morgan conducted the first scientific trials with peyote at what is known today as George Washington University, as described in Chapter 3.[11] A few months later, in November 1895, Erwin Ewell, a junior chemist who worked in the Department of Agriculture's chemistry division, took several buttons and reportedly saw angels and streets of gold. Despite being an agnostic and admirer of "the Great Agnostic," Robert G. Ingersoll, Ewell reportedly believed that his mescaline visions would convince Ingersoll that there is a heaven.[12] Of the same vein, but more consequential with respect to the written record, in 1897, Havelock Ellis published in *The Lancet* an account of his experience with mescaline, titled "Mescal: A New Artificial Paradise." As noted in Chapter 3, this began what could be described as the first wave of interest in psychedelics.

Later that year, mescaline was first isolated by Arthur Heffter, who noted that it was the agent responsible for peyote's effects. It was then synthesized in 1919 by Ernst Späth.[13] Starting in 1920, synthetic mescaline (mescaline sulfate) began being manufactured by Merck under the prosaic name Mescalinium-sulfat, which led to significantly more clinical research. The studies conducted by Kurt Beringer at Heidelberg University were extensive, involving over 60 subjects who received injections of mescaline in 200-, 400-, 500-, and 600-mg doses. It ultimately led to the publication of *Der Meskalinrausch* (Mescaline Intoxication) in 1927. Heinrich Klüver's 1928 *Mescal* attempted to more coherently organize the content of the visualizations produced by mescaline. Klüver's book had a significant influence on one of the most important American biologists of the 20th century and the father of ethnobotany, Richard Evan Schultes.[7(pp131-146)]

Interest in mescaline began to wane within the scientific community, as there did not seem to be any clear therapeutic use for the drug, and regulations passed in the 1930s restricted individuals' access to the drug.[14] Despite these restrictions, mescaline use continued in certain circles, particularly among artists and intellectuals like Walter Benjamin,

Stanisław Ignacy Witkiewicz, Gheorghe Marinescu, Antonin Artaud, and Maurice Merleau-Ponty.[7(pp147-223)]

By the time, when on one bright May morning, Aldous Huxley took "four-tenths of a gram of mescalin dissolved in half a glass of water,"[15] clinical researchers had already begun turning their attention toward a new, more potent psychedelic: LSD. As noted in Chapter 3, a similar phenomenon occurred with respect to the public's interest in psychedelics. If intellectuals of the Interwar Era had dipped a toe into the world of psychedelics, and the artists and poets of the Beat Era had waded up to their torso, the hippies of the 1960s took a full plunge. Moreover, whereas the first two groups had primarily used mescaline, the latter distinctly favored LSD. In fact, it is almost impossible to retell the cultural history of the decade within the United States without referring to LSD.

Despite its low profile, mescaline use has not entirely faded. A 2016 survey estimates that 8 million individuals in the United States 12 years of age and older had used mescaline in their lifetimes, which included 5.5 million who had specifically used peyote.[16] As the NAC has only a few hundred thousand members, nonceremonial use must be more widespread than would be implied in the media.

Unfortunately, little is known of the average mescaline user outside of the context of the NAC. What is known is that they are primarily White males and that they do not seem to be using mescaline in a purely recreational manner. A survey of worldwide use conducted by Uthaug and colleagues in 2019 that involved 452 individuals who had previously used mescaline found that 83% self-described as White or Caucasian and that 76% identified as male. According to the authors, "Almost all respondents reported being motivated to consume mescaline as a means to explore their spirituality or connect with nature (74%)." Furthermore, "Most believed that mescaline had potential applications for personal growth (90%), spiritual growth (87%), psychotherapeutic work (81%), enhancing creative abilities (76%), and enhancing cognitive abilities (61%)."[16]

Pharmacology

As noted earlier, mescaline (3,4,5-trimethoxyphenethylamine) is an alkaloid. It is synthesized from the amino acid phenylalanine, making it unique among the classic psychedelics, which are more similar in structure to tryptophan.[7(p19)] Mescaline is of the phenethylamine class and is found in several species of cacti. The primary sources of mescaline are from two cacti: peyote (*L. williamsii*) and the San Pedro (*E. pachanoi*).

Mescaline is not the sole psychoactive compound in either cactus. Consequently, individuals will feel significantly different after taking isolated mescaline than after consuming a decoction made from San Pedro cacti or eating a button of peyote—even if the doses of mescaline are identical—because of the other alkaloids.

Within peyote, these alkaloids include pellotine, anhalonidine, anhalinine, and hordenine.[1] Hordenine is known to produce sympathomimetic effects and has a structural similarity to neurotransmitters adrenaline and dopamine.[9] Conversely, pellotine can cause sedation and was briefly marketed as a hypnotic agent by Boehringer & Sohn in Germany approximately 100 years ago.[9] Some of the alkaloids found in the San Pedro include tyramine, hordenine, 3-methoxytyramine, 3,4-dimethoxy-β-phenethylamine, 3,4-dimethoxy-4-hydroxy-β-phenethylamine, 3,5-dimethoxy-4-hydroxy-β-phenethylamine, anhalonidine, and anhalinine.[17]

Description

The molecular weight of mescaline is 211.26 g/mol. According to Shulgin, mescaline hydrochloride (247.71 g/mol) appears as glistening white crystals. It may also be found in the form of mescaline sulfate (309.34 g/mol), which also looks like white crystals.[18] The chemical structure of mescaline is shown in Figure 12.3.

Peyote (*peyotl* in Nahuatl) is a slow-growing cactus of blue-green, yellow-green, or reddish-green color that may be found in clumps of crowded shoots that spread up to 1 m. Dinis-Oliveira and colleagues describe these shoots as being "mostly flattened spheres with sunken shoot tips without sharp spines" and note that they can range from 2 to 7 cm in height and 4 to 12 cm in diameter.[9] Their flowers are white, slightly yellow, pink, or even reddish, whereas the fruit of the cactus is pink when fresh. The crown of the shoot barely emerges above the ground and consists of disc-shaped buttons that are harvested for use. If done properly, the cactus will recover and grow more buttons, but if done

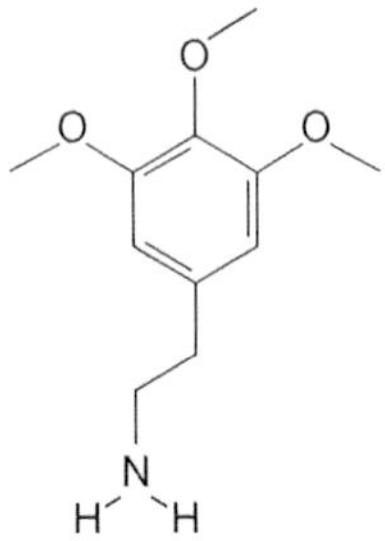

Figure 12.3 The chemical structure of mescaline.

improperly, the cactus will die. Poor harvesting techniques by people who are unfamiliar with peyote and urban sprawl have both contributed to the decline of wild peyote, which already had a relatively limited habitat ranging from central Mexico to southern Texas.[9] Calls for better conservation and more protections have been ongoing in the United States and Mexico.

The preparation of peyote buttons is relatively easy. Fresh or dried buttons can be chewed or boiled to make psychoactive tea. The mescaline content of peyote buttons is typically 0.4% when fresh and 3% to 6% when dried.[9]

San Pedro cacti (*achuma* or *huachuma* in Quechua and Aymara, respectively) are columnar cacti native to the Andes, particularly Peru, Ecuador, and Columbia.[7(p15)] They tend to grow best at 2,000 to 3,000 m. Unlike peyote, San Pedro cacti can grow quite fast and can be kept as ornamental plants in appropriate conditions.

The mescaline content of the San Pedro is significantly lower than peyote, so it is often prepared as a decoction. Slices of the cactus' stem are boiled for hours with additional herbs to make a bitter and viscous liquid. According to Mike Jay, author of *Mescaline: A Global History of the First Psychedelic*, "The dose is typically no more than mildly psychedelic in its effects: a languid, dreamy state, accompanied by mild nausea."[7(p26)]

Route of Administration

Synthetic mescaline can be swallowed, snorted, smoked/vaporized, injected, or administered rectally or sublingually. Despite the wide variety in routes of administration, it most commonly comes in the form of a tablet and is taken orally.[9] According to Uthaug and colleagues' study on the epidemiology of worldwide mescaline use, oral administration is the most common route of administration whether one is ingesting synthetic or a natural product that contains mescaline.[i] Of the 452 participants who reported previous mescaline use and took part in Uthaug's online survey, 97% of individuals said they ingested mescaline through oral ingestion.[16]

Uthaug also found that the most commonly encountered form of mescaline was the San Pedro cactus (66%), followed by peyote (36%), and then synthetic mescaline (31%).[16]

---

[i] It should be noted that there are some notable limitations with the study by Uthaug and colleagues. First, it was conducted online, which means many individuals without an internet connection or familiarity with the internet did not participate. Second, the survey assessed respondents' "most memorable experience with mescaline," so it is entirely possible (albeit doubtful) that other routes of administration produced less memorable experiences. Finally, the study included less than 10 individuals who identified as either Native American or Indigenous.

Pharmacokinetics

Mescaline is a long-acting (10-12 hours), low-potency psychedelic. It has a relatively delayed onset of action when compared to either LSD or psilocybin, with the average time of onset occurring approximately 1 hour after ingestion.[2]

Absorption

Mescaline is absorbed quickly in the gastrointestinal tract. According to Ley and colleagues, the effects may sometimes be felt in as little as 30 minutes after ingestion, though the time of onset after a 300-mg dose and 500-mg dose was found to be 0.8 ± 0.5 hour and 0.9 ± 0.6 hour.[2] Some have reported that peak effects are reached in 2 hours, but Ley and colleagues found the average time to maximal effect was 4.0 ± 1.3 hours and 3.4 ± 1.2 hours following administration of 300 mg and 500 mg, respectively.[1,2] The authors also found the mean maximum concentrations (C_{max}) in plasma for 300 mg and 500 mg doses of mescaline to be 858 ng/mL (range: 600-1,284 ng/mL) and 1,217 ng/mL (range: 721-1,822 ng/mL), respectively; the corresponding T_{max} values were 2.3 hours (range: 1.5-4.0 hours) and 2.3 hours (range: 1.5-4.0 hours), respectively; and elimination half-lives were 3.6 hours (range: 2.7-4.2 hours) and 3.6 hours (range: 2.6-4.3 hours), respectively.[2]

Distribution

Mescaline is primarily distributed to the liver where it interacts with proteins and to the kidneys, delaying its passage into the bloodstream. Mescaline has poor lipid solubility, so it does not readily transport across the blood-brain barrier, a significant reason psychedelic effects are only felt when relatively high doses are ingested.[9]

Bioavailability

The bioavailability of mescaline has not been determined.

Metabolism

Mescaline is poorly metabolized by the liver. Instead, its primary metabolic route is through oxidative deamination into 3,4,5-trimethoxyphenylacetaldehyde, which is then oxidized to form 3,4,5-trimethoxyphenylacetic acid (TMPA). Of note, both are nonpsychoactive. The enzyme responsible for deamination is unclear, though the two most likely candidates are monoamine oxidase or diamine oxidase. TMPA is then metabolized to 3,4-dihydroxy-5-methoxyphenylacetic acid via demethylation or 3,4,5-trimethoxybenzoic acid. Within the brain, mescaline is metabolized through N-acetylation into metabolites N-acetylmescaline and O-demethylated metabolites N-acetyl-3,4-dimethoxy-5-hydroxyphenylethylamine and N-acetyl-3, 4-dimethoxy-5-hydroxyphenethylamine.[9]

Elimination and Excretion

The half-life of mescaline is approximately 6 hours, with over 80% being eliminated unchanged via urine within 1 hour of ingestion, and 87% and 92% of the parent compound being found in urine within 24 hours and 48 hours of administration, respectively. The elimination of TMPA follows a similar timeline, with 87% being excreted within 24 hours and 96% being excreted within 48 hours.[9]

Pharmacodynamics

Mescaline is estimated to be 2,500 to 4,000 times less potent than LSD.[19] Consequently, doses are typically in the hundreds of milligrams rather than hundreds of micrograms, the latter being common for LSD. Surprisingly, Ley and colleagues found the disparity to be even higher. Their study indicates that similar subjective effects with LSD and mescaline were reached with doses of 100 µg and 500 mg, respectively.[2]

Peak effects occur approximately 2 to 4 hours after administration of an oral dose and may persist for a total of 8 to 12 hours, though some individuals report feeling the lingering effects of mescaline for upward of 24 hours.[2] Nausea and vomiting are common when consuming peyote and to a lesser extent San Pedro cactus. The discomfort is minimized or even eliminated with synthetic mescaline.[16]

Mechanism of Action

Like all classic psychedelics, mescaline is an agonist at serotonin 2A receptors ($5\text{-}HT_{2A}$). It also binds with $5\text{-}HT_{1A}$, $5\text{-}HT_{2B}$, and $5\text{-}HT_{2C}$ (see Table 12.1). Beyond serotonin receptors, mescaline binds with adrenergic α_{2A} receptors (as an antagonist), where it has a relatively high affinity, and at the adrenergic α_{1A} receptor (as an agonist), where it has a moderate affinity. Mescaline also demonstrates agonist activity at dopamine receptors (D_1, D_2, and D_3) and trace amine-associated receptor 1 (TAAR1). Additionally, mescaline influences intercellular levels of neurotransmitters serotonin, dopamine, and norepinephrine by binding to their transporters—serotonin transporter (SERT), dopamine transporter (DAT), and NET, respectively.[1]

Interestingly, Ley and colleagues found that mescaline and LSD significantly increased oxytocin levels in plasma when compared to

TABLE 12.1 Receptor and Monoamine Transporter–Binding Affinity of Mescaline

Receptor	Activity	Binding Affinity (K_i; μM)
5-HT$_{1A}$	Agonist	4.1
5-HT$_{2A}$	Agonist	6.3
5-HT$_{2B}$	Agonist	0.8
5-HT$_{2C}$	Agonist	17
α$_{1A}$	Agonist	>15
α$_{2B}$	Antagonist	1.4
D$_1$	Agonist	>14
D$_2$	Agonist	>10
D$_3$	Agonist	>17
TAAR1 (mouse)	Agonist	>4.2
TAAR1 (rat)	Agonist	>3
DAT	Agonist	>30
NET	Agonist	>30
SERT	Agonist	>30

5-HT, serotonin receptor; α, alpha-adrenergic receptor; D, dopamine receptor; DAT, dopamine transporter; NET, norepinephrine receptor; SERT, serotonin transporter; TAAR1, trace amine-associated receptor 1.
Adapted from Vamvakopoulou IA, Narine KAD, Campbell I, Dyck JRB, Nutt DJ. Mescaline: the forgotten psychedelic. *Neuropharmacology*. 2023;222:109294. doi:10.1016/j.neuropharm.2022.109294

placebo, but they did not observe a similar effect with psilocybin. Even more surprising, none of the substances tested in their experiment (LSD, psilocybin, or mescaline) had any effect on plasma brain-derived neurotrophic factor (BDNF) when compared to placebo.[2]

Therapeutic Index

The LD$_{50}$ for mescaline varies widely across species and routes of administration, as shown in Table 12.2. In 1962, Wolbach determined the lowest published toxic dose of mescaline to be 2.5 mg/kg (intramuscular injection) in humans.[20] However, for mice, the LD$_{50}$ for orally administered mescaline approached 1 g/kg, indicating that it is quite safe.[21]

TABLE 12.2 Mescaline LD$_{50}$ by Species

Species	Route	Dose (mg/kg)
Rhesus macaque	Intravenous	30
Dog	Intravenous	54
Rat	Intravenous	132
Rat	Subcutaneous	534
Mouse	Intravenous	157
Mouse	Oral	880

LD$_{50}$, lethal dose sufficient to kill 50% of tested animals.
Vamvakopoulou IA, Narine KAD, Campbell I, Dyck JRB, Nutt DJ. Mescaline: the forgotten psychedelic. *Neuropharmacology*. 2023;222:109294. doi:10.1016/j.neuropharm.2022.109294

Tolerance, Dependence, and Withdrawal

Tolerance to mescaline develops rapidly but dissipates within 3 to 4 days, whereas cross-tolerance to LSD and psilocybin has been widely reported in animals and humans.[9]

There is very little evidence in the literature to suggest that repeated use can lead to dependence or physical symptoms of withdrawal, though 9% of the individuals surveyed by Uthaug and colleagues reported experiencing cravings for mescaline and 3% responded that they had tried to quit or reduce their consumption of mescaline at least once.[16] Contrarily, 0% reported seeking medical treatment as a result of mescaline use, less than 1% reported having been in therapy/psychiatric treatment due to mescaline use, and 1% reported encounters with law enforcement due to their use of mescaline.[16]

Subjective Effects

The qualitative differences in nonordinary states of consciousness are similar for mescaline, LSD, and psilocybin.[2] Similar to LSD, synesthesia is quite common with mescaline, as is "geometrization" of objects, which may become distorted or flattened in a manner similar to a Cubist painting.[9] The colors of existing objects are said to become significantly brighter, and individuals may see kaleidoscopic imagery when their eyes are closed and, in some cases, open. Time distortion, ego dissolution, and experiences of transcendence or communication with perceived spiritual beings (eg, God, spirits, demons, souls of ancestors) may also occur.[7]

Like other psychedelics, patients may experience feelings ranging from euphoria to terror, with anxiety and panic attacks being reported as the effects of the drug intensify. Uthaug's survey, while uncontrolled for the route of administration or dose, found that most individuals experienced "moderate" mystical-type effects and "slight" ego dissolution, though many reported that the experience was spiritually significant (especially among those who had consumed peyote).[16]

Mescaline also had enduring effects on individuals' prior psychiatric conditions, with reported symptom improvements in depression and anxiety, as well as reductions in symptoms for disorders like posttraumatic stress disorder (PTSD) and substance use disorders.[16] Flashbacks have been reported only rarely. However, after a mescaline session in 1935, Jean-Paul Sartre, the French philosopher and Nobel-winning novelist, reportedly felt as though some kinds of mutant crustaceans were following him for several years following an experiment with mescaline.[7(pp149-168)] He evidently spoke with his good friend Jacques Lacan about it.[22]

Somatic Effects

Somatic effects are similar to other classic psychedelics. Following the administration of mescaline, individuals experience increases in body temperature, higher systolic blood pressure, and pupil dilation (mydriasis). Additionally, individuals may experience sleep difficulty for many hours even after the acute effects have dissipated.

Therapeutic Indications

Mescaline is a Schedule I drug, and currently has no established use for any clinical condition.

Potential Uses

Despite its use within indigenous communities and its historical use within clinical settings, mescaline has attracted very little attention from clinicians within the last two decades. However, anecdotal reports from members of the NAC say that individuals with substance use disorders, particularly alcohol use disorder, who participate in peyote ceremonies have experienced improvements in symptoms.[7] Unsurprisingly, these ceremonies parallel the psychedelic paradigm described by Bravo and Grob that was discussed in previous chapters.[23]

Individuals who took part in Uthaug's survey reported improvements in several conditions as well. Of those with preexisting depression ($n = 184$), 86% reported symptom improvement, while 80% of those with preexisting anxiety ($n = 167$) reported symptom improvement. Among those with PTSD ($n = 55$), 76% reported symptom improvement, while 76% of those with alcohol use disorder ($n = 48$) reported symptom improvement. Lastly, 68% of those with an unspecified drug use disorder ($n = 48$) reported symptom improvement.[16] However, clinical trials are needed to confirm these findings.

Precautions and Adverse Effects

As is the case with any psychedelic, individuals with a personal or family history of severe and persistent mental illnesses or existing psychiatric comorbidities that make them more susceptible to psychosis should be extremely cautious when using psychedelics. Even in healthy individuals who view psychedelics in a positive light, difficult experiences can happen.

According to Ley and colleagues, the most common acute adverse effects of mescaline include fatigue, nausea, headache, lack of energy, loss of appetite, difficulty concentrating, and feelings of weakness (see Table 12.3). Symptoms of overintoxication from mescaline can resemble sympathomimetic toxidrome—hyperreflexia, tachycardia, sialorrhea, agitation, ataxia, muscle stiffness, seizures, hyperthermia, and paresthesia.[9] Given the potential for increased cardiovascular stress, individuals with heart disease may not be good candidates for psychedelic therapy with mescaline.

Among healthy individuals, repeated use of mescaline does not appear to be associated with neurocognitive or psychological problems. Navajo members of the NAC who reported long-term peyote use ($n = 61$) showed no deficits when compared to members of the Navajo tribe who reported limited use of peyote, alcohol, or other substances ($n = 79$).[19]

Risk of Overdose

For mescaline, the risk of overdose is low, especially when it is administered as part of a religious ceremony or in a clinical setting. At this time, only two human deaths have been attributed to mescaline. One individual died as a consequence of bronchial aspiration of vomit during a Peyote ceremony. Their antemortem blood concentration of mescaline was 0.48 µg/mL.[21] The second individual fell off a cliff while under the

TABLE 12.3 Acute Adverse Drug Effects in Mescaline Versus Placebo

	Mescaline[a] (n = 32)			Placebo (n = 32)		
	0 h	0-12 h	12-24 h	0 h	0-12 h	12-24 h
Fatigue	15	26	26	15	21	20
Headache	0	20	19	2	10	9
Lack of energy	0	20	10	0	3	2
Lack of concentration	0	18	5	0	0	1
Dullness	2	15	9	0	3	1
Nausea	0	21	2	0	1	1
Inner tension	1	15	5	3	1	1
Feeling of weakness	0	17	3	0	1	1
Inner restlessness	1	12	7	0	1	2
Loss of appetite	0	19	6	0	1	1
Freezing	0	16	0	1	1	1
Troubled balance	0	12	1	0	0	0
Dry mouth	0	11	1	1	0	1
Exhaustibility	0	13	4	0	0	1
Trembling	0	16	0	0	0	0
Bruxism, jaw rigidity	1	12	2	0	0	1
Hypersensitivity to certain smells	0	8	2	1	0	0
Abdominal bloating or fullness	0	9	4	0	0	1
Dizziness	0	7	1	0	0	0
Shortness of breath	0	6	0	0	0	0
Heart palpitations	0	6	0	0	1	0
Ravenous appetite	0	5	0	1	0	0
Perspiration	0	4	0	0	0	0
Chest pain	0	2	1	0	0	0

[a]Figures include two different doses of mescaline: one 300 mg and one 500 mg.
Ley L, Holze F, Arikci D, et al. Comparative acute effects of mescaline, lysergic acid diethylamide, and psilocybin in a randomized, double-blind, placebo-controlled cross-over study in healthy participants. *Neuropsychopharmacology.* 2023;48(11):1659-1667. doi:10.1038/s41386-023-01607-2

TABLE 12.4 Drugs Associated With Elevated Serotonin Levels and Serotonin Syndrome

Drug Type	Examples
Analgesics	Fentanyl, meperidine, pentazocine, tramadol
Antibiotics	Linezolid, ritonavir
Anticonvulsants	Valproate
Antidepressants	Buspirone, clomipramine, nefazodone, trazodone, venlafaxine
Antiemetics	Granisetron, metoclopramide, ondansetron
Antimigraine medications	Sumatriptan
Bariatric drugs	Sibutramine
Monoamine oxidase inhibitors	Clorgiline, isocarboxazid, moclobemide, phenelzine
Over-the-counter drugs	Dextromethorphan
Selective serotonin reuptake inhibitors	Citalopram, fluoxetine, fluvoxamine, paroxetine, sertraline

influence of mescaline. Concentrations in the blood, liver, and urine were 9.7, 70.8, and 1,163 µg/mL, respectively.[21] For reference, among the 16 individuals in the Ley study, the mean C_{max} for a 500-mg dose of mescaline was reported to be 1,217 ng/mL (1.217 µg/mL).[2]

Drug Interactions

There is very little clinical evidence about drug-drug interactions with mescaline. As mescaline targets serotonin receptors, individuals who are on antidepressant drugs that affect serotonin (see Table 12.4) may be at risk of developing serotonin syndrome if mescaline is taken concurrently. There is also some evidence to suggest that the coadministration of classic psychedelics with lithium may increase the risk of seizure.[24]

Pregnant and Nursing Women

There is insufficient evidence indicating that mescaline is safe for pregnant or nursing individuals. Consequently, it is not advised that individuals who are pregnant, may become pregnant, or are currently nursing consume mescaline.

Dosage and Administration

According to some accounts, an effective oral dosage of synthetic mescaline falls within the range of 200 to 400 mg.[16] This is approximately equivalent to the mescaline content found in three to six buttons or 10 to 20 g of dried peyote.[9] That said, Ley and colleagues found that a dose of 300 mg was insufficient to compare to the experience of psilocybin or LSD at doses of 20 mg or 100 µg, respectively, but found that a dose of 500 mg was comparable to the aforementioned doses of psilocybin and LSD.[2]

Conclusion

Clinical research into the potential applications of mescaline has been inadequate, and other psychedelics have received significantly more attention. However, like other psychedelics, mescaline appears to be capable of producing mystical-type experiences, it is safe when administered in controlled settings, and there is evidence to suggest that it can help treat psychiatric disorders that are notoriously resistant to conventional treatments. Additionally, mescaline has an exceptionally long history of regular use among indigenous individuals throughout the Americas without leading to widespread problems, strongly suggesting that it is largely free of insidious effects. What remains to be seen is what unique therapeutic qualities mescaline possesses with respect to other classic psychedelics like LSD and psilocybin. To better understand this, more clinical research will be necessary.

REFERENCES

1. Vamvakopoulou IA, Narine KAD, Campbell I, Dyck JRB, Nutt DJ. Mescaline: the forgotten psychedelic. *Neuropharmacology*. 2023;222:109294. doi:10.1016/j.neuropharm.2022.109294
2. Ley L, Holze F, Arikci D, et al. Comparative acute effects of mescaline, lysergic acid diethylamide, and psilocybin in a randomized, double-blind, placebo-controlled cross-over study in healthy participants. *Neuropsychopharmacology*. 2023;48(11):1659-1667. doi:10.1038/s41386-023-01607-2

3. Clement BA, Goff CM, Forbes TDA. Toxic amines and alkaloids from *Acacia rigidula*. *Phytochemistry*. 1998;49(5):1377-1380. doi:10.1016/S0031-9422(97)01022-4
4. Pawar RS, Grundel E, Fardin-Kia AR, Rader JI. Determination of selected biogenic amines in *Acacia rigidula* plant materials and dietary supplements using LC-MS/MS methods. *J Pharm Biomed Anal*. 2014;88:457-466. doi:10.1016/j.jpba.2013.09.012. PMID: 24176750.
5. Pinto Nde C, Duque AP, Pacheco NR, Mendes Rde F, Motta EV, Bellozi PM, Ribeiro A, Salvador MJ, Scio E. *Pereskia aculeata*: a plant food with antinociceptive activity. *Pharm Biol*. 2015;53(12):1780-1785. doi:10.3109/13880209.2015.1008144. PMID: 26084799.
6. Lynch TF. *Guitarrero Cave: Early Man in the Andes*. Academic Press; 1980.
7. Jay M. *Mescaline: A Global History of the First Psychedelic*. Yale University Press; 2021.
8. El-Seedi HR, De Smet PA, Beck O, Possnert G, Bruhn JG. Prehistoric peyote use: alkaloid analysis and radiocarbon dating of archaeological specimens of Lophophora from Texas. *J Ethnopharmacol*. 2005;101(1-3):238-242. doi:10.1016/j.jep.2005.04.022. PMID: 15990261.
9. Dinis-Oliveira RJ, Pereira CL, da Silva DD. Pharmacokinetic and pharmacodynamic aspects of peyote and mescaline: clinical and forensic repercussions. *Curr Mol Pharmacol*. 2019;12(3):184-194. doi:10.2174/1874467211666181010154139. PMID: 30318013; PMCID: PMC6864602.
10. Coulter JM. A preliminary revision of the North American species of cactus, *Anhalonium* and *Lophophora*. Accessed April 8, 2024. https://www.living-rocks.com/coulter.htm
11. Prentiss DW, Morgan FP. Anhalonium lewinii (mescal buttons). A study of the drug, with especial reference to its physiological action upon man, with report of experiments. *Ther Gnz*. 1895;11(9). Accessed February 6, 2024. https://collections.nlm.nih.gov/bookviewer?PID=nlm:nlmuid-101751140-bk
12. United States Congress. Peyote: hearings before a subcommittee of the Committee on Indian Affairs of the House of Representatives on H.R. 2614 to amend sections 2139 and 2140 of the revised statutes and the acts amendatory thereof, and for other purposes pt. 1-2. 1918. Accessed April 6, 2024. https://babel.hathitrust.org/cgi/pt?id=coo1.ark:/13960/t8qc0mc72&seq=59
13. Hoffman A. *LSD: My Problem Child*. Multidisciplinary Association for Psychedelic Studies (MAPS); 2009:70.
14. United Nations Division of Narcotics. Bulletin on Narcotics. 1959;11(2) . Accessed April 6, 2024. https://www.unodc.org/documents/data-and-analysis/bulletin/BullOnNarc-XI-No-2-June-1959.pdf
15. Huxley A. *The Doors of Perception & Heaven and Hell*. HarperCollins Publishers; 2009:12.
16. Uthaug MV, Davis AK, Haas TF, et al. The epidemiology of mescaline use: pattern of use, motivations for consumption, and perceived consequences, benefits, and acute and enduring subjective effects. *J Psychopharmacol*. 2022;36(3):309-320. doi:10.1177/02698811211013583. PMID: 33949246; PMCID: PMC8902264.
17. Crosby DM, McLaughlin JL. Cactus alkaloids. XIX. Crystallization of mescaline HCl and 3-methoxytyramine HCl from *Trichocereus pachanoi*. *Lloydia*. 1973;36(4):416-418. PMID: 4773270.
18. Shulgin A, Shulgin A. *PiHKAL: A Chemical Love Story*. Transform Press; 2022:703.
19. Halpern JH, Sherwood AR, Hudson JI, Yurgelun-Todd D, Pope HG Jr. Psychological and cognitive effects of long-term peyote use among Native Americans. *Biol Psychiatry*. 2005;58(8):624-631. doi:10.1016/j.biopsych.2005.06.038. PMID: 16271313.
20. Wolbach AB Jr, Miner EJ, Isbell H. Comparison of psilocin with psilocybin, mescaline and LSD-25. *Psychopharmacologia*. 1962;3:219-223.
21. Henríquez-Hernández LA, Rojas-Hernández J, Quintana-Hernández DJ, Borkel LF. Hofmann vs. Paracelsus: do psychedelics defy the basics of toxicology?—a systematic review of the main ergolamines, simple tryptamines, and phenylethylamines. *Toxics*. 2023;11(2):148. doi:10.3390/toxics11020148

22. New York Times. When Sartre talked to crabs (it was mescaline). Published November 14, 2009. Accessed April 6, 2024. https://www.nytimes.com/2009/11/15/weekinreview/15grist.html
23. Bravo G, Grob C. Shamans, sacraments, and psychiatrists. *J Psychoactive Drugs*. 1989;21(1):123-128. doi:10.1080/02791072.1989.10472149
24. Nayak SM, Gukasyan N, Barrett FS, Erowid E, Erowid F, Griffiths RR. Classic psychedelic coadministration with lithium, but not lamotrigine, is associated with seizures: an analysis of online psychedelic experience reports. *Pharmacopsychiatry*. 2021;54(5):240-245. doi:10.1055/a-1524-2794. PMID: 34348413.

13

Ibogaine

Ibogaine is a tryptamine psychedelic derived from the root bark of *Tabernanthe iboga*, a shrub that grows naturally in Central and West Africa. It is an indole alkaloid that has been used by indigenous peoples for centuries primarily in modern-day Gabon as an entheogen, as well as a medicine to treat both acute conditions like fatigue and chronic conditions like diabetes.[1] During the 20th century, anecdotal evidence began to emerge that ibogaine could be characterized as an "addiction interrupter" that facilitated opioid detoxification.[2] In addition to mitigating some of the most severe symptoms associated with withdrawal, the psychotropic effects of ibogaine felt while under its influence helped many people abstain from heroin use following detoxification. These anecdotal reports were eventually backed up by preliminary studies, and there is now interest in ibogaine's potential applications not only in treating opioid withdrawal and substance use disorders but also in treating posttraumatic stress disorder (PTSD).

Ibogaine is not regulated in many African countries, which has led to some degree of ibogaine tourism, particularly in Gabon. Similarly, ibogaine's use is unregulated in countries like the Netherlands, Portugal, Costa Rica, Panama, Mexico, and several nations in the Caribbean, where a handful of clinics offering ibogaine treatment and supportive services have sprung up. The ibogaine experience is more protracted than most other drugs discussed in this book. Many describe it as being physically unpleasant, but spiritually rewarding. It occurs over the course of multiple days and is accompanied by trance-like states, ataxia, and excessive vomiting, which have traditionally been incorporated into a ritualization of death and rebirth by practitioners of the Bwiti religion, for whom the iboga plant is considered a sacrament. The subjective effects of ibogaine are strongly oneiric (dream-like), and the content of the visions tends to resemble Jungian archetypes. Consequently, ibogaine is sometimes referred to as a "oneirophrenic" drug.[2]

Even though ibogaine was first isolated well over a century ago, the pharmacology of the compound has not been well studied, and many questions persist about its mechanisms of action and safety. Ibogaine presents significant risks to those who take it, as cardiac complications have been reported following use. Consequently, individuals with cardiovascular disease may not be ideal candidates for treatment with ibogaine. Another concern is that the effects of ibogaine primarily derive from the action of the pharmacologically active metabolite noribogaine, which is produced following first-pass metabolism of the parent compound in the liver via cytochrome P450 (CYP) enzyme CYP2D6. Testing to confirm if individuals are poor metabolizers prior to administering ibogaine is strongly encouraged, as ingestion of standard doses of ibogaine may result in extremely long-lasting effects.[3]

History

Ibogaine is an alkaloid found in the iboga plant (*Tabernanthe iboga*), with the highest concentrations occurring in the plant's root bark. The iboga plant has a long history of ceremonial and medicinal use in Central and West African nations like the Republic of Congo, Cameroon, and especially Gabon. Archaeological evidence indicates that the iboga plant has been used medicinally by people within present-day Gabon for at least 2,000 years.[4] It is unclear if use elsewhere dates back that far.

Within the oral tradition of the region, the first people to discover the effects of the iboga plant were Pygmy hunters from the Mbenge ethnic group, who recognized that chewing on the roots of the plant had a pronounced effect on mountain gorillas.[5] The Mbenge realized that lower doses could be used to ward off hunger, thirst, and fatigue, while larger amounts of the root could induce profound changes in perception and nonordinary states of consciousness. They then passed this knowledge on to Bantu peoples in modern-day Gabon.

Iboga and the Bwiti Tradition

Ibogaine experiences have become central to practitioners of Bwiti, which is a loosely defined belief system that has spread throughout the region, though it is primarily practiced in Gabon and formally recognized as a religion by the Gabonese government. It is estimated that 5% of the nation's 2.3 million people formally practice the religion, and many more practice it in a more casual manner.[4] It is also possible that many of the individuals who profess to practice Bwiti also claim to practice Christianity or another religion because Bwiti lacks specific doctrines or hierarchies and, moreover, is decentralized and focused on self-improvement and spiritual discovery rather than adherence to strict dogmas.[5] Bwiti may include elements of Christianity, Islam, and indigenous religious traditions in syncretized form.[5] On account of this lack of hierarchy, Goutarel and colleagues report that there are distinctions between Bwiti initiation ceremonies among different ethnic groups such as the Mitsogo and the Fang. As an example, for the Mitsogo, full participation in iboga ceremonies is reserved only for men, though women are allowed to take smaller doses capable of producing milder or less revelatory visions. For the Fang, there are no restrictions placed on women.[6]

In practice, there are significant parallels between the Bwiti religion's relationship with iboga and the Native American Church's relationship with peyote (*Lophophora williamsii*). Perhaps most saliently, the iboga plant is often conceptualized as a spiritual entity or teacher plant capable of revealing to the initiate a separate realm where one can experience visions and gain insights about themselves and their place in the universe. According to Alper, the ritualistic consumption of iboga should be conceptualized as a means of connecting the individual to the tapestry of the community through a shared psychedelic experience. This connection extends not only to currently living people but also to one's ancestors and has helped cement the iboga plant as part of the Gabonese national identity following colonialization.[7] Despite its centrality to Gabonese identity, individuals from outside of the region can participate in Bwiti initiation ceremonies, which is why iboga tourism has been growing in Gabon and nearby nations.

Bwiti initiation rituals typically involve ceremonial purification/death of the initiate, followed by a rebirth once the peak effects of the drug have subsided.[5] During iboga ceremonies, the scrapings of the root bark of the iboga plant are consumed in a preparation referred to locally as *eboga* or *eboka* that is high in ibogaine and induces a trance-like state.[7] During the height of the ceremony when the drug's effects peak, individuals tend to describe the experience as oneiric or likened to a waking dream. They may also lose consciousness. Individuals frequently report interacting with the spirit of the iboga plant, Jungian archetypes, specific deities like Jesus Christ, their own ancestors, and versions of themselves from previous lives. Some have also reported experiencing an autobiographical and often chronologic slideshow of their life in vivid detail ("panoramic memory") and near-death experiences.[7] Although symbolic death is central to the ritual, practitioners of Bwiti believe that those who enter the ceremony with impure intentions may not survive.[8] Adverse cardiac events leading to death have been reported (as described in the "Pharmacology" section).

Like peyote in the Native American Church, individuals may continue to take iboga during communal ceremonies, to treat medical conditions, or for spiritual development.[5] Ceremonies oftentimes involve rhythmic drumming, singing, and dancing, and the acute effects of the drug may be felt for upward of 24 to 36 hours. A "residual phase" may persist for as long as 72 hours. Individuals may have trouble sleeping following the ceremony and may need several days to recover. In some cases, sleep difficulties may persist for months.[6]

Ibogaine in Europe

Europeans became aware of the iboga plant and its religious and medicinal purposes during the 19th century, but ibogaine was not synthesized until 1901 (by Dybowski and Landrin).[6] Initial interest in ibogaine among French pharmacologists was short lived, lasting only the first decade of the 20th century. There was a resurgence in interest in the 1930s, culminating in the introduction of Lambarène, a product sold in France starting in 1939 that contained 8 mg of ibogaine (doses that induce the psychedelic effects described throughout this chapter are several orders of magnitude higher, often in the range of 500-1,000 mg).[6]

The formulation was marketed as a "neuromuscular stimulant" to treat fatigue, depression, and infectious diseases.[2] Following World War II, Lambarène became known for its stimulating effects among athletes and was eventually banned by the International Olympic Committee, as well as other athletic organizations.[6] Lambarène was removed from the French market in 1966 and was classified by the World Health Assembly in 1968 as a drug capable of producing dependency or impairing human health.[6]

The Legacy of Howard Lotsof

In June 1962, Howard Lotsof was a 19-year-old film student and regular heroin user with no medical background. One day, he and several friends decided to experiment with a drug they had heard very little about, ibogaine. During the time that he was under the influence of the drug, he did not use heroin. In fact, to Lotsof's surprise, he emerged from the experience without sensing the oncoming symptoms of withdrawal and without the desire to continue using heroin. Remarkably, Lotsof would remain opioid free for the rest of his life.[2]

To see if the experience was a unique instance of serendipity or a characteristic of ibogaine, Lotsof gave 500-mg doses of ibogaine to six friends who were also regular heroin users. Five of them managed to quit using heroin.[9] As is the case with other drugs discussed in this book, many people walk away from the experience with insight into their addictive and self-destructive tendencies, which is believed to be at least partially responsible for ibogaine's efficacy.[10]

Even though ibogaine was among the many hallucinogenic substances made illegal in the 1960s before being classified as Schedule I drugs by the Controlled Substances Act of 1970, Lotsof worked tirelessly to investigate the efficacy of ibogaine and lobby for the end of its prohibition over the next two decades. His work led him to believe that ibogaine could help individuals with a variety of substance use disorders (eg, cocaine use disorder, alcohol use disorder) and end their addictions. In the 1980s, Lotsof began working with a Belgian drug company to manufacture ibogaine, which was then administered to patients in the Netherlands.[9] Lotsof's work also led the National Institute on Drug Abuse (NIDA) to conduct preclinical studies in the 1980s and into the early 1990s.[11]

In 1993, the Food and Drug Administration (FDA) gave approval to Dr Deborah C. Mash of the Leonard M. Miller School of Medicine at the University of Miami to run a clinical trial to assess the safety of ibogaine in treating patients diagnosed with cocaine use disorder. Unfortunately, a nonstudy-related death following ibogaine administration in the Netherlands disrupted the investigation, and a lack of private and public funding led to the discontinuation of the trial.[10] The death, possibly attributable to posttreatment heroin use, exacerbated existing safety concerns about ibogaine's potential to cause arrhythmia, leading NIDA to cease research into ibogaine in 1995.[12] To date, no clinical trials involving ibogaine in the United States have been completed.[11] However, Mash and others operate clinics outside of the United States, where individuals can receive treatment with ibogaine.

Like all drugs discussed in his book, interest in ibogaine has surged in recent years. Among Americans, there has been some interest in using the drug to grow spiritually, but this is often secondary to using it as a means to treat substance use disorders or PTSD. Interest in iboga alkaloids like ibogaine has been accompanied by the development of synthetic ibogaine congeners that include 18-methoxycoronaridine (18-MC) and tabernanthalog.[12]

The Iboga Trade

As noted earlier, interest in ibogaine has spread well beyond Africa, and many rehabilitation clinics in nations where iboga is not regulated currently use ibogaine in a medical setting. As noted in the introduction to this chapter, some of these countries include the Netherlands, Portugal, Costa Rica, Panama, Mexico, and nations in the Caribbean, such as St. Kitts and Nevis. Unfortunately, the increase in demand has led to an illicit trade in iboga that involves smuggling the whole plant out of Gabon and then selling the root via the internet at an inflated price. There are concerns that growing international demand for iboga, whether harvested legally or not, will ultimately push its price beyond the range of individuals in Gabon or the surrounding nations, potentially disrupting the lives of Bwiti practitioners.[4]

Within recent years, there have been attempts to make the iboga market more beneficial to Gabonese farmers and to use proceeds from the sale of iboga to benefit rural areas within Gabon.[4] The hope is that a better-regulated iboga market will ensure a sustainable and affordable supply of iboga for future practitioners of the Bwiti religion.

Pharmacology

Ibogaine belongs to a family of several dozen related monoterpene indole alkaloids known as iboga alkaloids, which are primarily found in West Africa.[13] These compounds are derived from tryptamine and occur in plants within the *Apocynaceae* family. Iboga alkaloids have been found in plants from the *Apocynaceae* family in Asia, Australia, and the Americas.[13] While ibogaine has attracted the most attention, other iboga alkaloids of note that appear in the iboga plant include ibogamine and voacangine. The former may have a pharmacology similar to ibogaine, while the latter can be used to produce ibogaine via semi-synthesis.[13]

Ibogaine's active metabolite, noribogaine, is believed to significantly contribute to the psychotropic and therapeutic effects of ibogaine.

Description

Tabernanthe iboga is believed to have the highest concentrations of ibogaine of any plant. It is an evergreen shrub and may grow up to 2 m

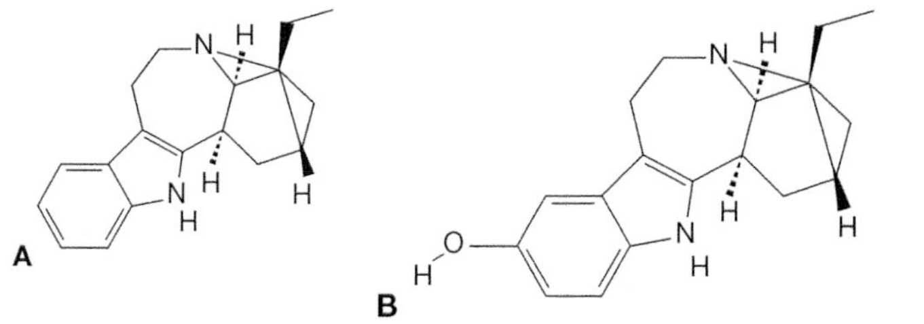

Figure 13.1 The chemical structures of ibogaine (left) and noribogaine (right).

in height, and it produces clusters of yellow or pinkish flowers and small fruits that resemble bulbous chili peppers. The fruits may be yellow or orange in color and are edible but contain very little or no iboga alkaloids.

Traditional preparations of iboga come in the form of a powder derived from the dried shavings of the root bark of *T. iboga*, as the root bark contains the highest concentrations of ibogaine. Unfortunately, these concentrations are still quite small—ibogaine accounts for between 0.3% and 1.93% of the root bark by dry weight.[1,13]

Isolated ibogaine appears as a white to off-white powder and has a molecular weight of 310.4 g/mol and 346.9 for its hydrochloride salt. Noribogaine's molecular weight is 296.4 g/mol, while its hydrochloride salt is 332.9 g/mol.[10] The chemical structure of both molecules is shown in Figure 13.1.

Route of Administration

Ibogaine is typically consumed orally by ingesting the root bark of the *T. iboga*. In a traditional setting, the root may be consumed whole, powdered, or within a mixture. It is possible that some traditional mixtures may contain other psychotropic substances.

Single doses of ibogaine in clinical settings typically come in the form of pills and range from 500 to 1,000 mg.

Pharmacokinetics

Absorption

Ibogaine reaches peak plasma levels (C_{max}) 2 hours after oral administration, reaching a free maximum plasma concentration of 300 to 1,250 ng/mL.[12] The active metabolite noribogaine is first detected in the brain within 15 minutes of oral administration and reaches a C_{max} of 700 to 1,200 ng/mL approximately 5 hours after ingestion.[12]

Distribution

Ibogaine is lipophilic and concentrates in adipose tissue at levels higher than in plasma or the central nervous system (CNS) and is rapidly distributed to organ tissue, including the spleen, liver, heart, and kidneys.[10] The highest concentrations of noribogaine are in the spleen following intragastric administration of ibogaine and in the liver following the intragastric administration of noribogaine.[10] The parent compound has a plasma protein binding of 65%.[14]

Bioavailability

Preclinical studies indicate that the bioavailability of ibogaine has a nonlinear association with dosing. In rats, bioavailability was 7% in males and 16% in females when ibogaine was administered orally in doses of 5 mg/kg, while oral doses of 50 mg/kg resulted in bioavailability of 43% in males and 71% in females.[15] Mean area under curves (AUCs) were 45 to 59 times greater at 50 mg/kg than 5 mg/kg.[15]

Although there were clear disparities between sexes in rodent models, it is not clear to what extent these disparities exist in humans.

Metabolism

Ibogaine is converted to the active metabolite noribogaine during first-pass metabolism in the liver through *O*-demethylation via cytochrome P450 liver enzyme 2D6 (CYP2D6) and to a lesser extent CYP2C9 and CYP3A4.[15] Metabolization also occurs via the gut wall and potentially the kidney and brain.[10]

Elimination and Excretion

The half-life of ibogaine is 4 to 7 hours, and it is estimated that 90% of the parent compound is eliminated within 24 hours.[15] Noribogaine has a significantly longer half-life of 28 to 49 hours, suggesting the active metabolite plays a significant role in the subjective experience and some of the pharmacologic actions attributed to ibogaine. Less than 5% of ibogaine is believed to be excreted unchanged in urine (according to rat models) and 15% is excreted after 24 hours, most likely as noribogaine.[10] It remains unclear how ibogaine is excreted.

Pharmacodynamics

The pharmacodynamics of ibogaine and noribogaine are complex. Although each drug discussed in this book has a unique mechanism of action, ibogaine and noribogaine are distinct from the classic psychedelics (eg, psilocybin, lysergic acid diethylamide [LSD], and mescaline), empathogens like 3,4-methylenedioxymethamphetamine (MDMA), and arylcyclohexylamines like ketamine and phencyclidine (PCP).

However, as this section will reveal, there are some overlaps. Similar to ketamine, ibogaine and noribogaine are active at *N*-methyl-D-aspartate (NMDA) receptors. Ibogaine and noribogaine also block the reuptake of serotonin (like MDMA), by binding to serotonin transporters (SERTs), though ibogaine shows limited affinity for serotonin receptors while noribogaine shows no activity at serotonin receptors. As noted in previous chapters on classic psychedelics, their primary mechanism of action is agonistic activity at 5-HT_{2A} receptors. For ibogaine, it is believed that the psychoactive/oneiric effects are mediated through activity at κ opioid receptors.

In animal and human models, the drug decreases the rewarding effects of opioids and appears to reduce the severity of opioid withdrawal. Some studies have found that withdrawal signs are more pronounced when ibogaine is administered in a manner that bypasses first-pass metabolism, thus avoiding the conversion of ibogaine to noribogaine. This suggests that noribogaine plays a central role in blocking withdrawal signs.[10] Animal studies have also shown that ibogaine dose-dependently blocks self-administration of nicotine, ethanol, and stimulants, strongly suggesting that the antiaddictive properties of ibogaine are mediated across multiple receptor systems.

Mechanism of Action

The mechanism of action of ibogaine and noribogaine remains only partially understood, but research has found both compounds interact with a variety of receptor systems (see Table 13.1). Ibogaine inhibits dopamine transporters (DATs), SERTs, and vesicular monoamine transporters, leading to increases in extracellular dopamine and serotonin. The blockade of SERTs is a similar mechanism of action for selective serotonin reuptake inhibitors (SSRIs), which are among the most widely used antidepressant medications in the world. Of note, ibogaine's inhibition of SERT is noncompetitive, which is unique, as all other known inhibitors are competitive with substrate.[10] Meanwhile, the blockade of DATs is believed to play a role in altering reward pathways and could help curb cravings in substance use disorders.[10]

Ibogaine also demonstrates open-channel antagonism at NMDA receptors. This antagonism of NMDA receptors is central to the dissociative effects of ketamine and is believed to account for some of its antidepressant effects, suggesting that ibogaine may have similar potential as a treatment for depressive disorders, though clinical evidence is currently lacking.[10]

TABLE 13.1 Binding-Site Affinities of Ibogaine and Noribogaine

Target	Ibogaine (K_i; IC_{50} (μM))	Noribogaine (K_i; IC_{50} (μM))	Pharmacodynamics
Monoamines			
SERT ([^{3}H]5-HT reuptake; rat)	0.5	0.3	Serotonin reuptake blocker
SERT (Paroxetine binding; human)	2.0	0.9	Serotonin reuptake blocker
SERT (RTI-55-cocaine analog binding; human)	0.5	0.04	Serotonin reuptake blocker
SERT (RTI-55-cocaine analog; rat)	0.2	0.2	Serotonin reuptake blocker
SERT (RTI-55-cocaine analog; HeLa cells)	2.5	N/A	Serotonin reuptake blocker, noncompetitive
5-HT2 (Ketanserin binding; rat cortex)	4.8; >100	Inactive	Unknown
5-HT3 (GR65630; N1 E-115 cells; area postrema)	3.8; >100	Inactive	Unknown
DAT (RTI-55-cocaine analog; human)	1.5-4.0	3.4	Dopamine reuptake blocker
Opioid Receptors			
μ (Naloxone binding, mouse forebrain; rat thalamus)	0.13-3.6	5.8	Agonist; partial agonist; mixed agonist-antagonist
μ (DAMGO binding, rat; DAGO calf cortex; human cortex)	5.6-11.0	1.5	Antagonist
HEK MOR cells; DAMGO	19	1.1; 0.2	
κ (U69,593 binding, human)	2.0-4.0	0.7	Partial agonist; biased agonist

Receptor/Assay	Value	Classification
δ (DPDPE, calf caudate)	>100	Unknown
σ Receptors		
σ-1 (guinea pig brain membranes; Pentazocine binding, human cerebellum)	24.7	Unknown
σ-1 (guinea pig brain membranes; Pentazocine binding, human cerebellum)	10	Inactive
σ-2 (rat liver membranes; guinea pig brain membranes)	0.10; 0.2–0.3	Inactive
Nicotinic Ionotropic Receptors		
Ganglionic (PC-12 cell line, human; NA+ influx)	0.02	Inhibitor, noncompetitive
$\alpha_3\beta_4$ nAChR (HEK cells, human)	0.22–1.0; 3.7	Inhibitor, noncompetitive antagonist (desensitized and resting state)
$\alpha_3\beta_4$ nAChR (SH-SY5Y cells)	5.2; 9.8	Inhibitor, noncompetitive antagonist (desensitized and resting state)
NMDA Receptors		
MK-801 (rat cortex; rat forebrain)	1.0; 2.3; 3.2	Channel blocker
MK-801 (human caudate; frog spinal cord)	5.2; 9.8	Channel blocker
Voltage dependent (rat hippocampal cells)	3.2	Channel blocker

DAGO: [D-Ala2,N-Me-Phe4,Gly-ollenkephalin; DAMGO: [D-Ala2,NMePhe4,Gly-ollenkephalin]; DAT, dopamine transporter; DPDPE: d-Pen2,d-Pen5 enkephalin; IC$_{50}$, half-maximal inhibitory concentration; HEK MOR: human embryonic kidney (HEK) 293 cells expressing human mu opioid receptors (MOR); K_i, inhibitory constant; N/A: Not applicable; nAChR, nicotinic acetylcholine receptor; RTI: research trial item; SERT, serotonin transporter.

The K_i or IC$_{50}$ values from ligand binding and functional assays and the agonist/antagonist classifications are taken from DemeRx Laboratory studies, Caliper Safety Pharmacology screen for binding-site activity, and published references cited in Mash DC. IUPHAR—invited review—ibogaine—a legacy within the current renaissance of psychedelic therapy. *Pharmacol Res*. 2023;190:106620. doi:10.1016/j.phrs.2022.106620

Courtesy of Mash DC. IUPHAR—invited review—ibogaine—a legacy within the current renaissance of psychedelic therapy. *Pharmacol Res*. 2023;190:106620. doi:10.1016/j.phrs.2022.106520

Other sites of activity for ibogaine include opioid, nicotinic acetylcholine, and σ receptors.[12] Agonistic or partial agonistic activity at μ, κ, and δ opioid receptors may account for the mitigation of opioid withdrawal symptoms, as well as treating substance use disorders.[12] Inhibitory activity at nicotinic receptors, specifically $α_3β_4$ receptors, may contribute to ibogaine's antiaddictive properties.[10] Ibogaine has a high affinity for σ-2 receptors, and to a lesser extent σ-1 receptors, but the pharmacologic effects of this relationship are not well understood. σ-2 ligands have been proposed as treatments for cancer and Alzheimer disease, and they may also play a role in cholesterol homeostasis.[16]

Ibogaine has also been found to increase the expression of brain-derived neurotrophic factor (BDNF) transcripts in multiple brain regions and glial cell–derived neurotrophic factor (GDNF) in the ventral tegmental area.[17] These effects on BDNF and GDNF could promote neuroplasticity and may play a role in reducing depressive symptoms and fostering long-term behavioral changes.[12]

Noribogaine shows a 10-fold higher affinity at SERTs when compared to the parent compound and is active at DATs, as well as κ and μ opioid and ionotropic nicotinic receptors.[12] Noribogaine's affinity for κ opioid receptors is significantly greater than that of the parent compound and may account for its antiaddictive properties.[12] Noribogaine is a full agonist at μ opioid receptors, which may suppress the subjective distress and autonomic effects associated with opioid withdrawal.[15] Noribogaine also appears to play a role in promoting neuroplasticity via routes similar to the parent compound.[17]

Therapeutic Index

In mouse models, the median lethal dose of ibogaine is 263 mg/kg, while the median lethal dose of noribogaine is 630 mg/kg, indicating that the toxicity of ibogaine is 2.4 times that of its active metabolite.[18] Studies into the chronic toxicity of ibogaine revealed that doses of 10 mg/kg administered intraperitoneally for 30 consecutive days caused no liver, kidneys, heart, or brain damage, while doses of 40 mg/kg for 12 days led to no pathologic changes in the liver, kidneys, heart, or brain in rats.[6] Other animal data have contradicted these findings, suggesting that ibogaine may have excitotoxic effects on Purkinje cells within the cerebellum.[19]

Tolerance, Dependence, and Withdrawal

There is currently no evidence to suggest that ibogaine use is habit-forming or that individuals who regularly use ibogaine develop a tolerance to its effects.

Subjective Effects

The subjective effects of ibogaine are oftentimes divided into three phases. The onset of the first phase occurs within 1 to 2 hours of ingestion and is described as a "waking dream" (oneiric). Individuals frequently claim that they experience watching something akin to a chronologic slideshow that rapidly documents their life. Visions are most intense when the individual's eyes are closed and may be suppressed when their eyes are open.[2] This phase lasts 4 to 8 hours and may be accompanied by ataxia and profuse vomiting.[2]

The second phase is less intense than the first, as the oneiric effects of the drug begin to subside. In most cases, the individual's focus turns inward, as they become less interested in visual stimuli and more introspective and reflective. This phase lasts 8 to 20 hours.[2]

The third and final phase is a residual phase that can last upward of 72 hours and is characterized by a heightened sense of awareness, mild stimulation, and sleep problems, which may persist for several weeks or even months after the experience.[12]

According to a survey of 60 individuals with cocaine or opioid use disorders, some of the most common interpretations to emerge once the acute effects of the drug subside are a sense of insight into one's destructive behaviors (86.7%), a need to become abstinent (68.3%), a sense of being cleansed or reborn (50.0%), the belief that they have a second chance at life (40.0%), and a feeling of increased self-confidence (33.3%). Meanwhile, 91.7% of this group said that ibogaine was useful for treating drug problems, while only 16.7% said that they would be willing to repeat the ibogaine experience.[20]

Therapeutic Indications

According to the FDA, there are currently no accepted uses for ibogaine, nor can one use ibogaine off-label, as it is not available in the United States. However, as mentioned earlier, there are potentially numerous uses for ibogaine that will be described below.

Potential Uses

As noted in the "History" section, researchers have long been interested in ibogaine's ability to minimize the difficulties of overcoming substance use disorders and going through opioid withdrawal. Lotsof's informal experiments in the early 1960s eventually led to more sophisticated research that has stretched from the 1980s to the present day, but most studies have lacked rigorous clinical designs. Studies suggest that ibogaine reduces the rewarding effects of opioids and shows a dose-dependent decrease in the self-administration of stimulants, ethanol, and nicotine in animal models, and numerous open-label clinical trials have demonstrated efficacy in treating substance use disorders (especially opioid use disorder and cocaine use disorder), but far more studies are needed.

The use of ibogaine has also been used in conjunction with 5-methoxy-N,N-dimethyltryptamine (5-MeO-DMT), which is a methoxylated derivative of N,N-dimethyltryptamine (DMT). The former will be covered in Chapter 16, while the latter was covered in Chapter 11. Polytherapy may be beneficial across multiple mental health domains, including substance use, depressive, and trauma- and stressor-related disorders. However, reports of ibogaine's efficacy in treating traumatic brain injury (TBI) and PTSD, with or without additional use of 5-MeO-DMT, are based on small studies.

Opioid Withdrawal

Doses of ibogaine capable of inducing oneirophrenic states appear to mitigate or even block opioid withdrawal symptoms in individuals with opioid use disorder. According to Mash, "Patients commonly report sustained resolution of their withdrawal symptoms within 12-18 h of dosing and a reduction in drug craving and improved mood for prolonged periods of up to several weeks or months."[10]

A retrospective study involving 33 subjects reported that 25 (76%) experienced complete resolution of opioid withdrawal and did not experience subsequent drug-seeking behavior, 4 (12%) did not experience withdrawal symptoms but used opioids within 72 hours of treatment, 2 (6%) reported attenuated signs of withdrawal without subsequent drug-seeking behavior, data were unavailable for 1 (3%) participant, while 1 (3%) participant experienced clear signs of opioid withdrawal and used heroin within 8 hours of treatment.[12]

The largest open-label trial to date involving ibogaine was conducted by Mash at her facility in St. Kitts and involved 191 individuals with opioid use and cocaine use disorders. Of those with opioid use disorder, physician-rated opioid withdrawal scores at 24 hours following administration of ibogaine were mild (0-2 on a scale ranging from 0 to 13) and did not increase at any other subsequent point.[10]

Substance Use Disorders

Although there have not been any controlled clinical efficacy trials on ibogaine and substance use disorders, retrospective and observational studies, as well as open-label trials, have all suggested that ibogaine disrupts the pathology of addiction in a way that allows patients to recover. Of note, efficacy is not just limited to opioid use disorder. Evidence suggests it is true of cocaine use disorder, cannabis use disorder, and alcohol use disorder, as well.[21] Patients experience not only less desire and cravings for substances but also a decline in depressive symptoms, which may contribute to the overall benefits of ibogaine.[12]

Ibogaine is efficacious with a single dose and may be even more beneficial in treating substance use disorders when administered in multiple doses. Schenberg and colleagues found that, of 75 individuals with substance use disorders (72% of whom had polysubstance use), the median period of abstinence following single-dose administration of ibogaine was 5.5 months and that multiple ibogaine sessions resulted in 8.4 months of abstinence.[21]

Meanwhile, a case report of a 31-year-old male veteran with alcohol use disorder who was treated with a combination of ibogaine and 5-MeO-DMT reported improved mood, alcohol cessation, and reduced alcohol cravings for at least 1 month.[22]

Posttraumatic Stress Disorder

Unfortunately, PTSD is very common among US veterans who may also experience comorbid depressive, anxiety, and substance use disorders. Psychedelic-assisted psychotherapy has shown to be effective in treating the kind of multidimensional pathology that frequently develops following traumatic experiences, including those that occur in combat situations resulting in TBI and those that do not. Though treatment with ibogaine is relatively novel, the results have been promising.

A study published in 2024 involving 30 special operations forces veterans who had suffered TBI examined the use of ibogaine in treating the multidimensional sequelae of TBI. Diagnosed conditions affecting the 30 patients included PTSD ($n = 23$), PTSD with dissociative symptoms ($n = 6$), major depressive disorder ($n = 15$), unspecified anxiety disorder ($n = 14$), alcohol use disorder ($n = 15$), and other substance use disorder ($n = 6$). Moreover, 19 patients reported suicidal ideation in their lifetimes. Following administration of a single dose of ibogaine, which was given in conjunction with magnesium to protect against cardiovascular complications, the authors reported a precipitous reduction in symptoms with large effect sizes that were sustained over the course of 1 month. World Health Organization Disability Assessment Schedule 2.0 dropped from 30.2 ± 14.7 (mild-to-moderate disability) at baseline to 19.9 ± 16.3 (borderline no-to-mild disability) following treatment and to 5.1 ± 8.1 (no disability). Similar responses were noted using the Clinician-Administered PTSD Scale for DSM-5 (CAPS-5), the Montgomery-Åsberg Depression Rating Scale (MADRS), and the Hamilton Anxiety Ratings Scale (HAM-A). Additionally, no serious or unexpected adverse events were reported.[23]

Polytherapy with ibogaine and 5-MeO-DMT produced similarly powerful results in a group of 51 veterans with similar backgrounds and pathologies. Perhaps the most impressive results highlight the decline in PTSD checklist (PCL-5) scores among the 38 participants diagnosed with PTSD. Mean baseline scores were 46.2 but dropped to 12.0 (a decline of 34.2) 30 days after treatment.[24]

Separately, 86 trauma-exposed special operations forces veterans took part in an open-label study involving psychedelic-assisted psychotherapy with the consecutive use of ibogaine and 5-MeO-DMT at a facility in Mexico. Those involved reported symptom improvement for not only PTSD but also individual symptoms like depression, anxiety, and insomnia. Participants also reported improved psychological flexibility, satisfaction with life, and cognitive functioning from baseline to 1-month follow-up.[25]

Precautions and Adverse Events

More than perhaps any other drug covered in this book, ibogaine use has been associated with very serious and even fatal complications—even in clinical settings. In addition to its activity in the CNS, ibogaine affects the cardiovascular system and its use can induce a QT interval prolongation, increasing the risk of torsade de pointes (TdP) arrhythmia.[14] Among 39 patients who received a single dose of ibogaine in the range of 500 to 1,000 mg, 6 experienced significant bradycardia and 1 had significant hypotension.[14] These patients were being treated for cocaine or heroin use disorder and may have had existing cardiovascular disorders. Ibogaine and possibly its active metabolite noribogaine may also lead to QT interval prolongation and potentially fatal TdP arrhythmias, possibly via the modulatory effects on cardiac ion channels.[14]

A systematic literature review from 2022 by Köck and colleagues identified 60 ibogaine-associated emergencies or deaths (20 and 40, respectively). "In 34.5% of these cases concomitant drug use was documented and in 70.7% ibogaine was administered with the intention of treating OUD [opioid use disorder]."[12] While the majority of these emergencies were related to cardiac events, one concerned a patient with schizophrenia who experienced an exacerbation of psychosis, and in two other instances, individuals experienced symptoms of mania.[12]

Less severe adverse events include dizziness, confusion, lack of coordination, nausea, vomiting, dry mouth, and headache. In most cases, these side effects are transient and resolve within a few days of drug administration.[10]

Drug Interactions

No drug interaction studies have been published on ibogaine at this time, but drugs that are CYP2D6 substrates will interact with ibogaine, requiring dose adjustment.

Special Populations

Pregnant and Nursing Women

Pregnant and nursing women should not ingest ibogaine.

Individuals With Cardiovascular Disease

If any cardiovascular risk factors are identified, the patient should be discouraged from using ibogaine, as it may cause QT interval prolongation and potentially fatal TdP arrhythmias.

CYP2D6 Polymorphism

Individuals who are CYP2D6-poor metabolizers may experience protracted effects of ibogaine. Significant adjustments in dosing may be necessary, especially if a patient is taking other medications subject to CYP2D6 metabolism.

Dosage and Administration

Within clinical settings, ibogaine is administered in the form of pills and doses range from 500 to 1,000 mg.

There are no existing guidelines for the administration of ibogaine. At a bare minimum, continuous medical observation and electrocardiographic monitoring are advised. The latter should continue for at least 24 hours after administration, given the extraordinarily long half-life of noribogaine. Baseline screening is also strongly encouraged and should include a physical evaluation, a medical examination, bloodwork, and an electrocardiogram recording. Koenig and Hilber also note that hypokalemia and hypomagnesemia may predispose patients to ibogaine cardiotoxicity, so replenishment of these electrolytes is advised.[14]

Recent use of alcohol, cocaine, and opioids may increase the risk of adverse cardiovascular events. This is a significant concern because individuals who are using ibogaine to treat substance use disorders may attempt to sneak off before the treatment to have "one last hurrah," and this may lead to complications. Recent methadone use, in particular, can be dangerous on account of its exceptionally long plasma half-life (up to 55 hours).

Conclusion

Ibogaine is unique among the drugs discussed in this book for several reasons. Its mechanism of action is truly distinct, it has very little potential of abuse, and its ability to blunt the most torturous aspects of opioid withdrawal in many patients could afford it a place within many clinicians' armamentarium. However, the extended nature of the ibogaine experience makes administration resource intensive, and its use is potentially dangerous, especially in populations with existing cardiovascular disease.

Although these dangers must be taken seriously, one cannot help but balance them against the destructive nature of addiction, the wide-reaching effects of the opioid crisis, and the lack of treatment options available to people struggling with substance use disorders. Although it is unlikely that therapy with ibogaine will become as common as ketamine or even MDMA, it could still be a treatment of last resort. Moreover, research into ibogaine congeners like 18-MC and tabernanthalog may eventually produce drugs that have similar therapeutic utility but are shorter-acting and devoid of ibogaine's adverse effects.

REFERENCES
1. Bading-Taika B, Akinyeke T, Magana AA, et al. Phytochemical characterization of *Tabernanthe iboga* root bark and its effects on dysfunctional metabolism and cognitive performance in high-fat-fed C57BL/6J mice. *J Food Bioact*. 2018;3:111-123. doi:10.31665/JFB.2018.3154. PMID: 30582133; PMCID: PMC6301038.

2. Brown TK. Ibogaine in the treatment of substance dependence. *Curr Drug Abuse Rev.* 2013;6(1):3-16. doi:10.2174/15672050113109990001. PMID: 23627782.
3. Martins MLF, Heydari P, Li W, et al. Drug transporters ABCB1 (P-gp) and OATP, but not drug-metabolizing enzyme CYP3A4, affect the pharmacokinetics of the psychoactive alkaloid ibogaine and its metabolites. *Front Pharmacol.* 2022;13:855000. doi:10.3389/fphar.2022.855000. PMID: 35308219; PMCID: PMC8931498.
4. Nuwer R. This psychoactive plant could save lives—and everyone wants to cash in. National Geographic. Published March 8, 2023. Accessed February 27, 2024. https://www.nationalgeographic.com/animals/article/ibogaine-pschedelic-drug-root-fair-trade-gabon
5. Havelka O. The syncretism of the Gabonese Bwiti religion and Catholic Christianity from a theological and theological-ethical perspective. *Theologica.* 2022;12(1):143-159. Accessed February 28, 2024. https://karolinum.cz/data/clanek/10749/Theol_12_1_0143.pdf
6. Goutarel R, Gollnhofer O, Sillans R. Pharmacodynamics and therapeutic applications of iboga and ibogaine (Gladstone WJ, trans). *Psychedelic Monogr Essays.* 1993;6:71-111.
7. Alper K. The ibogaine project: urban ethnomedicine for opioid use disorder. In: Prance G, ed. *Ethnopharmacologic Search for Psychoactive Drugs: 50th Anniversary Symposium June 6-8, 2017.* Vol II. Synergetic Press; 2018:160-174.
8. Alper KR, Stajić M, Gill JR. Fatalities temporally associated with the ingestion of ibogaine. *J Forensic Sci.* 2012;57(2):398-412. doi:10.1111/j.1556-4029.2011.02008.x. PMID: 22268458.
9. Hevisi D. Howard Lotsof dies at 66; saw drug cure in a plant. *New York Times.* Published February 17, 2010. Accessed March 19, 2024. https://www.nytimes.com/2010/02/17/us/17lotsof.html
10. Mash DC. IUPHAR—invited review—ibogaine—a legacy within the current renaissance of psychedelic therapy. *Pharmacol Res.* 2023;190:106620. doi:10.1016/j.phrs.2022.106620
11. Ovalle D, Gilbert D. Psychedelic drug ibogaine hailed as healing. U.S. patients ask why it's illegal. Washington Post. Published March 14, 2024. Accessed March 19, 2024. https://www.washingtonpost.com/health/2024/03/14/ibogaine-psychedelic-ptsd-veterans/
12. Köck P, Froelich K, Walter M, Lang U, Dürsteler KM. A systematic literature review of clinical trials and therapeutic applications of ibogaine. *J Subst Abuse Treat.* 2022;138:108717. doi:10.1016/j.jsat.2021.108717. PMID: 35012793.
13. Iyer RN, Favela D, Zhang G, Olson DE. The iboga enigma: the chemistry and neuropharmacology of iboga alkaloids and related analogs. *Nat Prod Rep.* 2021;38(2):307-329. doi:10.1039/d0np00033g. PMID: 32794540; PMCID: PMC7882011.
14. Koenig X, Hilber K. The anti-addiction drug ibogaine and the heart: a delicate relation. *Molecules.* 2015;20(2):2208-2228. doi:10.3390/molecules20022208. PMID: 25642835; PMCID: PMC4382526.
15. Mash DC, Kovera CA, Pablo J, et al. Ibogaine in the treatment of heroin withdrawal. *Alkaloids Chem Biol.* 2001;56:155-171. doi:10.1016/s0099-9598(01)56012-5. PMID: 11705106.
16. Yang K, Zeng C, Wang C, Sun M, Yin D, Sun T. Sigma-2 receptor-A potential target for cancer/Alzheimer's disease treatment via its regulation of cholesterol homeostasis. *Molecules.* 2020;25(22):5439. doi:10.3390/molecules25225439. PMID: 33233619; PMCID: PMC7699687.
17. Marton S, González B, Rodríguez-Bottero S, et al. Ibogaine administration modifies GDNF and BDNF expression in brain regions involved in mesocorticolimbic and nigral dopaminergic circuits. *Front Pharmacol.* 2019;10:193. doi:10.3389/fphar.2019.00193. PMID: 30890941; PMCID: PMC6411846.

18. Kubiliene A, Marksiene R, Kazlauskas S, Sadauskiene I, Razukas A, Ivanov L. Acute toxicity of ibogaine and noribogaine. *Medicina (Kaunas)*. 2008;44(12):984-988. PMID: 19142057.
19. Litjens RP, Brunt TM. How toxic is ibogaine? *Clin Toxicol (Phila)*. 2016;54(4):297-302. doi:10.3109/15563650.2016.1138226. PMID: 26807959.
20. Mash DC, Duque L, Page B, Allen-Ferdinand K. Ibogaine detoxification transitions opioid and cocaine abusers between dependence and abstinence: clinical observations and treatment outcomes. *Front Pharmacol*. 2018;9:529. doi:10.3389/fphar.2018.00529. PMID: 29922156; PMCID: PMC5996271.
21. Schenberg EE, de Castro Comis MA, Chaves BR, da Silveira DX. Treating drug dependence with the aid of ibogaine: a retrospective study. *J Psychopharmacol*. 2014;28(11):993-1000. doi:10.1177/0269881114552713. PMID: 25271214.
22. Barsuglia JP, Polanco M, Palmer R, Malcolm BJ, Kelmendi B, Calvey T. A case report SPECT study and theoretical rationale for the sequential administration of ibogaine and 5-MeO-DMT in the treatment of alcohol use disorder. *Prog Brain Res*. 2018;242:121-158. doi:10.1016/bs.pbr.2018.08.002. PMID: 30471678.
23. Cherian KN, Keynan JN, Anker L, et al. Magnesium-ibogaine therapy in veterans with traumatic brain injuries. *Nat Med*. 2024;30(2):373-381. doi:10.1038/s41591-023-02705-w. PMID: 38182784; PMCID: PMC10878970.
24. Davis AK, Averill LA, Sepeda ND, Barsuglia JP, Amoroso T. Psychedelic treatment for trauma-related psychological and cognitive impairment among US Special Operations Forces Veterans. *Chronic Stress (Thousand Oaks)*. 2020;4:2470547020939564. doi:10.1177/2470547020939564. PMID: 32704581; PMCID: PMC7359647.
25. Davis AK, Xin Y, Sepeda N, Averill LA. Open-label study of consecutive ibogaine and 5-MeO-DMT assisted-therapy for trauma-exposed male Special Operations Forces Veterans: prospective data from a clinical program in Mexico. *Am J Drug Alcohol Abuse*. 2023;49(5):587-596. doi:10.1080/00952990.2023.2220874. PMID: 37734158.

14

Ketamine

Ketamine hydrochloride (hereafter "ketamine") is a racemic mixture consisting of (S)- and (R)-ketamine. At high doses, ketamine induces dissociative anesthesia and amnesia. Subanesthetic doses of ketamine exert analgesic, anti-inflammatory, and rapid antidepressant actions. Ketamine can also induce nonordinary states of consciousness (NOSCs) and psychedelic experiences that are relatively brief, powerful, and uniquely dissociative. Even at relatively low doses of ketamine or when emerging out of ketamine-induced anesthesia, some individuals may experience dissociation, an out-of-body experience that may feel extremely strange or uncomfortable. Stanislav Grof, a psychiatrist who has been researching NOSCs since the 1960s, once wrote that it is "the strangest psychoactive substance I have ever experienced in the 50 years of my consciousness research. The effects of this compound are so extraordinary that they stand out even in the group of psychedelics."[1]

The short-term antidepressant effects of ketamine have been recognized for several decades (referred to as an "afterglow"), but they were not given serious attention by researchers until the late 1990s. In 2019, esketamine (Spravato), a nasal spray consisting of only the (S)-ketamine enantiomer, received approval from the U.S. Food and Drug Administration (FDA) for the treatment of treatment-resistant depression for individuals who failed prior trials or are suicidal. As of now, it is the only form of ketamine approved for the treatment of depression along with an oral antidepressant, while intravenous (IV) ketamine infusion, though not FDA approved, remains an off-label treatment option for treatment-resistant depression and/or suicidality.

Esketamine is only available through a restricted distribution system and may only be administered under the supervision of a health care provider in a *Risk Evaluation and Mitigation Strategy (REMS)*-certified medical facility. These extra precautions have been deemed necessary because ketamine can be used as a recreational drug on account of its euphoric and dissociative effects, and individuals can put themselves in harm's way when left unsupervised by a caregiver or medical professional. The very public 2023 death of actor Matthew Perry, which was attributed to the acute effects of ketamine intoxication, serves as a reminder that use outside of a clinical setting is dangerous, even though ketamine has a good safety profile.[2]

This chapter explores ketamine's beneficial effects for a myriad of conditions like treatment-resistant depression, as well as posttraumatic stress disorder (PTSD), anxiety disorders, eating disorders, and substance use disorders. Like other psychedelics, ketamine's therapeutic effects appear to be mediated through its mechanism of action, particularly but not limited to *N*-methyl-D-aspartate (NMDA) receptors, as well as induction of psychedelic experience. As noted elsewhere, the therapist's assistance and guidance are beneficial because they help the patient process the experience. Without this guidance, the experience is frequently bereft of therapeutic value.

History

Ketamine falls under the chemical class of drugs known as arylcyclohexylamines. Developed as anesthetics by Parke-Davis, these drugs induce a sense of dissociation between the mind and the body, hence the reason they are often referred to as dissociative anesthetics.

Precursors

The first arylcyclohexylamine to be developed was phencyclidine (also known as PCP or angel dust). Initially synthesized at Göttingen University by Kötz and Merkel in 1926,[3] the drug was rescued from obscurity by Parke-Davis, where it was developed as an anesthetic agent for use in animals and humans, patented, and briefly marketed under the name Sernyl during the 1950s.[4] "Sernyl" was evidently an allusion to the Latin *serenus*, which is the source of the English word "serenity" (though any clinician who has been tasked with treating a patient on PCP would probably pick virtually any other word in the English language *besides* "*serene*" to describe the experience!).[4] Animal studies of PCP conducted by Dr Edward Domino, who was a psychopharmacology pioneer at the University of Michigan's Department of Pharmacology, indicated that it was a potentially safe anesthetic for humans.[5]

Early trials in humans indicated that PCP was a potent anesthetic that did not cause depression in cardiovascular or respiratory systems, but many patients experienced protracted emergence delirium following surgery.[6] Further clinical studies made it increasingly evident that PCP was not suitable for humans, particularly as several studies looking into its effects found parallels to the positive symptoms of schizophrenia (eg, delusions, paranoia, hyperactivity). The parallels were so salient that it was referred to as a "schizophrenomimetic drug."[7] Consequently, clinical use was discontinued in 1965.[8] Today, PCP is classified as a Schedule II drug with a high risk of abuse but is used occasionally by veterinarians and researchers.

Despite the clear problems of using PCP in a clinical setting, the head of pharmaceutical research at Parke-Davis was convinced that a shorter-acting derivative of PCP had the potential to be an effective anesthetic for humans.[6] This led to the development of another drug of the arylcyclohexylamine class, eticyclidine, which is more potent than PCP. Testing of eticyclidine was brief, and experiments were discontinued by Parke-Davis following the discovery of the third arylcyclohexylamine, ketamine.[4]

Ketamine's Early Days

Ketamine was first synthesized in 1962 by Calvin Stevens.[4] Originally known as CI-581, animal testing suggested that the compound was a safe anesthetic agent that was also short acting. The head of clinical pharmacology at Parke-Davis requested that Domino conduct the first tests of ketamine on human participants, which occurred on August 3, 1964.[6] Domino and his University of Michigan colleague, Dr Guenter Corssen, administered the drug intravenously to 20 volunteers from Jackson Prison in Michigan.[6] During these tests, Domino recalled that "Guenter and I gradually increased the dose from no effect, to conscious but 'spaced out,' and finally to enough for general anesthesia."[6]

The results of the study were published in 1965.[9] This article also featured the first instance of the description "dissociative anesthetic," which had been proposed by Domino's wife, Toni, as a means of articulating how the participants involved in the study had felt as though they were "dreaming" or "disconnected" from their environments.[6] "Most of our subjects described strange experiences like a feeling of floating in outer space and having no feeling in their arms or legs," Domino later recalled, but noted that "frank emergence delirium was minimal."[6]

The term "dissociative anesthetic" was also believed to be a more palatable alternative to "schizophrenomimetic" or "psychomimetic," two words that had extremely negative connotations and could have derailed research into ketamine. According to Domino, it is likely that Parke-Davis would have abandoned its development due to the belief that its use would never gain FDA approval had the drug been described as schizophrenomimetic instead of a "dissociative anesthetic."[6]

More recent studies have corroborated the initial stance that ketamine, as well as other drugs of the arylcyclohexylamine class like PCP, do have schizophrenomimetic properties. One of the ligands at NMDA receptors is glutamate, and ketamine's antagonistic activity at these receptors disrupts glutamatergic pathways in a manner that is believed to lead to abnormal functional connectivity within the thalamus hub, producing ketamine's dissociative effects. Patients with schizophrenia appear to experience similar alterations of glutamatergic pathways and corticothalamic connectivity, suggesting that glutamatergic dysfunction is implicated in the pathology of schizophrenia.[10] Studies by Krystal and colleagues in the 1990s revealed that a single infusion of subanesthetic ketamine was capable of producing transient symptoms of psychosis in otherwise healthy adults, including feelings of persecution, sensory illusions, and disruptions in cognition evidenced by problems finding words, learning difficulties, and poor attention.[11] In other words, the concern that ketamine could have very easily been described as "schizophrenomimetic" was well founded.

As it stood, research continued, and in 1966 Domino and Corssen published findings on the clinical use of ketamine.[12] It was shown to be not only fast acting and to diminish the frequency of emergence delirium, it also produced minimal cardiovascular and respiratory events at modest doses, could be easily titrated, and had a very solid safety profile.[13] Consequently, it was patented by Parke-Davis that same year under the name Ketalar. Four years later, in 1970, the FDA approved the use of ketamine as a rapid-acting IV anesthetic.

From "Buddy Drug" to Club Drug

Most Americans first became acquainted with ketamine in the jungles of Vietnam, where it quickly became the most widely used battlefield anesthetic, analgesic, and sedative on account of its safety profile and ease of use. Many soldiers carried ketamine with them and could easily administer an intramuscular injection of the drug if a compatriot was injured. As a result, it earned the name the "buddy drug." In addition to soldiers, military anesthesiologists and surgeons became intimately familiar with the drug. It also proved to be a lifesaving medicine. The use of ketamine is believed to have helped decrease the mortality rate of wounded soldiers who made it to medical treatment from 4.5% during the Korean War to 2.6% during the Vietnam War.[4]

Ketamine also became popular off the battlefield. Shortly after approval by the FDA, it began to be used to provide preoperative sedation, reduce preoperative anxiety, facilitate the induction of general anesthesia, and provide postoperative analgesia. For these reasons, ketamine continues to enjoy wide use outside of the United States and Global North, which is why it is included on the World Health Organization's List of Essential Medicines. However, in the United States, ketamine's role within anesthesiology and most other fields of medicine has diminished. It is now primarily used for procedural sedation and as an analgesic for chronic and acute pain, oftentimes with a combination of a benzodiazepine and propofol to limit emergence delirium.[4]

Soon after ketamine was approved by the FDA, it began to be used for recreational purposes. At lower doses, its effects are relatively mild and may be compared to ethanol, though its effects are shorter acting. Psychedelic effects appear at higher (though still subanesthetic) doses and can also be experienced as patients emerge from anesthesia—something that was noted in the literature as early as 1972 by Collier.[14] Clinicians also noted that patients frequently experienced an antidepressant "afterglow" that would persist for up to 2 weeks.[15]

By the late 1970s, the psychedelic effects of ketamine had become more widely known, especially after the publication of books celebrating its use by the likes of neuroscientist John Lilly (*The Scientist*, 1978) and writer Marcia Moore (*Journeys into the Bright World*, 1978).[6] Both ultimately became obsessed with the psychedelic experiences occasioned by ketamine use. Moore died under mysterious circumstances in 1979, while Lilly's use of ketamine became increasingly problematic as he came to regard it as a necessary means of exploring realms of NOSCs.[16]

Ketamine use also became popular within dance clubs during the 1980s. Its popularity grew throughout that decade and into the 1990s, which is when the U.S. Drug Enforcement Agency (DEA) named ketamine a Schedule III drug. It has also become a popular recreational drug in other countries, including East Asia and Europe, which has resulted in a multitude of nations placing additional restrictions on ketamine's use and distribution.[4] Despite these limitations, ketamine continues to be a popular recreational drug.

Acceptance in Psychiatry

Ketamine's reputation was never as tarnished as many of the other drugs mentioned in this book, largely because its clinical utility as an anesthetic was never questioned. However, very few people considered that it could have applications outside of anesthesiology or to treat acute pain. For decades, the antidepressant "afterglow" was largely considered to be clinically irrelevant except among very few members of the medical community.

One of these individuals was Salvador Roquet, who pioneered psychedelic-assisted psychotherapy in Mexico during the late 1960s and early 1970s. Roquet used not only ketamine but several psychedelic substances (including but not limited to lysergic acid diethylamide [LSD], mescaline, psilocybin, morning glory seeds [of the family *Convolvulaceae*], and ayahuasca). These drugs were often administered in a group setting. The 1970s also saw the use of ketamine as an adjunct to psychotherapy in Argentina (Fontana) and Iran (Khorramzadeh and Lofty).[4]

In the former Soviet Union, Krupitsky used ketamine in psychedelic-assisted therapy to treat alcohol use disorder during the 1980s and 1990s. His work continued into the 2000s, and his early findings indicated that ketamine-assisted therapy could effectively treat opioid use disorder, stimulant use disorder, and a wide array of comorbid psychiatric conditions, including PTSD, mood and anxiety disorders, and avoidant personality disorder. It should be noted that Krupitsky developed a detailed and comprehensive course of ketamine psychedelic psychotherapy (KPP) that involved an extensive preparation stage before administration of the drug. It was then followed by group psychotherapy sessions to integrate the experience. Krupitsky's model was largely borrowed by Eli Kolp, who continues to practice in the United States. Kolp has found that Krupitsky's KPP program effectively treats a host of psychiatric illnesses, including treatment-resistant depression.[4]

Mainstream psychiatry has taken a more cautious approach to ketamine, even though ketamine had been identified as an NMDA antagonist in the early 1980s by David Lodge and colleagues, and preclinical tests of NMDA antagonists throughout the 1990s had shown putative antidepressant effects.[17] It was only in the 2000s that medical literature on ketamine and psychiatry began to be published. It started in the year 2000 when Berman and colleagues published the first placebo-controlled study showing rapid antidepressant effects that were superior to placebo following a 40-minute IV infusion of

0.5 mg/kg ketamine.[18] Zarate and colleagues replicated these findings in double-blind, placebo-controlled, randomized clinical trial involving 18 patients with treatment-resistant depression that was published in 2006.[19] Zarate and colleagues also noted that single-dose ketamine's antidepressant effects did not persist for long. Symptom improvement lasted for an average of 7 days for the 18 participants.[13]

Since that time, an enormous number of studies have been conducted showing ketamine's efficacy in reducing the severity of suicidal ideation, depression in unipolar and bipolar depressions, and countless other conditions in psychiatry that will be explored below (see Therapeutic Indications and "Off-Label Uses").[13] Regular ketamine infusions were also shown to be effective as a maintenance therapy among patients with treatment-resistant depression.[20] Consequently, during the 2010s, many health care providers began offering off-label subanesthetic doses of IV ketamine to patients with depressive disorders. This was well before the FDA's approval of esketamine, which consists of only the (S)-ketamine enantiomer, and often without any regulatory framework.[21] The practice has continued into the 2020s, still without official protocols and despite the fact that insurers are more likely to reimburse for esketamine treatment instead of ketamine infusions.[21] More recently, the American Psychiatric Association (APA) has voiced its concern about the proliferation of ketamine clinics without appropriate mental health professional supervision.

In the wake of the FDA's approval of intranasal esketamine in 2019 for treatment-resistant depression, several studies have questioned whether esketamine is actually more effective than IV, racemic ketamine in the treatment of depressive disorders.[17] Although there is little doubt that the former possesses antidepressant qualities, a systematic review and meta-analysis first published online by Bahji and colleagues in 2020 found IV ketamine to be superior to esketamine with respect to overall responses and remission rates, and there were fewer drop-outs and adverse events.[22] One other notable difference between racemic ketamine and the (S)-ketamine enantiomer is that the former patent has expired and the latter was patented by Janssen in 2013.

Pharmacology

Ketamine (Ketalar) is a racemic mixture of (S)- and (R)-ketamine enantiomers. Esketamine (Spravato) consists solely of the (S)-ketamine enantiomer. Both these formulations are Schedule III controlled substances.

Description

Ketamine is a white crystalline substance that is hydro- and liposoluble with a molecular mass of 238 g/mol and a pKa of 7.5.[23] All FDA-approved formulations of ketamine come in aqueous solutions that can be stored at room temperature. Powder formulations of ketamine—none of which are FDA approved—may be white or light brown. The structure of ketamine is shown in Figure 14.1.

Injectable formulations of ketamine, like Ketalar, are clear aqueous solutions that are slightly acidic (pH 3.5-5.5) and may contain concentrations of 10, 50, or 100 mg of ketamine per milliliter. If exposed to sunlight for extended periods of time, the color of the solution may darken and become slightly yellow. Change in color will not affect the efficacy of the drug. However, if precipitate is present, the solution should be discarded.[24]

Devices designed for the nasal administration of esketamine, as is the case with Spravato, contain 0.2. mL of colorless and clear aqueous solution with a pH of 4.5 designed to deliver two sprays and a total dosage of 32.3 mg of esketamine hydrochloride (= 28 mg of esketamine).[25]

Route of Administration

Ketamine can be administered via several routes that include IV, intramuscular, intranasal, oral, sublingual, and rectal. Intravenous, intramuscular, and intranasal are the most commonly used routes within a clinical setting.

Pharmacokinetics

Absorption

Ketamine is highly lipophilic. Effects are felt within 1 minute when administered intravenously, in 3 to 4 minutes when administered intramuscularly, within 5 to 10 minutes when administered intranasally, and within 20 to 30 minutes when given orally.[4] Ketamine reaches peak

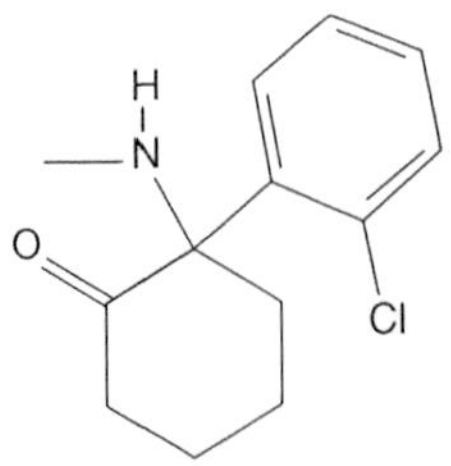

Figure 14.1 The molecular structure of ketamine.

plasma concentrations rapidly except when taken orally, in which case peak concentration levels may not be achieved for 45 minutes.[4]

Peak plasma concentrations of 1,200 to 2,400 ng/mL are needed to induce dissociative anesthesia.[13] Awakening occurs when ranges drop to 640 to 1,100 ng/mL.[13] Analgesic effects are associated with plasma concentrations of 70 to 160 ng/mL.[13] The most common dose for treating depression (0.5 mg/kg; 40-minute infusion) results in maximal plasma concentrations of approximately 185 ng/mL, though plasma concentrations of 75 ng/mL may be enough to produce an antidepressant response.[4] This level may not induce a full psychedelic/dissociative state capable of producing a transcendent experience.

Bioavailability

Depending on the route of administration, ketamine may have a bioavailability ranging from as low as 16% (oral administration) to as high as 100% (IV infusion)[26] (see Table 14.1).

Distribution

Ketamine has a plasma protein binding between 10% and 50%, so it is rapidly distributed into highly perfused tissues like the brain.[13]

Metabolism

Ketamine undergoes significant first-pass metabolism. Approximately 80% of ketamine is metabolized into norketamine primarily by cytochrome P450 liver enzymes CYP2B6 and CYP3A4. Norketamine is an active metabolite that retains the anesthetic qualities of the parent compound at approximately one-third the potency.[13]

Continuing with the major metabolic pathways, norketamine is then hydroxylated into the hydroxynorketamines (primarily 6-hydroxy-norketamine, but also 4-hydroxy-norketamine and 5-hydroxy-norketamine)

TABLE 14.1 Ketamine Bioavailability by Route of Administration

Route of Administration	Bioavailability (%)
Intravenous	100
Intramuscular	93
Intranasal	45-50
Intrarectal	25-30
Oral	16-29

and dehydronorketamine. Metabolism of 6-hydroxy-norketamine is carried out by CYP2A6 and CYP2B6; metabolism of 4-hydroxy-norketamine is carried out by CYP3A4 and CYP3A5; and metabolism of 5-hydroxy-norketamine is carried out by CYP2B6. Dehydronorketamine is metabolized by the CYP2B6 enzyme from norketamine.[13]

There are also minor metabolic pathways that occur within the liver.

Elimination and Excretion

Ketamine has a high rate of clearance ($\approx$95 L/h/70 kg) and a short elimination half-life (2-4 hours) and is primarily excreted in bile and urine.[13] Though a small percentage of the drug is excreted unchanged (2%) or as norketamine (2%), ketamine and norketamine have been detected in urine 11 and 14 days following anesthetic doses.[13] Repeated administration may prolong elimination time.[13]

Pharmacodynamics

Ketamine increases arterial pressure and heart rate at subanesthetic and anesthetic doses. At higher doses, it can lead to myocardial depression. Direct relaxation of vascular smooth muscle is another effect of ketamine. Of note, ketamine does not cause clinically significant pulmonary depression at anesthetic doses, and at subanesthetic doses it may stimulate respiration. Ketamine may increase intercranial pressure on account of increased cerebral metabolism.[8]

As has been noted earlier, ketamine produces dissociative anesthetic effects that are characterized by catatonia, catalepsy, and amnesia at high doses (1-2 mg/kg of an IV infusion). Ketamine is also an analgesic and at lower doses (0.5-1 mg/kg) it may be used to treat acute pain and shares many similar properties with opioids but with notably less respiratory depressive effects. Similar doses have been shown to have antidepressant effects, as well as anti-inflammatory and neuroprotective effects. Although ketamine's antagonistic effects at NMDA receptors are believed to be the primary reason for the observed antidepressant effects, its anti-inflammatory properties and activity at glutamate-independent sites could also play a role in its psychiatric applications. In fact, it has been demonstrated that the antagonism of opioid receptors blocks the antidepressant effects of ketamine.[27]

Mechanism of Action

Ketamine's mechanism of action is complex. Primarily, ketamine is a noncompetitive NMDA antagonist that is not selective at specific subtypes of NMDA receptors.[28] NMDA receptors play a significant role in the formation of memory and synaptic plasticity. Its ligands are glycine and glutamate, the latter being the most predominant excitatory neurotransmitters in the central nervous system (CNS). Blockade of NMDA receptors is believed to account for ketamine's dissociative and amnesic effects. There is also some evidence to suggest that, although ketamine is not selective at specific subtypes of NMDA receptors, it may possess 3 to 4 times the potency at NMDA receptors expressing GluN1/GluN2C subunits that are preferentially expressed on GABAergic (γ-aminobutyric acid) interneurons in the presence of Mg^{2+}. Ketamine's interactions with Mg^{2+} at NMDA receptors may be crucial to understanding why it possesses antidepressive effects, whereas other NMDA antagonists like memantine do not.[28]

Activity at NMDA receptors may not be all there is to ketamine. Some have suggested that, although NMDA antagonism may account for the dissociative or psychedelic effects of ketamine, as well as some of the drug's antidepressive effects, activation of α-amino-3-hydroxy-5-methyl-4-isoxazolepropionic acid (AMPA) receptors by ketamine and its active metabolite, 6-hydroxy-norketamine, results in glutamate release and downstream effects that result in synaptogenesis and elevated levels of brain-derived neurotrophic factor (BDNF).[29] Additionally, ketamine has been shown to be an inhibitor on HCN1-HCN2 heteromeric channels, which may account not only for ketamine's anesthetic but also for some of its antidepressant properties, as HCN1 activity in the hippocampus is associated with antidepressant effects in rodents. Additional targets that may play a role in ketamine's antidepressant properties include muscarinic and nicotinic acetylcholine receptors, dopamine receptors (D_2), subtypes of serotonin receptors (5-HT_1, 5-HT_2, and 5-HT_3), opioid receptors (δ, κ, and μ), sigma receptors (σ-1 and σ-2), and L-type voltage-dependent calcium channels (see Table 14.2).[17]

Therapeutic Index

Ketamine has a wide therapeutic index, with an average lethal dose (LD_{50}) of approximately 600 mg/kg in rodents.[4] Anesthesia can be achieved with doses of 1 to 2 mg/kg.

Tolerance, Dependence, and Withdrawal

Repeated use of ketamine can lead to the development of tolerance, dependence, and withdrawal, though this is extremely rare in a clinical setting. Dependence may affect memory and the ability to concentrate, as well as lead to abdominal pain (sometimes referred to as "K cramps" or "K pains"). This pain is believed to be associated with sterile ulcerative cystitis, which is difficult to distinguish from a urinary tract or bladder infection.[30] Uropathy due to chronic ketamine use is often referred to as "ketamine bladder."

TABLE 14.2 Ketamine Targets

Target	Action
N-methyl-D-aspartate (NMDA)	Antagonist
Muscarinic acetylcholine	Antagonist
α-7 nicotinic acetylcholine	Antagonist
δ-type opioid	Binder
κ-type opioid	Agonist
μ-type opioid	Binder
Dopamine (D2)	Partial agonist
5-Hydroxytryptamine (5-HT_1 5-HT_2)	Antagonist
5-Hydroxytryptamine (5-HT3A)	Potentiator
Sigma-1 (σ-1)	Agonist
Sigma-2 (σ-2)	Agonist
Neurokinin 1	Antagonist
Hyperpolarization-activated cyclic nucleotide-gated channels (HCN-1 and HCN-2)	Inhibitor
Cholinesterase	Inhibitor
Nitric oxide synthase	Inhibitor
Sodium-dependent noradrenaline transporter	Inhibitor

Withdrawal is characterized by cravings for the drug, lack of appetite, tiredness, difficulty sleeping, chills, irritability, restlessness, and irregular heartbeat.

Subjective Effects of Ketamine

Ketamine can produce drastically different subjective effects based on dose, and some individuals may not experience a psychedelic or NOSC. At very low doses (0.10-0.25 mg/kg), ketamine may induce a sense of relaxation, disinhibition, or sedation similar to ethanol in some individuals. Other individuals may experience a stimulant effect with the same dosage.

At slightly higher doses, ketamine can induce one of four NOSCs as described by Kolp and colleagues (see Table 14.3). Each NOSC is

TABLE 14.3 Ketamine-Induced Nonordinary States of Consciousness (NOSCs)

	Empathogenic Experience	Out-of-Body Experience	Near-Death Experience	Ego-Dissolving Transcendental Experience
Features	Awareness of body; comfort and relaxation; reduced ego defenses; empathy, compassion, and warmth; love and peace; euphoria; mind is dreamy with nonspecific colorful visual effects; sense of forgiveness to self and others	Complete separation from one's body; visits to mythologic realms of consciousness; encounters with nonterrestrial beings; emotionally intense visions (eg, deceased relatives, spirits); vivid dreams of past and future incarnations; reexperiencing the birth process	Departure from one's body; complete ego dissolution/loss of identity; experienced physical (body) and psychological (mind) death; experience being a single point of consciousness simply aware of itself (a thought thinking itself); reliving one's life, aware of how actions have affected others, with moral judgment of self	Ecstatic state of the dissolution of boundaries between the self and external reality; complete dissolution of one's body and self (soul); transcending normal mass/time/space continuum; collective consciousness; unity with nature/universe; sacredness
Dosage	0.25-0.50 mg/kg IM	0.75-1.5 mg/kg IM	2.0-3.0 mg/kg IM	Possible but rare in low doses (0.25-0.5 mg/kg IM), more common in higher doses (2.0-3.0 mg/kg IM)

(*continued*)

TABLE 14.3 Ketamine-Induced Nonordinary States of Consciousness (NOSCs) (continued)

	Empathogenic Experience	Out-of-Body Experience	Near-Death Experience	Ego-Dissolving Transcendental Experience
Nonpsychedelic use	Anxiolysis and/or analgesia	Mild conscious dissociative sedation	Moderate to severe conscious dissociative sedation	N/A
Duration	45-60 min	45-60 min	45-60 min	45-60 min
Recall	Near total	Partial	Limited	Limited
Similar drug	Low doses of classic psychedelics (eg, LSD); moderate doses of empathogenic substances (eg, MDMA)	Moderate doses of classic psychedelics (eg, LSD)	High doses of classic psychedelics (eg, LSD)	High doses of classic psychedelics (eg, LSD)

IM, intramuscular; LSD, lysergic acid diethylamide; MDMA, 3,4-methylenedioxymethamphetamine.
Adapted from Kolp E, Friedman HL, Krupitsky E, et al. Ketamine psychedelic psychotherapy: focus on its pharmacology, phenomenology, and clinical applications. In: Wolfson P, Hartelius G, eds. *The Ketamine Papers: Science, Therapy, and Transformation*. Multidisciplinary Association for Psychedelic Studies; 2016:97-197.

distinguished by the degree of dissociation between body and mind and the degree of ego dissolution. One unique issue with ketamine is that antagonism of NMDA receptors disrupts memory formation, and patients oftentimes have a difficult time recounting their full experience after the acute effects of ketamine have dissipated. Like other psychedelics, these types of NOSCs can be affected by dose, as well as set and setting.[4]

The first state described by Kolp is "empathogenic," referring to a state of increased empathy. This experience may be beneficial when treating patients with intrapsychic conflicts, acute stress disorder, PTSD, or interpersonal problems with members of their family.

The second state is an "out-of-body experience," which can mean not only a sense of dissociation between mind and body but the sense that one's noncorporeal self has traveled to a different realm. Meeting with nonterrestrial beings (eg, space aliens), noncorporeal beings (eg, angels), archetypal beings (eg, Buddha), or deceased relatives may occur, and these experiences may seem extremely realistic and well organized into a single narrative. Some of the lessons learned from the out-of-body experience may encourage the patient to have breakthroughs in psychotherapy later.

The third state is a "near-death experience" (NDE), which often involves ego death and rebirth, as well as a review of one's life. Like the out-of-body experience, individuals may feel as though they have visited other realms or met with other beings. Ketamine-induced NDEs are reportedly similar to organic NDEs, which are known to lead to a desire to change. Kolp also notes that ketamine-induced NDEs possess patients with a greater sense of resolve than that which follows an out-of-body experience. Consequently, patients with personality disorders and addictive illnesses (either substance use or eating disorders) may experience remission after an NDE. Spontaneous spiritual conversion and improvements in moral character are also common.

The fourth state is "ego-dissolving transcendental," which is described as a perceived dissolution of the boundaries separating the self from external reality and a sense of oneness with the physical universe and the divine. It appears to be less dose dependent than the other NOSCs mentioned, though it is more common at higher doses. Like NDEs, patients who have an ego-dissolving transcendental experience frequently come away with a vastly different perception of their place in the universe, which can facilitate symptom improvement in mental illnesses, positive changes in lifestyle, and psychospiritual growth.[4] Kolp reports that these benefits are far more likely if patients have gone through an orientation program prior to taking ketamine and have guidance in processing the experience in the days and weeks after it.

Therapeutic Indications

Three indications for ketamine have been approved by the FDA:
1. As an anesthetic agent, oftentimes in conjunction with other anesthetic agents
2. For depressive symptoms in adults diagnosed with major depressive disorder (MDD) with acute suicidal ideation (esketamine only)
3. For treatment-resistant depression in adults (esketamine only)

Most patients seeking ketamine for depression have had treatment with four or more antidepressants and a myriad of nonpharmacologic interventions with no success. However, esketamine can be recommended in patients who have not responded to as few as two antidepressants.[31]

Treatment-Resistant Depression and Suicidal Ideation

Ketamine and esketamine have both shown efficacy in alleviating symptoms associated with treatment-resistant depression and MDD with acute suicidality, though only esketamine is currently approved by the FDA for use in treating this disorder. Racemic ketamine is only approved for use as an anesthetic agent, though several studies have shown it can be administered intravenously to produce similar antidepressant effects when compared to intranasal esketamine (see Table 14.4).[31]

In many cases, the antidepressant effects of esketamine occur within a manner of hours, though the effect is not sustained without maintenance doses of esketamine and continued treatment with conventional antidepressants. This makes esketamine extremely useful in instances where the patient may be overwhelmed by suicidality due to depressive symptoms. What remains an open question is the medium-term and long-term utility of intranasal esketamine. Currently, there is very little information available about the long-term effects of intranasal esketamine treatment.

One notable exception is the SUSTAIN-3 study (trial registration code: NCT02782104), *interim results* of which were published in May 2023 by Zaki and colleagues (the study was not completed until December 2022 and full results were not available while drafting this chapter).[32] The study had a 4-week induction phase that involved 458 enrollees, followed by an optimization/maintenance phase of variable length that included 420 participants from the induction phase and additional 690 who enrolled directly into the optimization/maintenance phase (total = 1,148). Of the 1,110 who participated in optimization/maintenance phase, 768 were still participating at the interim database lock on December 1, 2020. Reasons why enrollees discontinued the trial can be found in Table 14.5.

TABLE 14.4 Esketamine Efficacy and Tolerability

First Author (Year)	Methodology	Key Results	Trial Registration Code	Reference (See Bottom of Table)
Fedgchin et al (2019)	Phase III, DBL, RCT, 346 participants with moderate/severe MDD nonresponsive to ≥2 AD; ESK 56/84 mg vs placebo + AD, 4 wk	MADRS scores did not support any significant difference between ESK and placebo at the endpoint.	NCT02417064	1
Popova et al (2019) Floden et al (2022)	Phase III, DBL, RCT, 227 participants with moderate/severe MDD nonresponsive to ≥2 AD; ESK 56/84 mg vs placebo + AD, 4 wk	ESK differentiated itself from placebo on MADRS and PHQ-9 scales.	NCT02418585	2,3
Ochs-Ross et al (2020)	Phase III, DBL, RCT, 138 participants with TRD; ESK 28/56/84 mg vs placebo + AD, 4 wk	No significant difference in the decrease of MADRS scores between groups. Patients aged 65-74 y responded better; first MDE <55 y of age was a favorable prognostic factor.	NCT02422186	4
Correia-Melo et al (2020)	DBL, RCT, 63 participants with TRD; ESK vs KET IV, single dose	The remission rate was higher under ESK vs KET treatment at 24 h postadministration based on MADRS scores.	UMIN000032355	5

(continued)

TABLE 14.4 Esketamine Efficacy and Tolerability (*continued*)

First Author (Year)	Methodology	Key Results	Trial Registration Code	Reference (See Bottom of Table)
Singh et al (2016)	DBL, RCT, 30 participants with TRD; ESK vs placebo IV, single dose; second phase: Rerandomization of nonresponsive patients on ESK vs placebo, on day 4	ESK was superior to placebo (based on MADRS scores) on day 2 after therapy. The effect of ESK was rapid (2 h postinfusion).	NCT01640080	6
Souza-Marques et al (2022)	Retrospective analysis, 15 patients with PMD; ESK single dose IV	ESK improved MADRS scores 24 h postadministration. No difference was observed between patients with MDD and PMD in relation to ESK treatment.	N/A	7
Fu et al (2020)	Phase III, DBL, RCT, 226 participants with MDD + active suicidal ideation and intent; ESK 84 mg vs placebo + SOC (AD included), 4 wk	ESK was associated with significantly greater improvement after 24 h post first dose administration. No difference in the severity of suicide risk was reported. The favorable effect was detected earlier in patients who received ESK (4 h postadministration).	NCT03039192	8

Ionescu et al (2021)	Phase III, DBL, RCT, 230 patients with MDD + suicidal ideation with intent, ESK 84 mg vs placebo, 4 wk + SOC (AD included)	ESK led to significantly greater improvement in MADRS scores 24 h from the first dose. The CGI-S scores were improved in both groups, without differences between them. The positive effect was detected earlier in patients with ESK (4 h).	NCT03097133	9
Caruso et al (2021)	Post hoc analysis, ESK vs placebo + SOC, 24 h posttreatment administration, two trials	Patients with a history of suicide attempts had a significantly greater decrease in suicidal behavior and/or ideation (CGI-SS-R) posttreatment.	N/A	10
Takahashi et al (2021)	Phase IIb, DBL, RCT, 202 patients with MDD nonresponsive to 1-4 Ads; 4 wk	No differences between active and placebo groups were reported, based on the primary outcome of MADRS scores.	NCT02918318	11
Araújo-de-Freitas et al (2021)	DBL, RCT, 54 patients with TRD; ESK vs KET IV single dose	No difference between groups was observed in cognitive functioning following treatment, but both drugs improved cognitive performance in patients with TRD.	UMIN000032355	12

(continued)

TABLE 14.4 Esketamine Efficacy and Tolerability (continued)

First Author (Year)	Methodology	Key Results	Trial Registration Code	Reference (See Bottom of Table)
Pfenninger et al (2002)	RCT, DBL, healthy participants, crossover design; KET vs ESK vs *R*-KET IV	Multiple cognitive parameters improved significantly after 5 min post-isomer administration vs racemic KET.	N/A	13
Dijkstra et al (2022)	27 participants with mild/moderate MDD; ESK 84 mg vs placebo, 6 ± 0.5 and 18 ± 2 h postadministration, 3 wk	ESK did not negatively affect driving performance vs placebo.	NCT02919579	14
Daly et al (2019)	Phase III, 297 patients, ESK vs placebo + AD, 16 wk	The risk of relapse was decreased by 51%-70% in patients treated with ESK + AD vs placebo + AD.	NCT02493868	15
Wajs et al (2020)	Phase III, DBL, RCT, 802 patients with TRD; ESK 28/56/84 mg + AD, 4 wk (first phase) + OL second phase (48 wk)	MADRS scores improved compared with baseline up to the end of the second phase.	NCT02497287	16

AD, antidepressant; CGI-S, Clinical Global Impression-Severity; CGI-SS-R, Clinical Global Impression-Severity of Suicidality-Revised; DBL, double-blind; ESK, esketamine; IV, intravenous; KET, ketamine; MADRS, Montgomery-Asberg Depression Rating Scale; MDD, major depressive disorder; MDE, major depressive episode; N/A, not applicable; OL, open label; PHQ, Patient Health Questionnaire; PMD, persistent mood disorder; MDD, major depressive disorder with psychotic features; RCT, randomized controlled trial; SOC, standard of care; TRD, treatment-resistant depression.

Table adapted with permission from the author. Vasiliu O. Esketamine for treatment-resistant depression: a review of clinical evidence (Review). *Exp Ther Med.* 2023;25(3):111. doi:10.3892/etm.2023.11810. PMID: 36793329; PMCID: PMC9922941.

1. Fedgchin M, Trivedi M, Daly EJ, et al. Efficacy and safety of fixed-dose esketamine nasal spray combined with a new oral antidepressant in treatment-resistant depression: results of a randomized, double-blind, active-controlled study (TRANSFORM-1). *Int J Neuropsychopharmacol.* 2019;22:616-630. doi:10.1093/ijnp/pyz039
2. Popova V, Daly EJ, Trivedi M, et al. Efficacy and safety of flexibly dosed esketamine nasal spray combined with a newly initiated oral antidepressant in treatment-resistant depression: a random zed double-blind active-controlled study. *Am J Psychiatry.* 2019;176:428-438. doi:10.1176/appi.ajp.2019.19020172
3. Floden L, Hudgens S, Jamieson C, et al. Evaluation of individual items of the Patient Health Questionnaire (PHQ-9) and Montgomery-Asberg Depression Rating Scale (MADRS) in adults with treatment-resistant depression treated with esketamine nasal spray combined with a new oral antidepressant. *CNS Drugs.* 2022;36:649-658. doi:10.1007/s40263-022-00916-2
4. Ochs-Ross R, Daly EJ, Zhang Y, et al. Efficacy and safety of esketamine nasal spray plus an oral antidepressant in elderly patients with treatment-resistant depression—TRANSFORM-3. *Am J Geriatr Psychiatry.* 2020;28:121-141. doi:10.1016/j.jagp.2019.10.008
5. Correia-Melo FS, Leal GC, Vieira F, et al. Efficacy and safety of adjunctive therapy using esketamine or racemic ketamine for adult treatment-resistant depression: a randomized, double-blind, non-inferiority study. *J Affect Disord.* 2020;264:527-534. doi:10.1016/j.jad.2019.11.086
6. Singh JB, Fedgchin M, Daly E, et al. Intravenous esketamine in adult treatment-resistant depression: a double-blind, double-randomization, placebo-controlled study. *Biol Psychiatry.* 2016;80 424-431. doi:10.1016/j.biopsych.2015.10.018
7. Souza-Marques B, Telles M Leal GC, et al. Esketamine for unipolar major depression with psychotic features: a retrospective chart review and comparison with nonpsychotic depression. *J Cl n Psychopharmacol.* 2022;42:408-412. doi:10.1097/JCP.0000000000001571
8. Fu DJ, Ionescu DF, Li X, et al. Esketamine nasal spray for rapid reduction of major depressive disorder symptoms in patients who have active suicidal ideation with intent: double-blind, randomized study (ASPIRE I). *J Clin Psychiatry.* 2020;81(3):19m13191. doi:10.4088/JCP.19m13191
9. Ionescu DF, Fu DJ, Qiu X, et al. Esketamine nasal spray for rapid reduction of depressive symptoms in patients with major depressive disorder (ASPIRE II). *Int J Neuropsychopharmacol.* 2021;24:22-31. doi:10.1093/ijnp/pyaa068
10. Caruso CM, Ionescu DF, Li X, et al. Esketamine nasal spray for the rapid reduction of depressive symptoms in major depressive disorder with acute suicidal ideation or behavior *J Clin P-ychopharmacol.* 2021;41:516-524. doi:10.1097/JCP.0000000000001465
11. Takahashi N, Yamada A, Shiraishi A, Shimizu H, Goto R, Tominaga Y. Esketamine as add-on therapy to oral antidepressant in Japanese patients with treatment-resistant depression: a phase 2b randomized clinical study. *BMC Psychiatry.* 2021;21(1):526. doi:10.1186/s12888-021-03538-y
12. Araújo-de-Freitas L, Santos-Lima C, Mendoça-Filho E, et al. Neurocognitive aspects of ketamine and esketamine on subjects with treatment-resistant depression: a comparative, randomized and double-blind study. *Psychiatry Res.* 2021;303:114058. doi:10.1016/j.psychres.2021.114058
13. Pfenninger EG, Durieux ME, Himmelseher S. Cognitive impairment after small-dose ketamine isomers in comparison to equianalgesic racemic ketamine in human volunteers. *Anesthesiology.* 2002;96:357-366. doi:10.1097/00000542-200202000-00022
14. Dijkstra FM, van de Loo AJ, Abdulahad S, et al. The effects of intranasal esketamine on on-road driving performance in patients with major depressive disorder or persistent depressive disorder. *J Psychopharmacol.* 2022;36:614-625. doi:10.1177/02698811221078764
15. Daly EJ, Trivedi MH, Janik A, et al. Efficacy of esketamine nasal spray plus oral antidepressant treatment for relapse prevention in patients with treatment-resistant depression: a randomized clinical trial. *JAMA Psychiatry.* 2019;76:893-903. doi:10.1001/jamapsychiatry.2019.1189
16. Wajs E, Aluisio L, Holder R, et al. Esketamine nasal spray plus oral antidepressant in patients with treatment-resistant depression: assessment of long-term safety in phase 3, open-label study (SUSTAIN-2). *J Clin Psychiatry.* 2020;81(3):19m12891. doi:10.4088/JCP.19m12891

TABLE 14.5 SUSTAIN-3 Participant Disposition

Induction Phase		Optimization/Maintenance Phase	
Total discontinued	38 (8.3%)	Total discontinued	342 (30.8%)
Lack of efficacy	9 (2.0%)	Adverse events	59 (5.3%)
Day 28 nonresponder	9 (2.0%)	Lack of efficacy	49 (4.4%)
Adverse event	7 (1.5%)	Withdrawal by participant	46 (4.1%)
Withdrawal by participant	4 (0.9%)	Relocation	33 (3.0%)
Lost to follow-up	3 (0.7%)	Symptom improvement	29 (2.6%)
Other reasons	6 (1.3%)	Participant/family choice	24 (2.2%)
		Noncompliance	20 (1.8%)
		Lost to follow-up	17 (1.5%)
		Other reasons	65 (5.9%)

Adapted from Zaki N, Chen LN, Lane R, et al. Long-term safety and maintenance of response with esketamine nasal spray in participants with treatment-resistant depression: interim results of the SUSTAIN-3 study. *Neuropsychopharmacology*. 2023;48(8):1225-1233. doi:10.1038/s41386-023-01577-5. PMID: 37173512; PMCID: PMC10267177.

During the induction phase, the patients (under supervision) self-administered a flexible dose of esketamine twice weekly for 4 weeks. Doses were 28 mg (starting dose), 56 mg, or 84 mg. The dose during the optimization/maintenance phase varied depending on individual patient symptom severity. To assess symptom severity, the researchers used the Sheehan Disability Scale (SDS), the Patient Health Questionnaire 9-item (PHQ-9), and Clinical Global Impression-Severity (CGI-S). They also used the Montgomery-Åsberg Depression Rating Scale (MADRS) at baseline, every week during the induction phase, and every 8 weeks during the optimization/maintenance phase.

As of the December 2020 database lock, mean exposure to intranasal esketamine was 31.5 months (median 37.7, range 0-56 months). Of the total participants (1,148), 930 (81.0%) were exposed for 12 months or more, 830 (72.3%) for 24 months or more, 556 (48.4%) for 36 months or more, and only 6 (0.5%) for 48 months or more. The mean duration of intermittent esketamine treatment during the parent and

SUSTAIN-3 studies combined was 36.8 months (range 0-64 months). Of the total participants, 991 (86.3%) were treated for 12 months or more, 866 (75.4%) for 24 months or more, 726 (63.2%) for 36 months or more, and 173 (15.1%) for 48 months or more. Throughout this time, almost all (96.8%) reported adverse events were mild or moderate in severity. The most common severe events included dysgeusia, dissociation, and dizziness—all of which resolved within 90 minutes. Serious adverse events were reported by 171 (14.9%) participants, the most common of which were worsening depression (1.5% [17 participants]), suicide attempt (1.0% [11 participants]), and suicidal ideation (0.8% [9 participants]). Of the 66 participants who discontinued treatment with esketamine due to an adverse event, the most common reasons were depression (7 [0.6%]), blood pressure increase (6 [0.5%]), dissociation (5 [0.4%]), anxiety (3 [0.3%]), mania (3 [0.3%]), fatigue (2 [0.2%]), and suicidal ideation (2 [0.2%]).

The results are promising, with the proportion of responders (defined as a 50% or greater reduction in total MADRS score) increasing throughout the induction phase from 15% on the eighth day to 49.2% at the phase's endpoint. By this time, 35.6% of participants had a total MADRS score of 12 or less, which is defined as being in remission. The percentage of participants in remission increased to 50.9% and 46.1% after 1 year of the optimization/maintenance phase and at the end of the phase, respectively. It should also be noted that, while 49 patients (4.4%) discontinued during the optimization/maintenance phase due to esketamine's lack of efficacy, 29 (2.6%) discontinued because their symptoms improved.[32]

Off-Label Uses

Though only esketamine has been approved by the FDA for use in psychiatry, racemic ketamine has been used off-label to treat MDD, postpartum depression, bipolar disorders, anxiety disorders, obsessive-compulsive disorder (OCD), PTSD, substance use disorders, eating disorders, and borderline personality disorder. Research also suggests that ketamine may induce stress resilience in the aftermath of a traumatic event, thereby preventing the development of PTSD or other trauma- and stressor-related disorders.

Although there is no question that ketamine can be used within psychiatry, what remains unresolved is whether its full benefits can be realized without a full psychedelic experience or if the experience is necessary to gain the full effects of the drug. The clinical trials noted below have used subanesthetic doses that are designed to avoid the kinds

Major Depressive Disorder

Racemic ketamine has long been used off-label to treat MDD and treatment-resistant depression. The most common IV dose is 0.5 mg/g over 40 minutes. Single-dose ketamine has been repeatedly shown to produce extremely high response rates in patients with depressive disorders like MDD in the short term, but these rates decline quickly, oftentimes within a matter of just a few days. Two open-label investigations, one by Ibrahim and colleagues published in 2012 and one by Matthew and colleagues published in 2010, found that the majority of patients' MADRS scores declined by 50% within 24 hours (responded to treatment, by definition). In the Ibrahim study, 48% of patients responded to treatment within 24 hours before falling to 38% at 72 hours and then 14% at 28 days.[33] In the Matthew study, 65% of patients responded to treatment within 24 hours, but that the figure declined to 54% at 72 hours and to 27% at 32 days.[34]

Postpartum Depression

Postpartum depression often occurs within the first trimester following birth and may affect as many as 19.2% of new mothers.[35] Ketamine's rapid antidepressant onset and rapid clearance from maternal bloodstreams make it an ideal treatment for postpartum depression. A meta-analysis investigating the use of perioperative ketamine during cesarean delivery found that a single IV dose of subanesthetic ketamine significantly reduced postpartum depression scores.[36] Similarly, a randomized control trial involving 319 participants found that the use of perioperative, IV esketamine (0.2 mg/kg) significantly lowered the average postpartum depression scores when compared to the control group at 6 hours, 12 hours, 24 hours, and 4 days after surgery. At the subsequent follow-up (day 42), there was no clinical significance in postpartum depression scores between the control group and the esketamine group.[37]

What remains a question is if ketamine is a potential treatment for postpartum depression outside of the first few days following birth. Literature is currently lacking on this issue.

Bipolar Disorders

As is the case with unipolar depression, ketamine has been shown to mitigate the symptoms of depressive episodes in patients diagnosed with bipolar depressive disorders. Diazgranados and colleagues demonstrated efficacy in a randomized, placebo-controlled, double-blind, crossover study with a single infusion of ketamine as an adjunct to mood stabilizers.[38] Results were then replicated by Zarate and colleagues.[39] Meanwhile, Zheng and colleagues found that symptom improvement increased among a group of 19 patients with treatment-resistant bipolar depression with multiple (six) IV infusions of 0.5 mg/kg of ketamine (though only 16 received all six infusions). Following the first infusion, response and remission rates were 21.1% and 15.8%, respectively. Following the sixth infusion, response and remission rates were 73.7% and 63.2%, respectively. The authors note that the average times for response and remission were 9.1 and 12.5 days.[40]

Ketamine has also been shown to reduce suicidality in patients with either unipolar or bipolar depressive disorders with a single infusion, though a clear mechanism of action of ketamine for either suicidality or antisuicidal effects has yet to be elucidated.[41] More research into ketamine's potential to mitigate suicidal ideation or suicidal intentions (whether associated with bipolar disorders or not) is needed.

One area of concern whenever treating bipolar disorders is affective switch. The data on ketamine and depressive episodes in bipolar disorders may appear promising, but more studies are needed to better understand if there are potential risks of affect switch and to identify potential means of reducing those risks.[41]

Anxiety Disorders

In a 2022 systematic review, Tully and colleagues found 18 studies involving the use of ketamine and the treatment of refractory anxiety disorders. Of those 18 studies, 8 focused exclusively on refractory anxiety disorders, while 10 examined concomitant refractory anxiety disorders among patients with treatment-resistant depression.

Similar to depressive disorders, their findings suggest that a single dose of IV ketamine (0.5 mg/kg) can reduce the symptoms of generalized anxiety and social anxiety disorders immediately following administration. These effects can last for several days, but eventually, the patient's symptoms return—typically in approximately 14 days. Maintenance treatment with IV ketamine was also found to decrease anxiety symptoms, but the symptoms returned once ketamine therapy ended. Though the effects of these treatments appear to be transient, it should be noted that symptoms were typically less severe than prior to treatment with ketamine. Additionally, the results of using larger doses appeared to be somewhat mixed, as many patients experienced reduced anxiety scores with doses of 1 mg/kg, whereas others noted that a dose-dependent increase in dissociation was found to be anxiogenic.

Ultimately, the review suggests that ketamine therapy has the potential to help patients with anxiety disorders that exist in isolation or in conjunction with depressive disorders.[42]

Obsessive-Compulsive Disorders

Preliminary studies have shown that ketamine can dampen the symptoms of OCD, but these effects are short lived. Trials have found they last just a few hours, after which symptom severity begins to creep up and typically returns to baseline within 7 days.[43] These findings suggest that adjunctive ketamine therapy could be particularly beneficial in an emergency setting where patient obsessions and compulsions present a danger to themselves or others.

Though ketamine's effects are transitory when used as an adjunct to existing medication regimens, researchers have found that polytherapy involving maintenance infusions of ketamine and either deep brain stimulation or cognitive behavioral therapy (CBT) may prolong the effects of ketamine.[43] A case report published by Veraart and colleagues in 2021 describes a patient with treatment-resistant depression and comorbid psychotic and obsessive-compulsive symptoms, who had not responded to either electroconvulsive therapy or deep brain stimulation without ketamine, but experienced prolonged (18-month) symptom reduction when the deep brain stimulation was combined with ketamine therapy.[44]

Given that as many as one-third of patients with OCD do not respond to first-line treatments and that preliminary testing suggests that some patients may respond extremely well to ketamine therapy, it is an avenue of research that is worth pursuing.[45]

Posttraumatic Stress Disorder

The literature on ketamine and PTSD is less extensive than one might expect. Preclinical studies have suggested symptom improvement may be mediated through increases in BDNF, specifically in the hippocampus, as one potential mechanism of action. Disrupted consolidation of fear conditioning via antagonism of NMDA receptors in the hippocampus has been proposed as another.[46]

A handful of case reports have suggested that ketamine may temporarily reduce PTSD symptom severity, as well as symptom severity of comorbid MDD.[47] It is worth noting here that there is significant overlap in the symptoms of MDD and the negative thinking and anhedonia that are part of the pathology of PTSD (as outlined in Criterion D in the text revision of the fifth edition of the *Diagnostic and Statistical Manual of Mental Disorders* [DSM-5-TR]).[48] Given ketamine's antidepressant effects, it is not surprising that it would help with the symptoms.

Meanwhile, a double-blind, crossover, randomized controlled trial involving 41 patients with PTSD showed that ketamine was well tolerated and that it led to temporary symptom reduction. Patients were given either a single IV infusion of ketamine (0.5 mg/kg; $n = 22$) or active control midazolam (0.045 mg/kg; $n = 19$). Patients who received ketamine experienced rapid symptom reduction within 24 hours of infusion that was superior to the active control, as measured by the Impact of Event Scale-Revisited score. For 7 (32%) of the patients who received ketamine, compared to 1 (5%) who received midazolam, symptom improvement persisted for at least 2 weeks. The alleviation of comorbid depressive symptoms was also more pronounced among those who received ketamine, albeit temporarily.[49]

Preclinical trials have suggested that ketamine may impact the encoding of negative memories and could, consequently, have prophylactic utility.[50] At this time, no human studies have tested ketamine's ability to promote resiliency or to disrupt the development of trauma- and stressor-related disorders in the aftermath of a traumatic event.

Substance Use Disorders

One of the earliest uses of ketamine in psychiatry was to treat alcohol use disorder in the former Soviet Union. Krupitsky pioneered this work starting in the 1980s. Although his methodology was initially based on concomitant aversive therapies designed to produce strong negative emotions toward alcohol use, Krupitsky realized that patients showed better results when their ketamine experience was to a greater extent psychedelic.[4] Consequently, the manner in which he treated patients evolved to facilitate these experiences. His first study to use this methodology, published in 1992, involved 111 patients split between a ketamine group and a control group. At 1-year follow-up, 69.8% of the former had maintained abstinence, while only 24% of the control group were still sober.[51] Krupitsky's work also showed efficacy in treating opioid use disorder. Once again, the psychedelic/mystical-type experience, which is more likely to be induced at higher dosages of ketamine (typically 2.0-2.5 mg/kg, IM), is central to the therapeutic effect.[4]

Smaller doses of IV ketamine (0.5-0.8 mg/kg) have also been shown to be efficacious in the treatment of alcohol use disorder, though its effects on abstinence rates are mixed. Grabski and colleagues conducted a double-blind placebo-controlled phase 2 clinical trial involving 96 patients with severe alcohol use disorder and found a greater number of nondrinking days among the study's ketamine plus therapy group, but no significant difference in relapse rates after 6 months.[52] In that study, the ketamine group received three IV infusions (0.8 mg/kg over 40 minutes). Dakwar and colleagues, meanwhile, found that motivational enhancement therapy in conjunction with a single, 52-minute infusion of ketamine (0.71 mg/kg) was superior to a single infusion of midazolam (0.025 mg/kg) with respect to abstinence rates, delayed time to relapse, and number of heavy drinking days over the course of 21 days post infusion.[53] Results from a small pilot study involving four patients with MDD and comorbid alcohol use disorder indicate that naltrexone (Vivitrol, ReVia) combined with weekly ketamine infusions of 0.5 mg/kg over the course of 4 weeks dramatically improved depressive symptoms. Mean MADRS scores fell from 34.4 at baseline to 8.4 following the final measurement (240 minutes after the fourth infusion), though it should be noted that one patient left the study after the second infusion (their MADRS score fell from 46 at baseline to 5 at final reading). Four of the five patients reported reduced cravings for alcohol and consumption.[54]

Ketamine may also help with cocaine use disorder by increasing motivation to quit while reducing cravings for cocaine. As one example, a randomized clinical trial involving 55 individuals with cocaine use disorder found that a single IV infusion of ketamine (0.5 mg/kg) was superior to the active control midazolam (0.025 mg/kg) using a variety of metrics. The ketamine or midazolam was administered during a 5-day inpatient stay that was accompanied by and followed by a 5-week course of mindfulness-based relapse prevention. Of the ketamine group, 48.2% maintained abstinence compared with 10.7% of the midazolam group. Craving scores were also lower in the ketamine group (58.1%), and this group was 53% less likely to relapse.[55]

It seems likely that at the very least ketamine could be used to treat other substance use disorders.

Eating Disorders

The first trial involving the use of ketamine to treat eating disorders dates back to the 1990s and involved an IV infusion of ketamine (20 mg/h) for 10 hours with twice daily 20-mg doses of nalmefene, an opioid antagonist. Between two and nine infusions (average 5.8) were given at intervals of 5 to 21 days to a total of 15 patients with long-term and treatment-resistant anorexia. Nine patients responded to treatment, while six did not. What is interesting to note is that depressive scores dropped significantly in the nine patients who responded to treatment, while depressive scores remained high among nonresponders.[56]

More recently, three case studies and a longitudinal case series involving four patients have been published, each showing the efficacy of ketamine in treating anorexia nervosa with comorbid treatment-resistant depression. Patients diagnosed with eating disorder otherwise not specified (binge/purge subtype) were not particularly responsive to the treatment.[57] However, as the data apply only to seven patients (five with anorexia nervosa and two with eating disorder otherwise not specified [binge/purge subtype]), making any conclusions about the efficacy of ketamine seems extremely premature.

Borderline Personality Disorder

Ketamine may also help manage symptoms of borderline personality disorder, especially mood disturbances, social difficulties, and suicidal ideation. To date, there has been one randomized controlled trial showing that ketamine was well tolerated and that a single infusion of ketamine (0.5 mg/kg) performed better than the benzodiazepine midazolam (Dormicum or Versed) with respect to socio-occupational functioning, largely as a result of reduced depressive symptoms.[58]

Psychedelic-Assisted Psychotherapy With Ketamine

As discussed in this chapter, there is strong evidence to support the use of lower doses of ketamine (ie, 0.5 mg/kg) for a range of psychiatric conditions, but many of the benefits of ketamine are clearly transient. Practitioners of psychedelic-assisted psychotherapy who use significantly higher doses of ketamine, such as Krupitsky and Kolp, have reported significantly long-lasting benefits, especially when the experience results in NOSCs like near-death or ego-dissolving transcendental experiences. This is especially the case when this treatment modality is paired with the kind of preparatory and integrative sessions that are common in other types of psychedelic-assisted psychotherapies with LSD or psilocybin. In other words, the dissociative effects that many are attempting to subdue or perceive as an adverse effect may in fact serve as a psychological catalyst that results in long-term patient improvement in conditions like those described previously.[4]

Although promising, far more studies are needed to understand the risks and benefits of using higher doses of ketamine in treating psychiatric conditions.

Precautions and Adverse Effects

The effects of subanesthetic ketamine are not always predictable, nor are patients' responses uniform to these effects. Dissociation was reported by 61% to 75% of patients treated with esketamine during clinical trials.[25] Although some found it to be calming, others found it to be unsettling. In some cases, this experience can be unpleasant or too intense, but the effect can be mitigated by dose reductions or administration of lorazepam.

It should be noted that even low doses of ketamine can cause sedation, which was experienced by between 49% and 61% of patients treated with esketamine during clinical trials.[25] Patients may also experience dizziness and gait instability following ketamine infusion. Consequently, patients should be monitored until they have recovered, while older patients should not attempt to walk for at least 1 hour after the infusion. In most cases, patients fully return to baseline within 2 hours of completing their session with ketamine.

Precautions

Ketamine increases heart rate and blood pressure, so caution is warranted when considering treatment for those with comorbid cardiovascular disease. Patients with kidney disease and other genitourinary disorders may not be ideal candidates for ketamine treatment, as excessive ketamine use is associated with some urinary tract pathologies.[25]

Adverse Effects

Most adverse effects of ketamine resolve on their own after the acute effects have dissipated. These include anxiety, dissociation, dizziness, dysgeusia, headache, hypertension, hypoesthesia, lethargy, nausea, sedation, vertigo, and vomiting.[25] Frequent and long-term ketamine users may develop cognitive impairment, memory deficits, and genitourinary pathologies. In extreme cases, habitual users may develop ketamine bladder syndrome, which is characterized by a painful bladder, incontinence, hematuria, and papillary necrosis.

Risk of Overdose or Abuse

The risk of a fatal overdose of ketamine is extremely low, especially in a clinical setting. Outside of a clinical setting, ketamine does have the potential to be abused, which is why it is a Schedule III drug in the United States. Fatal overdose may be uncommon, but individuals who use ketamine in an unsupervised setting can put themselves at risk, as ketamine can cause sedation and impaired motor function. In addition to those taking ketamine on their own, and putting themselves at risk, the drug has been used to immobilize individuals, thereby facilitating rape or sexual assault. Street names for ketamine include "Vitamin K," "Super K," "Special K," or just the letter "K," and may be snorted, added to drinks, cigarettes, or injected. It has also been used by law enforcement agencies/emergency medical services to subdue violent individuals though lately this has come under scrutiny, especially after the death of an arrested man in Colorado in 2019.

Pregnant and Nursing Women

The use of ketamine during pregnancy is not advised, as it may harm the embryo or fetus.[59]

Very small percentages of ketamine and its active metabolites are ingested by nursing infants following the use of ketamine by the mother. The relative infant dose of ketamine is estimated to be between 0.34% and 0.57%, while the relative infant dose of norketamine is estimated to fall within the range of 0.29% and 0.95%, which are well below accepted safety protocols.[60] This suggests that the use of ketamine for the treatment of depressive disorders among new mothers is unlikely to adversely affect infants in clinically significant ways and that ketamine may be an acceptable treatment for postpartum depression and postpartum pain.

Use of ketamine in infants is not advised.[25]

Drug Interactions

Ketamine is metabolized by cytochrome P450 enzymes CYP3A4 and CYP2B6, while the active ketamine metabolite norketamine is primarily hydroxylated to 6-hydroxy-ketamine by CYP2A6. Inhibitors of CYP3A4 include clarithromycin, diltiazem, erythromycin, itraconazole, ketoconazole, ritonavir, verapamil, goldenseal, and grapefruit. Strong inhibitors of CYP2A6 include clotrimazole, letrozole, miconazole, pilocarpine, and tranylcypromine. Strong inhibitors of CYP2B6 include ticlopidine, orphenadrine, raloxifene, and rilpivirine.

Ketamine also inhibits many human UDP-glucuronosyltransferase (UGT) enzymes, particularly UGT2B4, UGT2B7, and UGT2B15. UGT2B7 metabolizes morphine and codeine.[61] Higher doses of ketamine may result in UGT2B7 inhibition that is clinically significant for the metabolism of these two opioids, while analgesic (subanesthetic) doses of ketamine are only clinically significant for the metabolism of codeine.

Drugs that cause sedation, including benzodiazepines, opioids, and ethanol, may compound sedative effects. Concomitant use of monoamine oxidase inhibitors and psychostimulants may increase blood pressure.[25]

Dosage and Clinical Guidelines

A typical dose of an IV ketamine infusion for depression is usually 0.5 mg/kg infused over 40 minutes for the initial 2 to 3 weeks of treatment with 1-week intervals between infusions. Dosage can be gradually increased by 0.1 to 1.0 mg/kg during subsequent sessions. Most patients receive treatment for 6 weeks but may need booster infusions depending on clinical need or may receive them periodically every few weeks or months.

As a matter of practical protocol, patients should fast for 3 hours prior to ketamine infusion to limit nausea. Clinicians should then obtain the patient's weight and baseline vitals, conduct a brief psychiatric interview, determine the dose, and then begin the 40-minute infusion. Vital signs should be taken 20 minutes after starting the infusion and upon completion of the treatment. In addition, the patient's vital signs should be checked again after the treatment at 20 and 40 minutes to monitor downtrends in heart rate and blood pressure. Thereafter, it is recommended to offer and assist the patient to the restroom and assess gait and any signs of dizziness.

Intranasal esketamine can be administered 2 times per week for the first 2 to 4 weeks, once per week for weeks 5 to 9, and then once every week or every other week thereafter. Patients should begin with the 56-mg dose and, if tolerated well, may increase to the 84-mg dose.[25] There is no standard guideline for maintenance treatment. A 4-week course of ketamine treatment with no response is considered a failed trial.

There are currently no formal guidelines issued by the FDA for alternative treatments involving ketamine.

Special Populations

Children

Ketamine is regularly used for procedural sedation and analgesia for neonates, infants, and young children in emergency departments due to its ease of administration and safety profile. However, esketamine is not indicated for use in individuals under the age of 18. Although studies have found that ketamine infusions may potentially help children and adolescents with treatment-resistant depression or mood disorders, more studies are needed to determine its long-term safety.[62]

Persons With Hepatic Insufficiency

Patients with moderate hepatic impairment may need to be monitored for adverse reactions for longer than those with no such impairment. Use of ketamine in patients with severe hepatic impairment is not recommended.

Esketamine Risk Evaluation and Mitigation Strategy

A REMS is required by the FDA to manage potential risks associated with esketamine, including dissociation and sedation. All inpatient and outpatient health care settings should be certified to receive or dispense esketamine. In addition, pharmacies must be certified, and all patients need to be enrolled with their prescriber to receive treatment.

Esketamine should be administered under the direct supervision of a health care provider and should be monitored for 2 hours post treatment. All patients should have a monitoring form completed by the health care provider that includes:

- Patients' demographic information
- Concomitant medications
- Health care provider and setting information
- Treatment session information, including:
  - Treatment date
  - Dose administered
  - Treatment duration
  - Vital signs monitoring
  - Adverse events
- A report of all serious adverse events

Approved REMS for esketamine can be explored in greater detail on the esketamine and FDA's website (https://www.spravatorems.com/).

Conclusion

Unlike many of the drugs discussed in this book, ketamine has enjoyed widespread clinical use for several decades, and multiple, well-designed trials have been conducted to test its efficacy in treating a myriad of conditions. However, perhaps nowhere else is it more evident that psychedelic drugs have two distinct mechanisms of action, one that is largely neurophysiologic and the other that is fundamentally existential. Ketamine clearly demonstrates activity at NMDA and opioid receptors, as well as multiple other sites, and this activity can lead to symptom reduction in a host of psychiatric disorders. One drawback is that symptom reduction is often short lived. Alternatively, many patients who have mystical-type experiences via higher doses of ketamine, coupled with guidance before and after by trained professionals, frequently enjoy long-term relief of symptoms. The major drawback is that this kind of treatment is resource intensive and expensive.

What will likely remain a challenge in psychiatry and for psychiatrists is deciding which treatment modality is most appropriate, given the patient, the condition, and the regulatory environment.

REFERENCES

1. Grof S. My ketamine journeys or ketamine and the enchantment of other worlds. Ketamine psychedelic psychotherapy: focus on its pharmacology, phenomenology, and clinical applications. In: Wolfson P, Hartelius G, eds. *The Ketamine Papers: Science, Therapy, and Transformation*. Multidisciplinary Association for Psychedelic Studies; 2016:39-45.
2. Stevens M, Taylor DB. Matthew Perry died of 'acute effects of ketamine,' autopsy says. *New York Times*. Published December 15, 2023. Accessed February 1, 2024. https://www.nytimes.com/2023/12/15/arts/matthew-perry-cause-death-friends.html
3. Kötz A, Merkel P. Zur Kenntnis Hydroaromatischer Alkamine. *J Prakt Chem*. 1926;113:49-76. Accessed January 29, 2024. https://gallica.bnf.fr/ark:/12148/bpt6k90883j/f57.item
4. Kolp E, Friedman HL, Krupitsky E, et al. Ketamine psychedelic psychotherapy: focus on its pharmacology, phenomenology, and clinical applications. In: Wolfson P, Hartelius G, eds. *The Ketamine Papers: Science, Therapy, and Transformation*. Multidisciplinary Association for Psychedelic Studies; 2016:97-197.
5. Krystal JH. Edward F. Domino, Ph.D. (1924-2021). *Neuropsychopharmacology*. 2022;47:1138-1139. doi:10.1038/s41386-022-01280-x
6. Domino EF, Warner DS. Taming the ketamine tiger. *Anesthesiology*. 2010;113(3):678-684. doi:10.1097/ALN.0b013e3181ed09a2
7. Luby ED, Cohen BD, Rosenbaum G, Gottlieb JS, Kelley R. Study of a new schizophrenomimetic drug—Sernyl. *AMA Arch Neurol Psychiatry*. 1959;81:363-369.
8. Li L, Vlisides PE. Ketamine: 50 years of modulating the mind. *Front Hum Neurosci*. 2016;10:612. doi:10.3389/fnhum.2016.00612
9. Domino EF, Chodoff P, Corssen G. Pharmacologic effects of CI-581, a new dissociative anesthetic, in man. *Clin Pharmacol Ther*. 1965;6:279-291.
10. Höflich A, Hahn A, Küblböck M, et al. Ketamine-induced modulation of the thalamo-cortical network in healthy volunteers as a model for schizophrenia. *Int J Neuropsychopharmacol*. 2015;18(9):pyv040. doi:10.1093/ijnp/pyv040. PMID: 25896256; PMCID: PMC4576520.
11. Krystal JH, Karper LP, Seibyl JP, et al. Subanesthetic effects of the noncompetitive NMDA antagonist, ketamine, in humans. Psychotomimetic, perceptual, cognitive, and neuroendocrine responses. *Arch Gen Psychiatry*. 1994;51(3):199-214. doi:10.1001/archpsyc.1994.03950030035004. PMID: 8122957.

12. Corssen G, Domino EF. Further pharmacologic studies and first clinical experience with the phencyclidine derivative CI-581. *Anesth Analg.* 1966;45(1):29-40.
13. Zanos P, Moaddel R, Morris PJ, et al. Ketamine and ketamine metabolite pharmacology: insights into therapeutic mechanisms. *Pharmacol Rev.* 2018;70(3): 621-660. doi:10.1124/pr.117.015198. Erratum in: *Pharmacol Rev.* 2018;70(4):879. PMID: 29945898; PMCID: PMC6020109.
14. Collier BB. Ketamine and the conscious mind. *Anaesthesia.* 1972;27(2):120-134. doi:10.1111/j.1365-2044.1972.tb08186.x. PMID: 5021517.
15. Wolfson P. Ketamine: its history, uses, pharmacology, therapeutic practice, and an exploration of its potential as a novel treatment for depression. In: Wolfson P, Hartelius G, eds. *The Ketamine Papers: Science, Therapy, and Transformation.* Multidisciplinary Association for Psychedelic Studies; 2016:1-23.
16. Wolfson P. Ketamine dependence: John Lilly as Explorer and as caveat. In: Wolfson P, Hartelius G, eds. *The Ketamine Papers: Science, Therapy, and Transformation.* Multidisciplinary Association for Psychedelic Studies; 2016:51-52.
17. Wei Y, Chang L, Hashimoto K. A historical review of antidepressant effects of ketamine and its enantiomers. *Pharmacol Biochem Behav.* 2020;190:172870. doi:10.1016/j.pbb.2020.172870
18. Berman RM, Cappiello A, Anand A, et al. Antidepressant effects of ketamine in depressed patients. *Biol Psychiatry.* 2000;47(4):351-354. doi:10.1016/s0006-3223(99)00230-9. PMID: 10686270.
19. Zarate CA Jr, Singh JB, Carlson PJ, et al. A randomized trial of an N-methyl-D-aspartate antagonist in treatment-resistant major depression. *Arch Gen Psychiatry.* 2006;63(8):856-864. doi:10.1001/archpsyc.63.8.856. PMID: 16894061.
20. Phillips JL, Norris S, Talbot J, et al. Single, repeated, and maintenance ketamine infusions for treatment-resistant depression: a randomized controlled trial. *Am J Psychiatry.* 2019;176(5):401-409. doi:10.1176/appi.ajp.2018.18070834. PMID: 30922101.
21. Wilkinson ST, Palamar JJ, Sanacora G. The rapidly shifting ketamine landscape in the US. *JAMA Psychiatry.* 2024;81(3):221-222. doi:10.1001/jamapsychiatry.2023.4945
22. Bahji A, Vazquez GH, Zarate CA Jr. Comparative efficacy of racemic ketamine and esketamine for depression: a systematic review and meta-analysis. *J Affect Disord.* 2021;278:542-555. doi:10.1016/j.jad.2020.09.071. Erratum in: *J Affect Disord.* 2020. PMID: 33022440; PMCID: PMC7704936.
23. Mion G, Villevieille T. Ketamine pharmacology: an update (pharmacodynamics and molecular aspects, recent findings). *CNS Neurosci Ther.* 2013;19(6):370-380. doi:10.1111/cns.12099
24. Ketalar. Package insert. JHP Pharmaceuticals, LLC; 2007. Accessed March 12, 2024. https://www.accessdata.fda.gov/drugsatfda_docs/label/2012/016812s039lbl.pdf
25. Spravato. Package insert. Janssen Pharmaceuticals, LLC; 2019. Accessed March 12, 2024. https://www.accessdata.fda.gov/drugsatfda_docs/label/2019/211243lbl.pdf
26. Marland S, Ellerton J, Andolfatto G, et al. Ketamine: use in anesthesia. *CNS Neurosci Ther.* 2013;19(6):381-389. doi:10.1111/cns.12072. PMID: 23521979; PMCID: PMC6493613.
27. Williams NR, Heifets BD, Bentzley BS, et al. Attenuation of antidepressant and antisuicidal effects of ketamine by opioid receptor antagonism. *Mol Psychiatry.* 2019;24(12):1779-1786. doi:10.1038/s41380-019-0503-4. PMID: 31467392.
28. Zorumski CF, Izumi Y, Mennerick S. Ketamine: NMDA receptors and beyond. *J Neurosci.* 2016;36(44):11158-11164. doi:10.1523/JNEUROSCI.1547-16.2016. PMID: 27807158; PMCID: PMC5148235.
29. Lazarevic V, Yang Y, Flais I, Svenningsson P. Ketamine decreases neuronally released glutamate via retrograde stimulation of presynaptic adenosine A1 receptors. *Mol Psychiatry.* 2021;26(12):7425-7435. doi:10.1038/s41380-021-01246-3. PMID: 34376822; PMCID: PMC8872981.

30. Beerten SG, Matheï C, Aertgeerts B. Ketamine misuse: an update for primary care. *Br J Gen Pract.* 2023;73(727):87-89. doi:10.3399/bjgp23X731997. PMID: 36702586; PMCID: PMC9888585.
31. Vasiliu O. Esketamine for treatment-resistant depression: a review of clinical evidence (Review). *Exp Ther Med.* 2023;25(3):111. doi:10.3892/etm.2023.11810. PMID: 36793329; PMCID: PMC9922941.
32. Zaki N, Chen LN, Lane R, et al. Long-term safety and maintenance of response with esketamine nasal spray in participants with treatment-resistant depression: interim results of the SUSTAIN-3 study. *Neuropsychopharmacology.* 2023;48(8):1225-1233. doi:10.1038/s41386-023-01577-5. PMID: 37173512; PMCID: PMC10267177.
33. Ibrahim L, Diazgranados N, Franco-Chaves J, et al. Course of improvement in depressive symptoms to a single intravenous infusion of ketamine vs add-on riluzole: results from a 4-week, double-blind, placebo-controlled study. *Neuropsychopharmacology.* 2012;37(6):1526-1533. doi:10.1038/npp.2011.338. PMID: 22298121; PMCID: PMC3327857.
34. Mathew SJ, Murrough JW, aan het Rot M, Collins KA, Reich DL, Charney DS. Riluzole for relapse prevention following intravenous ketamine in treatment-resistant depression: a pilot randomized, placebo-controlled continuation trial. *Int J Neuropsychopharmacol.* 2010;13(1):71-82. doi:10.1017/S1461145709000169. PMID: 19288975; PMCID: PMC3883127.
35. Gavin NI, Gaynes BN, Lohr KN, Meltzer-Brody S, Gartlehner G, Swinson T. Perinatal depression: a systematic review of prevalence and incidence. *Obstet Gynecol.* 2005;106(5 pt 1):1071-1083. doi:10.1097/01.AOG.0000183597.31630.db. PMID: 16260528.
36. Li Q, Wang S, Mei X. A single intravenous administration of a sub-anesthetic ketamine dose during the perioperative period of cesarean section for preventing postpartum depression: a meta-analysis. *Psychiatry Res.* 2022;310:114396. doi:10.1016/j.psychres.2022.114396. PMID: 35278826.
37. Xu S, Yang J, Li J, et al. Esketamine pretreatment during cesarean section reduced the incidence of postpartum depression: a randomized controlled trail. *BMC Anesthesiol.* 2024;24(1):20. doi:10.1186/s12871-023-02398-1. PMID: 38200438; PMCID: PMC10777554.
38. Diazgranados N, Ibrahim L, Brutsche NE, et al. A randomized add-on trial of an N-methyl-D-aspartate antagonist in treatment-resistant bipolar depression. *Arch Gen Psychiatry.* 2010;67(8):793-802. doi:10.1001/archgenpsychiatry.2010.90. PMID: 20679587; PMCID: PMC3000408.
39. Zarate CA Jr, Brutsche NE, Ibrahim L, et al. Replication of ketamine's antidepressant efficacy in bipolar depression: a randomized controlled add-on trial. *Biol Psychiatry.* 2012;71(11):939-946. doi:10.1016/j.biopsych.2011.12.010. PMID: 22297150; PMCID: PMC3343177.
40. Zheng W, Zhou YL, Liu WJ, et al. A preliminary study of adjunctive ketamine for treatment-resistant bipolar depression. *J Affect Disord.* 2020;275:38-43. doi:10.1016/j.jad.2020.06.020. PMID: 32658821.
41. Wilkowska A, Szałach Ł, Cubała WJ. Ketamine in bipolar disorder: a review. *Neuropsychiatr Dis Treat.* 2020;16:2707-2717. doi:10.2147/NDT.S282208. PMID: 33209026; PMCID: PMC7670087.
42. Tully JL, Dahlén AD, Haggarty CJ, Schiöth HB, Brooks S. Ketamine treatment for refractory anxiety: a systematic review. *Br J Clin Pharmacol.* 2022;88(10):4412-4426. doi:10.1111/bcp.15374. PMID: 35510346; PMCID: PMC9540337.
43. Budies GL, Tyagi H. Rapid anti-obsessive treatments of obsessive-compulsive disorder: reviewing effects of ketamine in OCD. *J Neurol Neurosurg Psychiatry.* 2021;92(8):A10. doi:10.13140/RG.2.2.21069.97769
44. Veraart JKE, Kamphuis J, Schlegel M, Schoevers RA. Oral S-ketamine effective after deep brain stimulation in severe treatment-resistant depression and extensive

comorbidities. *BMJ Case Rep.* 2021;14(1):e238135. doi:10.1136/bcr-2020-238135. PMID: 33495180; PMCID: PMC7839911.
45. Sharma LP, Thamby A, Balachander S, et al. Clinical utility of repeated intravenous ketamine treatment for resistant obsessive-compulsive disorder. *Asian J Psychiatr.* 2020;52:102183. doi:10.1016/j.ajp.2020.102183. PMID: 32554207.
46. Zhang LM, Zhou WW, Ji YJ, et al. Anxiolytic effects of ketamine in animal models of posttraumatic stress disorder. *Psychopharmacology (Berl).* 2015;232(4):663-672. doi:10.1007/s00213-014-3697-9. PMID: 25231918.
47. Liriano F, Hatten C, Schwartz TL. Ketamine as treatment for post-traumatic stress disorder: a review. *Drugs Context.* 2019;8:212305. doi:10.7573/dic.212305. PMID: 31007698; PMCID: PMC6457782.
48. American Psychiatric Association. *Diagnostic and Statistical Manual on Mental Disorders.* 5th ed. The American Psychiatric Association; 2013:271-280.
49. Feder A, Parides MK, Murrough JW, et al. Efficacy of intravenous ketamine for treatment of chronic posttraumatic stress disorder: a randomized clinical trial. *JAMA Psychiatry.* 2014;71(6):681-688. doi:10.1001/jamapsychiatry.2014.62. PMID: 24740528.
50. Evers AG, Murrough JW, Charney DS, Costi S. Ketamine as a prophylactic resilience-enhancing agent. *Front Psychiatry.* 2022;13:833259. doi:10.3389/fpsyt.2022.833259. PMID: 35966469; PMCID: PMC9365980.
51. Krupitsky EM, Grinenko AY, Berkaliev TN, et al. The combination of psychedelic and aversive approaches in alcoholism treatment: the affective contra-attribution method. *Alcohol Treat Q.* 1992;9(1):99-105. doi:10.1300/J020V09N01_09
52. Grabski M, McAndrew A, Lawn W, et al. Adjunctive ketamine with relapse prevention-based psychological therapy in the treatment of alcohol use disorder. *Am J Psychiatry.* 2022;179(2):152-162. doi:10.1176/appi.ajp.2021.21030277. PMID: 35012326.
53. Dakwar E, Levin F, Hart CL, et al. A single ketamine infusion combined with motivational enhancement therapy for alcohol use disorder: a randomized midazolam-controlled pilot trial. *Am J Psychiatry.* 2020;177(2):125-133. doi:10.1176/appi.ajp.2019.19070684. PMID: 31786934.
54. Yoon G, Petrakis IL, Krystal JH. Association of combined naltrexone and ketamine with depressive symptoms in a case series of patients with depression and alcohol use disorder. *JAMA Psychiatry.* 2019;76(3):337-338. doi:10.1001/jamapsychiatry.2018.3990. PMID: 30624551; PMCID: PMC6439824.
55. Dakwar E, Nunes EV, Hart CL, et al. A single ketamine infusion combined with mindfulness-based behavioral modification to treat cocaine dependence: a randomized clinical trial. *Am J Psychiatry.* 2019;176(11):923-930. doi:10.1176/appi.ajp.2019.18101123. PMID: 31230464.
56. Mills IH, Park GR, Manara AR, Merriman RJ. Treatment of compulsive behaviour in eating disorders with intermittent ketamine infusions. *QJM.* 1998;91(7):493-503. doi:10.1093/qjmed/91.7.493. PMID: 9797933.
57. Ragnhildstveit A, Slayton M, Jackson LK, et al. Ketamine as a novel psychopharmacotherapy for eating disorders: evidence and future directions. *Brain Sci.* 2022;12(3):382. doi:10.3390/brainsci12030382. PMID: 35326338; PMCID: PMC8963252.
58. Fineberg SK, Choi EY, Shapiro-Thompson R, et al. A pilot randomized controlled trial of ketamine in Borderline personality disorder. *Neuropsychopharmacology.* 2023;48(7):991-999. doi:10.1038/s41386-023-01540-4. PMID: 36804489; PMCID: PMC10209175.
59. Cheung HM, Yew DTW. Effects of perinatal exposure to ketamine on the developing brain. *Front Neurosci.* 2019;13:138. doi:10.3389/fnins.2019.00138. PMID: 30853884; PMCID: PMC6395450.
60. Majdinasab E, Datta P, Krutsch K, Baker T, Hale TW. Pharmacokinetics of ketamine transfer into human milk. *J Clin Psychopharmacol.* 2023;43(5):407-410. doi:10.1097/JCP.0000000000001711. PMID: 37683228.

61. Uchaipichat V, Raungrut P, Chau N, Janchawee B, Evans AM, Miners JO. Effects of ketamine on human UDP-glucuronosyltransferases in vitro predict potential drug-drug interactions arising from ketamine inhibition of codeine and morphine glucuronidation. *Drug Metab Dispos*. 2011;39(8):1324-1328. doi:10.1124/dmd.111.039727. PMID: 21551257.
62. Meshkat S, Rosenblat JD, Ho RC, et al. Ketamine use in pediatric depression: a systematic review. *Psychiatry Res*. 2022;317:114911. doi:10.1016/j.psychres.2022.114911. PMID: 37732856.

15

3,4-Methylenedioxymeth-amphetamine

3,4-Methylenedioxymethamphetamine (MDMA) is a psychoactive substance that promotes the release of neurotransmitters such as dopamine, serotonin, and norepinephrine, as well as neurohormones, most notably oxytocin. Its use in psychiatry dates back to the 1970s. Illicit use was not particularly common until the early 1980s, but a rapid increase in popularity led to its prohibition and classification as a Schedule I drug by the Drug Enforcement Agency (DEA) in the middle of the decade. Despite restrictions on its use, MDMA has become the focus of intense interest by veteran groups and practitioners who treat patients with posttraumatic stress disorder (PTSD). Once considered a fringe idea, preliminary trials involving MDMA in the treatment of PTSD have been shown to be successful, and the drug was granted "breakthrough therapy" status in 2017 by the U.S. Food and Drug Administration (FDA). Clinical trials to better establish efficacy are ongoing.

It has been known for several decades that MDMA produces euphoric effects, and individuals experience a heightened sense of connectivity to others. These prosocial features made it a popular drug in underground dance and rave communities, where illicit (and frequently adulterated) MDMA was referred to as ecstasy, E, X, XTC, or molly. However, these features also appear to be one of the most important therapeutic characteristics of MDMA since it allows therapists to help patients break down psychological barriers and to explore memories and emotions that might otherwise be deemed too painful or too private to be examined. On account of these prosocial characteristics, MDMA is frequently referred to as an *empathogen* or *entactogen*. The former was favored by Ralph Metzner.[1] The latter coinage came from researcher David E. Nichols in a 1986 paper which refers to the capacity of a substance such as MDMA to produce a "touching within."[2] Consequently, these two terms tend to be used interchangeably within literature. Given that MDMA not only induces an empathetic state but also attenuates fear and anxiety, even in the face of exposure to frightening or stressful stimuli such as negative or traumatic memories, entactogen seems to be the appropriate term and will be used throughout this chapter.

History

While many of the drugs described in this book have intriguing stories about their origin that verge on the mythologic, MDMA's history is largely one of elision. Originally known as "Methylsafrylamin," the drug was first synthesized in 1912 by the German pharmaceutical company Merck and patented in 1913. Some accounts claim that it was intended to be an appetite suppressant, but the patent did not mention any such intended use. Research conducted by Freudenmann and colleagues in Merck's historical archives found no indication that the company planned to develop an appetite suppressant at any point between 1900 and 1960. Instead, the reason for the patent is far more procedural. According to the authors, it was considered nothing more than an insignificant precursor that was necessary for the synthesis of hemostatic agents; "the new pathway was patented in order to evade an existing patent by a local competitor."[3]

Alexander Shulgin reportedly synthesized MDMA in 1965 while working at Dow Chemical Company, and notes that he met several individuals who experimented with the drug sometime after 1967. Shulgin's personal experience with the drug led him to describe it as not being a psychedelic "in the visual or interpretive sense, but the lightness and warmth of the psychedelic was present and quite remarkable."[4(p69)] Shulgin developed a respect for the drug and believed that doses in the range of 80 to 100 mg endowed him with the capacity for greater introspection: "It enabled me to see out, and to see my own insides, without distortion or reservations."[4(p72)] He also coauthored two papers on the pharmacology of MDMA in humans at doses of 80 to 160 mg that were both published in 1978.[5(p12)]

Shulgin may have also introduced the drug to psychiatry in the late 1970s. As he recounts in his memoir, he provided MDMA to a psychotherapist in the Bay Area who often used psychoactive materials in some scenarios to sand down particularly obstructive psychological barriers in patients. Shulgin mentions by name 3,4-methylenedioxyamphetamine (MDA), lysergic acid diethylamide (LSD), and ibogaine as just three examples utilized by this individual. After receiving MDMA from Shulgin, "Adam" (as he is referred to in Shulgin's memoir, though later identified as Leo Zeff[6]) introduced an estimated 4,000 individuals either directly or indirectly to MDMA's entactogenic properties.[4(pp73,74)]

The timeline described by Shulgin appears to be accurate, as independent sources verify that MDMA-assisted therapy became relatively common among a small group of therapists in the late 1970s and into the 1980s.[6] The drug was found to be a very useful tool during individual and group therapy, particularly in patients with poor emotional regulation who struggled to process painful or negative memories. MDMA allowed them to gain greater emotional insight into their conditions, relationships, or situations. According to Shulgin, one psychiatrist even referred to MDMA as "penicillin for the soul."[4(p74)]

According to Passie and Benzenhöfer, illicit use of MDMA appears to have begun in the 1960s but did not become widespread until the late 1970s.[7] The rise in popularity was largely due to its use in dance clubs, where it was commonly referred to as "ecstasy." One of the most well-documented hazards associated with MDMA is that it causes hyperthermia and hyperhidrosis, especially in settings like dance clubs, which may lead to dehydration and further complications, including rhabdomyolysis.[8] Additional concerns about its toxicity led the DEA to criminalize its use in 1985 and led to it being classified as a Schedule I drug in 1986.

Despite these restrictions, illicit MDMA use continued from the 1980s into the 2000s, when it became associated with the underground "rave" scenes of the era, and it continues to this day. Based on the 2015-2020 National Survey on Drug Use and Health, Yang and colleagues were able to determine that average past-year use from 2015 to 2020 for MDMA was 0.9% among individuals aged 12 years and older.[9] For reference, estimates from the 2022 National Survey on Drug Use and Health, which was released in late 2023, found that 22.0% of individuals aged 12 years or older used marijuana within the past year (lifetime use was 46.9%).[10] Unfortunately, MDMA use could not be determined from the 2022 survey because the published data lump all hallucinogens into one class without greater specificity. According to the survey, past-year hallucinogen use in 2022 among individuals aged 12 years and older was 3.0% (lifetime use was 17.3%).[10]

Even though MDMA use was stigmatized following its criminalization, interest in its clinical utility never faded entirely. After years of lobbying, research into MDMA's use in psychiatry resumed in the early 1990s at Harbor University of California Los Angeles (UCLA) Medical Center.[11] Charles Grob led the phase 1 study that began in 1994, and FDA-approved research into MDMA has continued ever since. Research has been primarily focused on how MDMA can be used to reduce symptoms of PTSD when administered in conjunction with psychotherapy. The underlying premise behind this course of treatment is that MDMA allows the patient to revisit the traumatic memory without triggering negative emotional symptoms characteristic of PTSD and to then work with the therapist to mitigate the fear or anxiety associated with the trauma. This model relies on fear extinction and memory reconsolidation, which is similar to theoretical principles used in conventional treatment modalities such as prolonged exposure therapy. While most of the research into MDMA-assisted psychotherapy has focused on its potential to treat symptoms associated with PTSD, some believe it could be useful for the treatment of anxiety, substance use, and eating disorders. Some have even suggested that MDMA may reduce suicidal thoughts, but this argument is based on observational evidence.[12]

In 2017, MDMA received breakthrough therapy designation from the FDA. Since then, numerous phase 2 and phase 3 trials have been conducted by the Multidisciplinary Association for Psychedelic Studies (MAPS), which suggest that MDMA is an effective treatment for PTSD.[5] Lykos Therapeutics (formerly known as MAPS Public Benefit Corporation) has applied for FDA approval to market MDMA for the treatment of PTSD. In early June 2024, a panel of advisors to the FDA voted against approval, citing concerns of improper blinding, researcher bias, failure to report some adverse effects, cardiovascular events, and abuse potential.[13] The FDA ultimately voted against approving MDMA for the treatment of PTSD in August 2024, though the agency has indicated it will reconsider the decision following additional phase 3 trials.

Pharmacology

The pharmacology of MDMA is similar to amphetamines and some psychedelics, as it shares the phenethylamine core of the former and structural similarities to mescaline (covered in Chapter 12). It is also similar to 2,5-dimethoxy-4-iodoamphetamine (DOI) and

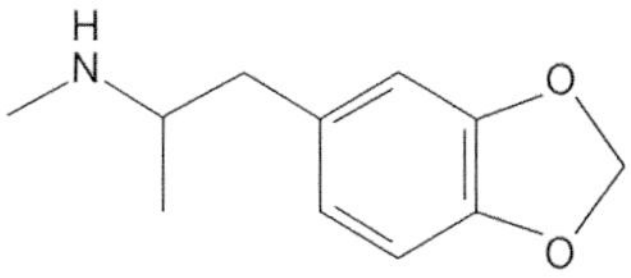

Figure 15.1 The structure of 3,4-methylenedioxymethamphetamine (MDMA). Courtesy of the National Institute on Drug Abuse.

2,5-dimethoxy-4-bromophenethylamine (2C-B), which will, both, be touched upon in Chapter 16. The structure of MDMA is shown in Figure 15.1.

Description

The base of MDMA is a colorless oil that is quite small, with a molecular weight of 193.24 g/mol.[1] Its more common form is a hydrochloride salt, which is a white or off-white powder or crystal that is soluble in water. One may also encounter bromide and phosphate salts.

Route of Administration

Outside of clinical settings, MDMA is typically consumed as a capsule or tablet. The latter may be adorned with a symbol or logo. MDMA may also occur as a powder that may be snorted or ingested orally. Outside of a clinical setting, it is common for drugs that are described as MDMA to be adulterated with inert and less costly substances or with other illicit drugs such as cocaine, amphetamines, or opioids (especially fentanyl).

In a clinical setting, MDMA is administered orally as a capsule or tablet.

Pharmacokinetics

MDMA follows a nonlinear pharmacokinetics in animal models and in humans. Active doses of MDMA may autoinhibit the function of cytochrome P450 enzyme 2D6 (CYP2D6) for an extended period, with enzyme function normalizing up to 10 days post-MDMA use. The enzymes CYP1A2, catechol-*O*-methyltransferase (COMT), and monoamine oxidase A (MAO-A) are also involved in the metabolism of MDMA. Consequently, monoamine oxidase inhibitors (MAOIs) are contraindicated with MDMA.

While the elimination half-life of active MDMA doses is 7 to 9 hours, the end of systemic exposure is up to 48 hours postdose.

Absorption

Following oral administration, MDMA is absorbed within 30 minutes in the intestinal tract and reaches peak plasma concentration in 1.5 to 2 hours. Peak blood concentrations of 106, 131, and 236 ng/mL are reached in healthy volunteers following oral doses of 50, 75, and 125 mg, respectively.[14] Following an oral dose of 125 mg, peak blood concentrations are reached within 2.4 ± 1 hours.[15]

Bioavailability

Absolute or relative bioavailability in humans is unknown.[5(p58)]

Distribution

In humans, MDMA is partially bound to plasma proteins, with the unbound fraction in plasma being 49% at 200 ng/mL, a volume that is above the therapeutic threshold and corresponds with a moderate dose of oral MDMA.[16] The volume of distribution at a dose of 1 mg/kg MDMA was observed to be 5.5 ± 1.1 L/kg, while a notably higher dose of 1.6 mg/kg produced a volume of distribution of 5.5 ± 1.3 L/kg.[17]

Metabolism

The most common metabolites of MDMA include MDA, 3,4-dihydroxymethamphetamine (HHMA), 3,4-dihydroxyamphetamine (HHA), 4-hydroxy-3-methoxymethamphetamine (HMMA), and 4-hydroxy-3-methoxyamphetamine (HMA). HMMA is the major metabolite of MDMA, and MDA is the sole metabolite confirmed to be pharmacologically active. 4-Hydroxyamphetamine, which is related to several metabolites of MDMA, has demonstrated activity at trace amine-associated receptor 1 (TAAR1), so there is a possibility that some metabolites may demonstrate weak activity at this receptor site.[1]

MDMA is primarily metabolized via N-demethylation in the liver by cytochrome P450 CYP2D6 into HHMA, an unstable compound that is converted into HMMA before being metabolized into HMA by CYP1A2.[18] In a secondary metabolic pathway, MDMA is N-demethylated by CYP3A4 to form MDA, which then undergoes further demethylation via CYP2D6 to form HHA.[18] COMT and MAO-A are also associated with the metabolism of MDMA.[5(p61)] Its inhibition of MAO-A makes it contraindicated with MAOI medications.

3,4-Methylenedioxyamphetamine

In addition to being a metabolite of MDMA, MDA has some history of also being used as a recreational drug. Derived from the oil of the sassafras plant, MDA is commonly referred to as sass or sally and will be described in Chapter 16.

Elimination and Excretion

The elimination half-life of MDMA is 7 to 9 hours,[15] and it may take upward of 5 half-lives (~40 hours) for 95% of the drug to be cleared following administration.[14] MDMA and its metabolites are excreted in urine, primarily as sulfate and glucuronide conjugates. After a single dose of MDMA, the maximum concentration in urine is highly variable (3.3-30.4 hours) and metabolites may be detected for more than 7 days following administration.[18]

Pharmacodynamics

The subjective and psychological effects of MDMA are typically felt 30 to 75 minutes following oral administration of doses in the range of 75 to 125 mg.[5(p11)] Patients are likely to become more appreciative of sensory stimuli or may observe alterations in perceptions (eg, colors are more vivid, time appears to move slower, and music is more enjoyable), while thoughts and memories may be given new or heightened significance. Peak subjective effects typically occur 75 to 125 minutes following administration, and effects may persist for 3 to 6 hours.[5(p11)] Throughout this time, patients may experience increasingly mild visual hallucinations, euphoria, anxiety, enhanced connectivity to others, and a wide range of emotional states. Adverse effects are noted below.

Mechanism of Action

MDMA acts by increasing the net release of monoamine neurotransmitters, which is accomplished through several mechanisms. MDMA binds to transporters (including serotonin transporters [SERTs], dopamine transporters [DATs], and norepinephrine transporters [NETs]), thereby preventing their reuptake of respective neurotransmitters.[1] These effects are most pronounced in serotonin, as well as norepinephrine, and to a lesser extent dopamine. The increase in net release of serotonin (and to some degree dopamine) is believed to be the primary mechanism of action for MDMA.[19] The net increase of norepinephrine results in effects akin to other amphetamines. MDMA also induces the release of serotonin, dopamine, and norepinephrine by reversing the flux of monoamines through their transporters, primarily via binding to vesicular amine transporters.[1]

MDMA also binds directly to multiple receptors, as noted in Table 15.1. It has an affinity for $5\text{-}HT_{2B}$ receptors at the submicromolar level (K_i = 500 nM), which is yet another mechanism through which MDMA causes the release of serotonin.[20] MDMA also has an affinity at the micromolar level for $5\text{-}HT_{2A}$. Though relatively weak, the

TABLE 15.1 Binding Affinity Profile for MDMA

Receptor	Ligand Classification	Species	K_i (nM)	Reference
5-HT$_{1A}$	Agonist	Human	>10,000	1
5-HT$_{1A}$	Agonist	Human	12,200	2
5-HT$_{1B}$	Antagonist	Human	>10,000	1
5-HT$_{1D}$	Antagonist	Human	>10,000	1
5-HT$_{1E}$	Agonist	Human	>10,000	1
5-HT$_{2A}$	Agonist	Rat	>10,000	1
5-HT$_{2A}$	Agonist	Human	7,800	2
5-HT$_{2B}$	Agonist	Human	500	1
5-HT$_{2C}$	Antagonist	Rat	>10,000	1
5-HT$_{2C}$	Antagonist	Human	>13,000	2
5-HT$_3$	Antagonist	Human	>10,000	1
5-HT$_5$	Agonist	Human	>10,000	1
5-HT$_6$	Agonist	Human	>10,000	1
5-HT$_7$	Agonist	Human	>10,000	1
α_{1A}	Antagonist	Human	>10,000	1
α_{1A}	Inverse agonist	Human	>6,000	2
α_{1B}	Antagonist	Human	>10,000	1
α_{2A}	Agonist	Human	2,532	1
α_{2A}	Antagonist	Human	15,000	2
α_{2B}	Agonist	Human	1,785	1
α_{2C}	Agonist	Human	1,123	1
β_1	Partial agonist	Rat	>10,000	1
β_2	Partial agonist	Rat	>10,000	1
CB$_1$	Agonist	Rat (brain)	>10,000	1

TABLE 15.1 Binding Affinity Profile for MDMA (*continued*)

Receptor	Ligand Classification	Species	K_i (nM)	Reference
M_1	Antagonist	Human	>10,000	1
M_2	Antagonist	Human	>10,000	1
M_3	Antagonist	Human	1,851	1
M_4	Antagonist	Human	8,245	1
M_5	Antagonist	Human	6,339	1
nACh $\alpha_1\beta_2$	Agonist	Human	>10,000	1
nACh $\alpha_2\beta_2$	Agonist	Human	>10,000	1
nACh $\alpha_2\beta_4$	Agonist	Human	>10,000	1
nACh $\alpha_3\beta_2$	Agonist	Human	>10,000	1
nACh $\alpha_3\beta_4$	Agonist	Human	>10,000	1
nACh α_7	Agonist	Human	>10,000	1
D_1	Antagonist	Human	>10,000	1
D_1	Antagonist	Human	>13,600	2
D_2	Antagonist	Human	>10,000	1
D_2	Antagonist	Human	25,200	2
D_3	Antagonist	Human	>10,000	1
D_3	Antagonist	Human	>17,700	2
D_4	Antagonist	Rat	>10,000	1
D_5	Antagonist	Human	>10,000	1
$GABA_A$	Agonist	Rat (forebrain)	>10,000	1
$GABA_B$	Agonist	Rat (forebrain)	>10,000	1
NMDA	Antagonist	Rat (forebrain)	>10,000	1
H_1	Antagonist	Human	2,138	1

(*continued*)

TABLE 15.1 Binding Affinity Profile for MDMA *(continued)*

Receptor	Ligand Classification	Species	K_i (nM)	Reference
H_1	Antagonist	Human	>14,400	2
H_2	Antagonist	Human	>10,000	1
Prostaglandin EP_3	Agonist	Human	>10,000	1
Prostaglandin EP_4	Agonist	Human	>10,000	1
NET	Inhibitor	Human	>10,000	1
NET	Inhibitor	Human	30,500	2
DAT	Inhibitor	Human	>10,000	1
DAT	Inhibitor	Human	6,500	2
SERT	Inhibitor	Human	>10,000	1
SERT	Inhibitor	Human	13,300	2
$TAAR_1$	Agonist	Rat	370	2
$TAAR_1$	Agonist	Mouse	2,400	2

5-HT, serotonin receptor; α, α-adrenergic receptor; β, β-adrenergic receptor; CB, cannabinoid receptor; D, dopamine; DAT, dopamine transporter; GABA, γ-aminobutyric acid; H, histamine; M, muscarinic acetylcholine receptor; MDMA, 3,4-methylenedioxymethamphetamine; nACh, nicotinic acetylcholine; NET, norepinephrine transporter; NMDA, N-methyl-D-aspartate; SERT, serotonin transporter; TAAR, trace amine-associated receptor.

References:
1. Setola V, Hufeisen SJ, Grande-Allen KJ, et al. 3,4-methylenedioxymethamphetamine (MDMA, "Ecstasy") induces fenfluramine-like proliferative actions on human cardiac valvular interstitial cells in vitro. *Mol Pharmacol.* 2003;63(6):1223-1229. doi:10.1124/mol.63.6.1223
2. Simmler L, Buser T, Donzelli M, et al. Pharmacological characterization of designer cathinones in vitro. *Br J Pharmacol.* 2013;168(2):458-470. doi:10.1111/j.1476-5381.2012.02145.x

Adapted from Dunlap LE, Andrews AM, Olson DE. Dark classics in chemical neuroscience: 3,4-methylenedioxymethamphetamine (MDMA). *ACS Chem Nurosci.* 2018;9(1):2408-2427. doi:10.1021/acschemneuro.8b00155

hallucinogenic properties of MDMA can be blocked by ketanserin, a selective 5-HT_{2A} antagonist.[21]

Drugs of the amphetamine and methamphetamine class have been shown to be potent agonists at TAAR1, which increases the production of cyclic adenosine 3,5-monophosphate (cAMP) and contributes to the increase in extracellular monoamine levels. While it is clear that MDMA is active at TAAR1 in rodent models, the same activity has not been demonstrated in humans.[22] At least some of the psychostimulant effects of MDMA are believed to be mediated through activity at σ receptors, particularly the $σ_1$ subtype, as it shows greater affinity for $σ_1$ than $σ_2$ (k_i = 3,057 ± 45 nM; k_i = 8,889 ± 500 nM, respectively).[23] The significance of MDMA's activity at σ receptors is unknown but could be associated with increased synaptic plasticity as mediated through brain-derived neurotrophic factor (BDNF).[24]

MDMA also increases plasma levels of the neurohormone oxytocin, which is believed to be associated with its prosocial effects.[25] It is also associated with increased plasma levels of cortisol, prolactin, and dehydroepiandrosterone (DHEA), which are believed to be associated with MDMA's autonomic effects (eg, increased heart rate, shortened pre-ejection period, pupil dilation) and its characteristic euphoria.[26-28]

The neurophysiologic mechanism behind MDMA's promotion of fear extinction is still not entirely understood, though it may be mediated via increased levels of BDNF and enhanced neural plasticity via σ receptors and other mechanisms.[29] It is also possible that MDMA's ability to reopen critical periods for social reward learning, a common characteristic of psychedelics, may play a significant role, as suggested by pioneering research by Dölen and colleagues. Most recently, Dölen's work has suggested that β-arrestin-2 signaling is required for MDMA- and LSD-induced reopening of these critical periods.[30]

Therapeutic Index

A relatively standard effective dose of MDMA for a 70-kg (154 lb) person would be 125 mg, while a potentially lethal dose would be 2 g (therapeutic index = 16).[31] Within a clinical setting, MDMA is remarkably safe and nontoxic.

Tolerance, Dependence, and Withdrawal

While extremely uncommon, MDMA dependence is possible and has been reported, suggesting that it does have some abuse potential.[32] Additionally, chronic users of MDMA appear to develop a tolerance to the psychoactive effects of the drug, while cross-tolerance with methamphetamines has been evidenced in rodent models.[33] It should be noted that real-world data about tolerance to MDMA in humans is difficult to establish because illicit MDMA tends to contain myriad impurities and other drugs.[34] Risk of dependence or abuse within a clinical setting is extremely unlikely because it is only administered a few times during treatment.

Withdrawal symptoms are typically felt after first-time use and appear to be mediated by depletions in serotonin. Following use, one may feel depressed, anxious, fatigued, and exhausted, though these negative effects tend to dissipate within a day or at most a few days. Unlike many other drugs, withdrawal tends to lack serious physical symptoms.[35] Chronic use of MDMA may result in more severe depletions of serotonin resulting in persistent emotional and cognitive impairments.[36]

Subjective Effects of 3,4-Methylenedioxymethamphetamine

Doses of MDMA may range from 75 to 150 mg and produce subjective effects lasting several hours. The most notable subjective effects of MDMA are of a prosocial nature. Patients feel increased closeness to and empathy with others, as well as a reduction in social inhibitions. Patients are also more likely to feel quite alert, focused, and euphoric. Auditory hallucinations are extremely uncommon and visual hallucinations tend to be relatively rare. Should they occur, they are not especially well formed. According to a survey of 100 individuals who had ingested MDMA, only 20 (20%) experienced visual hallucinations.[37] Rather than hallucinating, patients report that existing phenomena are given greater meaning.

Therapeutic Indications

As of this writing, MDMA is considered a Schedule I drug and is not indicated for any condition according to the FDA.

Potential Uses

Despite being a Schedule I drug, there have been close to 100 clinical trials involving MDMA, more than 20 of which have been conducted by MAPS.[5(pp43-55)] The majority of the clinical trials conducted by MAPS have involved patients with PTSD, and these studies (which have included phase 1, phase 2, and phase 3 trials) indicate that MDMA-assisted psychotherapy is an effective treatment for PTSD.[5(pp43-55)] In most cases, MDMA is administered in three different sessions over the course of several weeks. Patients meet for psychotherapy regularly before their first dose of MDMA, between doses, and following the final dose.

Studies have also suggested that MDMA may be used to help treat existential crises in terminally ill patients and social anxiety among adults with autism spectrum disorders. Additionally, there has been some interest in studying MDMA's effects on individuals with eating disorders.

While there has been some interest in using MDMA to treat suicidality, anxiety, and depressive disorders, studies on these conditions are wanting. At this time, there is no evidence to support the use of MDMA in treating social anxiety disorder outside the context of autism spectrum disorder. Moreover, there is no evidence to support the use of MDMA in treating mood disorders or as a form of prophylaxis in patients who have expressed a desire to end their lives. Though MDMA can induce states of acute euphoria, the long-term effects on patients who are suicidal or experiencing depressive episodes are not well understood at this time.

Within the context of PTSD treatment, studies have documented subclinical improvements in alcohol use disorders, indicating that MDMA does not appear to increase the risk of illicit drug use.[38] Moreover, clinical trials in patients with a primary diagnosis of PTSD have reported decline in the use of alcohol and improvements in symptoms associated with alcohol use disorder, suggesting that MDMA-assisted therapy may benefit patients with substance use disorders.[38] However, there is currently insufficient evidence to suggest that MDMA can treat patients with a primary diagnosis of substance use disorder.

Posttraumatic Stress Disorder

An evaluation of six phase 2 trials among patients who received active doses of MDMA (75-125 mg; $n = 72$) revealed steep declines in PTSD symptoms from baseline to primary end point (1 or 2 months following blinded MDMA sessions), as well as secondary end points (1 or 2 months following final dosing session and 12 months after last treatment) using the Clinician-Administered PTSD Scale (CAPS-IV). The randomized, double-blind controlled trials took place from 2004 to 2017, and MDMA showed superior effects compared to the placebo dose (40 mg MDMA). Active doses were administered to patients with PTSD in two or three 8-hour sessions spaced approximately 1 month apart. Mean CAPS-IV scores declined for both groups from baseline but were 22.0 points lower in the active group. Additionally, 54.2% of patients in the active group no longer met the criteria for PTSD following two dosing sessions with MDMA.[39] It should be noted that this paper was retracted in 2024 due to ethical and protocol violations by one of the researchers associated with the study.

A 2023 randomized phase 3 trial published by Mitchell and colleagues that enrolled 104 participants (53 in the MDMA group, 51 controls) produced similar results, though the study relied on the Clinician-Administered PTSD Scale for *DSM-5* (CAPS-5) rather than

CAPS-IV. At the end of the 18-week study, the mean CAPS-5 score for the placebo group had fallen by 14.8 from baseline, while the mean score for the MDMA group had fallen by 23.7 points. Of the 52 within the MDMA group, 45 (86.5%) achieved a clinically meaningful benefit (defined in this study as a 10-point decline in CAPS-5 score). Additionally, 37 (71.2%) no longer met the criteria for PTSD diagnosis. The team also noted that MDMA-assisted therapy reduced functional impairment as measured with the Sheehan Disability Scale (SDS), which ranges from 0 (unimpaired) to 30 (highly impaired). The MDMA group experienced an average decline in score of 3.3 while the placebo group saw an average decline of 2.1.[40]

The vast majority of participants (102/104) experienced at least one treatment-emergent adverse event. Most were minor, though there were a total of seven severe treatment-emergent adverse events reported, five in the MDMA group (including dissociation, flashback, and grief reaction) and two in the control group (agitation and anxiety). The most common adverse events included muscle tightness, nausea, decreased appetite, and hyperhidrosis.[40]

Palliative Care

Patients who have recently received a terminal diagnosis may benefit from MDMA-assisted psychotherapy. A small, phase 2 pilot study involving six patients each with a terminal illness found that the MDMA experience (125 mg MDMA initially with an optional 62.5 mg boost 90-150 minutes later) helped them process trauma, reconcile with their own mortality, and reclaim a sense of presence that had initially been lost after learning of their diagnosis. Additionally, five of the six participants reported a mystical-type experience, suggesting that entactogens such as MDMA are capable of easing existential duress through mechanisms that transcend pharmacology in ways that are distinct from classic psychedelics such as LSD and psilocybin. Even if entactogens are not typically associated with the kinds of mystical-type experiences that result from the use of classic psychedelics, ketamine, and ibogaine, the study suggests that a sense of unity or connectivity with others may induce experiences that can be categorized as mystical type. While all patients credited the treatment with positive changes in their lives, a qualitative analysis revealed more mixed results.[41]

Wolfson and colleagues performed a double-blind study involving 18 patients with anxiety due to a life-threatening illness that similarly utilized MDMA-assisted therapy. Both the MDMA group ($n = 13$, 125 mg) and the placebo group ($n = 5$) received two 8-hour psychotherapy sessions. While the researchers found that MDMA was well tolerated,

State-Trait Anxiety Inventory (STAI) trait scores did not reach clinical significance at the primary end point (1 month after the final session) when compared with the baseline. However, the group difference is still notable, as STAI trait scores declined 23.5 points in the MDMA group and 8.8 points in the controls.[42]

Social Anxiety Disorders in Adults With Autism Spectrum Disorders

A blinded placebo-controlled pilot study involving 12 individuals with autism spectrum disorder and severe social anxiety was randomized to receive either MDMA (n = 8, 75-125 mg) or a placebo (n = 4) during two 8-hour psychotherapy sessions (experimental sessions). Experimental sessions were approximately 1 month apart. Following each experimental session, three nonexperimental sessions were administered where patients received psychotherapy only.

Primary outcomes (1 month after the second experimental session) showed that the MDMA group experienced a significant decline in anxiety scores, as measured using the Liebowitz Social Anxiety Scale (LSAS; P = .037) and placebo-subtracted Cohen d effect size (d = 1.4, CI: −0.074, 2.874). Positive results were still apparent at the 6-month follow-up as measured by LSAS score (P = .036), with a Cohen d effect size of 1.1 (CI: −0.307, 2.527).[43]

Eating Disorders

A double-blind, placebo-controlled pivotal trial involving 89 individuals revealed that MDMA-assisted therapy may be beneficial in addressing the pathologies of both PTSD and eating disorders. All study participants had been diagnosed with PTSD and included 58 females (placebo = 31, MDMA = 27) and 31 males (placebo = 12, MDMA = 19), who were assessed using the CAPS-5, SDS, and Eating Attitudes Test 26 (EAT-26) at baseline and at the end of the study. At baseline, 13 (15%) of the 89 participants had total EAT-26 scores ($\geq$20) warranting a diagnosis of an eating disorder, while 28 (31.5%) had EAT-26 scores ($\geq$11) indicating high risk of developing an eating disorder. Among those who completed the study (n = 82), total EAT-26 scores had declined among the MDMA group by 3.04 but only 0.68 among controls.[44]

Despite clear limitations, especially generalizability to the treatment of eating disorders outside of a PTSD context, the study indicates that patients with eating disorders may benefit from MDMA-assisted psychotherapy.

Precautions and Adverse Effects

MDMA-assisted psychotherapy is usually contraindicated for people with a personal or family history of severe and persistent mental illnesses or existing psychiatric comorbidities that make them more susceptible to psychosis. Even those who are not predisposed to mental illness or psychosis may experience adverse psychological effects during the acute phase of the treatment, including confusion, agitation, fear, restlessness, paranoia, depersonalization, and panic attacks. These effects typically wear off within a few hours.

Beyond the psychological impact, common adverse effects include hyperthermia, dehydration, hyponatremia, headache, increased blood pressure, pupil dilation, nausea, involuntary jaw clenching or teeth grinding, and hyperhidrosis. If used in a recreational setting, particularly in a dance club, the combination of hyperthermia, hyperhidrosis, hyponatremia, and dehydration can become life threatening. It should be noted that hyperthermia has also been reported in clinical settings but has not risen to the level of being clinically significant.[5(pp63-68)]

MDMA may also cause tachycardia, posing a risk to patients with cardiovascular diseases. In rare instances, MDMA may cause liver injury or acute liver failure. It should be noted that these more severe events seem to have occurred solely in a recreational setting.[1] Within a clinical setting, panic attacks have been reported in rare instances.[1]

Long-term use of MDMA can lead to impairments in executive functioning, memory, and mood. There are also reports of deficits in visual processing.[45] Additionally, long-term use is associated with depleted serotonin, which can lead to depression, anxiety, irritability, and fatigue.

Risk of Overdose

The risk of overdose or misuse in a clinical setting is very low. MDMA overdose is possible in a recreational setting but still relatively rare unless used in conjunction with alcohol or other drugs.

Pregnant and Nursing Women

The safety of MDMA among pregnant and nursing individuals has not been established due to lack of data. Therefore, pregnant and nursing women are advised to not use MDMA.

Drug Interactions

Clinical studies on drug interactions between common pharmaceuticals and MDMA are currently lacking, though it is known that MDMA is primarily metabolized by cytochrome P450 CYP2D6 and that coadministration with other pharmaceuticals that are metabolized by this enzyme may lead to adverse events. Similarly, patients who have been prescribed antidepressant drugs that inhibit serotonin reuptake (see Table 15.2) should taper and discontinue use at least 2 weeks prior to administration of MDMA. Similarly, MDMA is contraindicated in those taking MAOIs. In the case of fluoxetine, patients should taper

TABLE 15.2 Drug-Drug Interactions Between Antidepressants and Classic Psychedelics

Drug Type	Examples
Monoamine oxidase inhibitors	Isocarboxazid, moclobemide, phenelzine, selegiline, tranylcypromine
Noradrenergic and specific serotonergic antidepressants	Mianserin, mirtazapine, setiptiline
Select serotonin reuptake inhibitors	Citalopram, escitalopram, fluvoxamine, fluoxetine,[a] paroxetine, sertraline
Serotonin modulators	Nefazodone, trazodone, vilazodone, vortioxetine
Serotonin norepinephrine reuptake inhibitors	Desvenlafaxine, duloxetine, levomilnacipran, venlafaxine
Serotonin partial agonist reuptake inhibitors	Vilazodone, vortioxetine
Tricyclic antidepressants	Amitriptyline, chlorpheniramine, clomipramine, desipramine, imipramine, nortriptyline
Other	Buspirone

Listed drugs should be tapered and discontinued at least 2 weeks prior to acute MDMA (3,4-methylenedioxymethamphetamine)-assisted psychotherapy.
[a]Fluoxetine should be tapered and discontinued at least 6 weeks prior to acute MDMA-assisted psychotherapy.

TABLE 15.3 Drugs Associated With Elevated Serotonin Levels and Serotonin Syndrome

Drug Type	Examples
Analgesics	Fentanyl, meperidine, pentazocine, tramadol
Antibiotics	Linezolide, ritonavir
Anticonvulsants	Valproate
Antidepressants	Buspirone, clomipramine, nefazodone, trazodone, venlafaxine
Antiemetics	Granisetron, metoclopramide, ondansetron
Antimigraine medications	Sumatriptan
Bariatric drugs	Sibutramine
Monoamine oxidase inhibitors	Clorgiline, isocarboxazid, moclobemide, phenelzine
Over-the-counter drugs	Dextromethorphan
Selective serotonin reuptake inhibitors	Citalopram, fluoxetine, fluvoxamine, paroxetine, sertraline

and discontinue use at least 6 weeks prior to administration of MDMA. Patients run a higher risk of developing serotonin syndrome if MDMA is taken in conjunction with other drugs that elevate serotonin levels (see Table 15.3).

Dosage and Clinical Guidelines

While there are no set guidelines at this time for administering MDMA, the protocol for MDMA-assisted psychotherapy established by MAPS recommends two to three sessions prior to the administration of MDMA to create a rapport between the patient and the therapist and to introduce the patient to the drug. This is followed by a session where the drug is administered, oftentimes with a 125-mg dose and a smaller, supplemental dose midway through the session (typically 62.5 mg). Following the session with the administered drug, the patient will be expected to attend follow-up sessions, often over the course of several weeks, to discuss their experience and to take steps to incorporate it into a larger psychotherapeutic framework. This may be repeated 2 to 3 times in total.

No clinical programs that utilize MDMA-assisted psychotherapy currently support the perpetual administration of MDMA.

Conclusion

Like other psychedelics, MDMA holds tremendous promise as an adjunctive to traditional treatment modalities for conditions that are notoriously difficult to treat, particularly trauma- and stressor-related disorders such as PTSD. Though MDMA was not initially approved by the FDA for use in the treatment of PTSD, there is a signal evidencing efficacy that is hard to ignore.

While there are receptor targets that may help partially explain the mechanisms of action, the entactogenic qualities of MDMA within the context of psychotherapy seem to be crucial to realize its full therapeutic potential. Developing more standardized procedures for administering psychotherapy in conjunction with MDMA will be a complex (but solvable) challenge, as such standardization will need to be not only strict enough to prioritize patient safety and ensure therapists' adherence to ethical guidelines, but also flexible enough to respect that all therapy sessions are unique and that therapists should be granted some degree of latitude when providing treatment, as there is no one-size-fits-all approach that will be effective for all patients.

REFERENCES

1. Dunlap LE, Andrews AM, Olson DE. Dark classics in chemical neuroscience: 3,4-methylenedioxymethamphetamine (MDMA). *ACS Chem Neurosci*. 2018;9(1):2408-2427. doi:10.1021/acschemneuro.8b00155
2. Nichols DE. Entactogens: how the name for a novel class of psychoactive agents originated. *Front Psychiatry*. 2022;13:863088. doi:10.3389/fpsyt.2022.863088
3. Freudenmann RW, Oxler F, Bernschneider-Reif S. The origin of MDMA (ecstasy) revisited: the true story reconstructed from the original documents. *Addiction*. 2006;101(9):1241-1245. doi:10.1111/j.1360-0443.2006.01511.x
4. Shulgin A, Shulgin A. *PiHKAL: A Chemical Love Story*. Transform Press; 2022.
5. Multidisciplinary Association for Psychedelic Studies. *MDMA Investigator's Brochure*. 15th ed. MAPS Public Benefit Corporation; 2023.
6. Passie T. The early use of MDMA ('Ecstasy') in psychotherapy (1977–1985). *Drug Sci Policy Law*. 2018;4. doi:10.1177/2050324518767442
7. Passie T, Benzenhöfer U. The history of MDMA as an underground drug in the United States, 1960-1979. *J Psychoactive Drugs*. 2016;48(2):67-75. doi:10.1080/02791072.2015.1128580. PMID: 26940772.
8. Parrott AC, Young L. Saturday night fever in ecstasy/MDMA dance clubbers: heightened body temperature and associated psychobiological changes. *Temperature (Austin)*. 2014;1(3):214-219. doi:10.4161/23328940.2014.977182. PMID: 27626048; PMCID: PMC5008707.

9. Yang KH, Kepner W, Nijum A, Han BH, Palamar JJ. Prevalence and correlates of past year ecstasy/MDMA use in the United States. *J Addict Med*. 2023;17(5):592-597. doi:10.1097/ADM.0000000000001188. PMID: 37788615; PMCID: PMC10593986.
10. U.S. Department of Health and Human Services, Substance Abuse and Mental Health Services Administration, Center for Behavioral Health Statistics and Quality. National Survey on Drug Use and Health 2022. Published November 13, 2023. Accessed March 22, 2024. https://www.samhsa.gov/data/report/2022-nsduh-detailed-tables
11. Grob C. MDMA research: preliminary investigations with human subjects. *Int J Drug Policy*. 1998;9(2):119-124. doi:10.1016/S0955-3959(98)00008-5
12. Jones GM, Nock MK. MDMA/ecstasy use and psilocybin use are associated with lowered odds of psychological distress and suicidal thoughts in a sample of US adults. *J Psychopharmacol*. 2022;36(1):46-56. doi:10.1177/02698811211058923. PMID: 34983249.
13. Jacobs A. F.D.A. panel rejects MDMA-aided therapy for PTSD. *New York Times*. Updated June 5, 2024. Accessed June 6, 2024. https://www.nytimes.com/2024/06/04/health/fda-mdma-therapy-ptsd.html
14. Kalant H. The pharmacology and toxicology of "ecstasy" (MDMA) and related drugs. *CMAJ*. 2001;165(7):917-928. PMID: 11599334; PMCID: PMC81503.
15. de la Torre R, Farré M, Ortuño J, et al. Non-linear pharmacokinetics of MDMA ('ecstasy') in humans. *Br J Clin Pharmacol*. 2000;49(2):104-109. doi:10.1046/j.1365-2125.2000.00121.x. PMID: 10671903; PMCID: PMC2014905.
16. Wan Aasim WR, Tan SC, Gan SH. Interspecies in vitro evaluation of stereoselective protein binding for 3, 4-methylenedioxymethamphetamine. *J Chem*. 2017;2017:8103726. doi:10.1155/2017/8103726
17. Kolbrich EA, Goodwin RS, Gorelick DA, Hayes RJ, Stein EA, Huestis MA. Plasma pharmacokinetics of 3,4-methylenedioxymethamphetamine after controlled oral administration to young adults. *Ther Drug Monit*. 2008;30(3):320-332. doi:10.1097/FTD.0b013e3181684fa0. PMID: 18520604; PMCID: PMC2663855.
18. Abraham TT, Barnes AJ, Lowe RH, et al. Urinary MDMA, MDA, HMMA, and HMA excretion following controlled MDMA administration to humans. *J Anal Toxicol*. 2009;33(8):439-446. doi:10.1093/jat/33.8.439. PMID: 19874650; PMCID: PMC3159864.
19. Müller F, Holze F, Dolder P, et al. MDMA-induced changes in within-network connectivity contradict the specificity of these alterations for the effects of serotonergic hallucinations. *Neuropsychopharmacology*. 2021;46:545-553. doi:10.1038/s41386-020-00906-2
20. Doly S, Valjent E, Setola V, et al. Serotonin 5-HT2B receptors are required for 3,4-methylenedioxymethamphetamine-induced hyperlocomotion and 5-HT release in vivo and in vitro. *J Neurosci*. 2008;28(11):2933-2940. doi:10.1523/JNEUROSCI.5723-07.2008. PMID: 18337424; PMCID: PMC6670669.
21. Liechti ME, Saur MR, Gamma A, Hell D, Vollenweider FX. Psychological and physiological effects of MDMA ("Ecstasy") after pretreatment with the 5-HT(2) antagonist ketanserin in healthy humans. *Neuropsychopharmacology*. 2000;23(4):396-404. doi:10.1016/S0893-133X(00)00126-3. PMID: 10989266.
22. Simmler LD, Buchy D, Chaboz S, Hoener MC, Liechti ME. In vitro characterization of psychoactive substances at rat, mouse, and human trace amine-associated receptor 1. *J Pharmacol Exp Ther*. 2016;357(1):134-144. doi:10.1124/jpet.115.229765. PMID: 26791601.
23. Brammer MK, Gilmore DL, Matsumoto RR. Interactions between 3,4-methylenedioxymethamphetamine and sigma1 receptors. *Eur J Pharmacol*. 2006;553(1-3):141-145. doi:10.1016/j.ejphar.2006.09.038. PMID: 17070798; PMCID: PMC1780037.
24. Barker SA. N, N-dimethyltryptamine (DMT), an endogenous hallucinogen: past, present, and future research to determine its role and function. *Front Neurosci*. 2018;12:536. doi:10.3389/fnins.2018.00536

25. Vizeli P, Liechti ME. Oxytocin receptor gene variations and socio-emotional effects of MDMA: a pooled analysis of controlled studies in healthy subjects. *PLoS One.* 2018;13(6):e0199384. doi:10.1371/journal.pone.0199384. PMID: 29912955; PMCID: PMC6005537.
26. Harris DS, Baggott M, Mendelson JH, Mendelson JE, Jones RT. Subjective and hormonal effects of 3,4-methylenedioxymethamphetamine (MDMA) in humans. *Psychopharmacology (Berl).* 2002;162(4):396-405. doi:10.1007/s00213-002-1131-1. PMID: 12172693.
27. Clark CM, Frye CG, Wardle MC, Norman GJ, de Wit H. Acute effects of MDMA on autonomic cardiac activity and their relation to subjective prosocial and stimulant effects. *Psychophysiology.* 2015;52(3):429-435. doi:10.1111/psyp.12327. PMID: 25208727; PMCID: PMC4634859.
28. Kolbrich EA, Goodwin RS, Gorelick DA, Hayes RJ, Stein EA, Huestis MA. Physiological and subjective responses to controlled oral 3,4-methylenedioxymethamphetamine administration. *J Clin Psychopharmacol.* 2008;28(4):432-440. doi:10.1097/JCP.0b013e31817ef470. PMID: 18626271; PMCID: PMC2587205.
29. Yazar-Klosinski BB, Mithoefer MC. Potential psychiatric uses for MDMA. *Clin Pharmacol Ther.* 2017;101(2):194-196. doi:10.1002/cpt.565. PMID: 27859039; PMCID: PMC5260336.
30. Nardou R, Sawyer E, Song YJ, et al. Psychedelics reopen the social reward learning critical period. *Nature.* 2023;618:790-798. doi:10.1038/s41586-023-06204-3
31. Gable RS. Acute toxic effects of club drugs. *J Psychoactive Drugs.* 2004;36(3):303-313. doi:10.1080/02791072.2004.10400031. PMID: 15559678.
32. Jansen KL. Ecstasy (MDMA) dependence. *Drug Alcohol Depend.* 1999;53(2):121-124. doi:10.1016/s0376-8716(98)00111-2. PMID: 10080038.
33. Zacny JP, Virus RM, Woolverton WL. Tolerance and cross-tolerance to 3,4-methylenedioxymethamphetamine (MDMA), methamphetamine and methylenedioxyamphetamine. *Pharmacol Biochem Behav.* 1990;35(3):637-642. doi:10.1016/0091-3057(90)90301-w. PMID: 1971112.
34. Parrott AC. Chronic tolerance to recreational MDMA (3,4-methylenedioxymethamphetamine) or ecstasy. *J Psychopharmacol.* 2005;19(1):71-83. doi:10.1177/0269881105048900. PMID: 15671132.
35. Degenhardt L, Bruno R, Topp L. Is ecstasy a drug of dependence? *Drug Alcohol Depend.* 2010;107(1):1-10. doi:10.1016/j.drugalcdep.2009.09.009. PMID: 19836170.
36. Meyer JS. 3,4-methylenedioxymethamphetamine (MDMA): current perspectives. *Subst Abuse Rehabil.* 2013;4:83-99. doi:10.2147/SAR.S37258. PMID: 24648791; PMCID: PMC3931692.
37. Peroutka SJ, Newman H, Harris H. Subjective effects of 3,4-methylenedioxymethamphetamine in recreational users. *Neuropsychopharmacology.* 1988;1(4):273-277. PMID: 2908020.
38. Nicholas CR, Wang JB, Coker A, et al. The effects of MDMA-assisted therapy on alcohol and substance use in a phase 3 trial for treatment of severe PTSD. *Drug Alcohol Depend.* 2022;233:109356. doi:10.1016/j.drugalcdep.2022.109356. PMID: 35286849; PMCID: PMC9750500.
39. Mithoefer MC, Feduccia AA, Jerome L, et al. MDMA-assisted psychotherapy for treatment of PTSD: study design and rationale for phase 3 trials based on pooled analysis of six phase 2 randomized controlled trials. *Psychopharmacology (Berl).* 2019;236(9):2735-2745. doi:10.1007/s00213-019-05249-5. PMID: 31065731; PMCID: PMC6695343.
40. Mitchell JM, Ot'alora G M, van der Kolk B, et al. MDMA-assisted therapy for moderate to severe PTSD: a randomized, placebo-controlled phase 3 trial. *Nat Med.* 2023;29(10):2473-2480. doi:10.1038/s41591-023-02565-4. PMID: 37709999; PMCID: PMC10579091.

41. Barone W, Mitsunaga-Whitten M, Blaustein LO, Perl P, Swank M, Swift TC. Facing death, returning to life: a qualitative analysis of MDMA-assisted therapy for anxiety associated with life-threatening illness. *Front Psychiatry*. 2022;13:944849. doi:10.3389/fpsyt.2022.944849. PMID: 36238946; PMCID: PMC9552520.
42. Wolfson PE, Andries J, Feduccia AA, et al. MDMA-assisted psychotherapy for treatment of anxiety and other psychological distress related to life-threatening illnesses: a randomized pilot study. *Sci Rep*. 2020;10(1):20442. doi:10.1038/s41598-020-75706-1. PMID: 33235285; PMCID: PMC7686344.
43. Danforth AL, Grob CS, Struble C, et al. Reduction in social anxiety after MDMA-assisted psychotherapy with autistic adults: a randomized, double-blind, placebo-controlled pilot study. *Psychopharmacology (Berl)*. 2018;235(11):3137-3148. doi:10.1007/s00213-018-5010-9. PMID: 30196397; PMCID: PMC6208958.
44. Brewerton TD, Wang JB, Lafrance A, et al. MDMA-assisted therapy significantly reduces eating disorder symptoms in a randomized placebo-controlled trial of adults with severe PTSD. *J Psychiatr Res*. 2022;149:128-135. doi:10.1016/j.jpsychires.2022.03.008. PMID: 35272210.
45. White C, Brown J, Edwards M. Altered visual perception in long-term ecstasy (MDMA) users. *Psychopharmacology (Berl)*. 2013;229(1):155-165. doi:10.1007/s00213-013-3094-9. PMID: 23609769.

16
Miscellaneous Psychedelics

In addition to the drugs covered in previous chapters, there are hundreds, if not thousands, of psychedelic compounds that have been discovered. The vast majority of these drugs have not been studied extensively. As this book is focused on the clinical utility of psychedelics, only a few will be mentioned here in detail, including salvinorin A, 5-methoxy-N,N-dimethyltryptamine (5-MeO-DMT), 5-hydroxy-N,N-dimethyltryptamine (5-OH-DMT or bufotenin), ibotenic acid, and muscimol.

Bufotenin is one of the two compounds excreted by the Colorado River toad (*Incilius alvarius*, also known as *Bufo alvarius*); the other being 5-MeO-DMT. The inclusion of bufotenin in this chapter is due to the rise in popularity of toad-derived 5-MeO-DMT among recreational users. Ibotenic acid and muscimol, the psychoactive compounds found in *Amanita muscaria*, have also been included in this chapter given the rising popularity of *A. muscaria* among recreational users and its nebulous legal status.

Another 11 psychedelics will be described in less detail. This latter group will include five of Shulgin's "magical half dozen" (the sixth member of the half dozen, mescaline, was covered in Chapter 12). Many of these substances could be characterized as entactogens with subjective effects that are similar to 3,4-methylenedioxymethamphetamine (MDMA). Clinical work involving most of these compounds has been extremely limited.

With the exception of salvinorin A, muscimol, and ibotenic acid, all of the drugs covered in this chapter are considered illicit and Schedule I substances. Salvinorin A is a Schedule IV drug. Muscimol and ibotenic acid are not considered controlled substances.

Salvinorin A

While most compounds discussed in this book are alkaloids, salvinorin A is a diterpenoid found in *Salvia divinorum*, which grows wildly in Mexico and is a member of the sage family.[1] The leaves of the plant may be chewed or smoked to allow for absorption through oral mucosa or the respiratory tract, respectively. Of note, salvinorin A is quickly degraded by enzymes in the digestive tract, and oral use renders the drug inactive.[1]

Salvinorin A is a selective agonist of κ-opioid receptors (KORs) and is surprisingly potent, producing subjective effects with doses as low as 200 μg. When smoked, peak effect occurs at 2 minutes before rapidly dissipating. The effects are more akin to dreaming than classic psychedelics, dissociative psychedelics, or marijuana, with MacLean and colleagues identifying five consistent themes: "Disruptions in vestibular and interoceptive processing (eg, feeling of movement in a particular direction, spinning, stretching), communication and interaction with entities or beings, revisiting childhood memories, cartoonlike visual imagery and auditory experiences (often associated with childhood), and recurring content across sessions."[2]

Unlike the vast majority of psychedelics described in this book, salvinorin A demonstrates no activity at 5-HT$_{2A}$ receptors.[2] Given its unique pharmacology, salvinorin A may be beneficial in the treatment of depressive disorders, pain, and drug dependence.[1] Research into the therapeutic utility of salvinorin A is still in its infancy.

5-Methoxy-*N*,*N*-Dimethyltryptamine

5-MeO-DMT was first synthesized in 1936 by Hoshino and Shimodaira.[3] However, the compound has a long history of use among indigenous peoples from South America and the West Indies, as it is found in a variety of plant sources, which served as ingredients for psychoactive snuffs.[4] 5-MeO-DMT is also secreted by the Colorado River toad and is believed to be endogenous in mammals, including humans, like its relative, *N*,*N*-dimethyltryptamine (DMT).[3]

While the primary route of administration among indigenous peoples is traditionally insufflation, most people today smoke 5-MeO-DMT, which results in rapid onset (5-10 seconds) and brief but extremely intense psychoactive effects that peak within a matter of minutes and last approximately 30 minutes.[5] Online surveys suggest that 5-MeO-DMT is capable of producing both non-ordinary states of consciousness and mystical experiences, which could serve as a nonpharmacologic mechanism of therapeutic importance. Surveys also suggest that toad-derived 5-MeO-DMT and plant-based 5-MeO-DMT may be more conducive to these kinds of experiences than synthetic 5-MeO-DMT.[6]

As 5-MeO-DMT is a tryptamine psychedelic, it should come as no surprise that it acts as an agonist at several serotonin receptors, including $5-HT_{1A}$, $5-HT_{1B}$, $5-HT_{1D}$, $5-HT_6$, and $5-HT_7$.[3] It also inhibits the reuptake of serotonin.[6] What is surprising is that it has demonstrated 300-fold selectivity for $5-HT_{1A}$ (3 ± 0.2 nM) when compared to $5-HT_{2A}$ receptors (907 ± 170 nM).[3]

Though 5-MeO-DMT and DMT are both short-acting psychedelics with similar chemical structures, their mechanisms of action appear to be distinct, suggesting that their therapeutic and safety profiles may also be different. At this time, clinical trials of 5-MeO-DMT are still years behind DMT and perhaps a decade behind other psychedelics described in this book.

As of spring 2024, a phase 1/2 trial involving eight participants showed that a vaporized formulation of 5-MeO-DMT, developed by GH Research and known as GH001, showed efficacy in the short-term treatment of treatment-resistant depression and that the drug was well tolerated.[5] Additional phase 1 trials by the GH Research team have shown that adverse events in healthy volunteers were typically mild and resolved spontaneously; that no notable somatic side effects were reported; and that no negative impact on participants' well-being, mood, or cognition occurred.[7]

As noted in Chapter 13, 86 trauma-exposed special operations forces veterans took part in an open-label study involving psychedelic-assisted psychotherapy with the consecutive use of ibogaine and 5-MeO-DMT at a facility in Mexico. Those involved reported symptom improvement for not only posttraumatic stress disorder (PTSD), but also individual symptoms like depression, anxiety, and insomnia. Participants also reported improved psychological flexibility, satisfaction with life, and cognitive functioning from baseline to 1-month follow-up.[8]

5-Hydroxy-*N,N*-Dimethyltryptamine (Bufotenin)

Bufotenin was first isolated from toad skin by Hans Handovsky in 1920, and it is excreted from the parotoid glands of several species of toad, including the Colorado River toad. It is structurally similar to psilocybin, DMT, and 5-MeO-DMT.[9]

While it is no doubt psychoactive and capable of inducing hallucinations when taken in isolation, these experiences (which last 1-2 hours) tend to be quite unpleasant and accompanied by adverse somatic effects that may include face flushing, burning sensations, lightheadedness, nausea, and increased respiratory rate.[10(pp474,475)] Classifying bufotenin as a psychedelic, however, remains controversial. Even after self-administering bufotenin several times and at varying doses, Shulgin was equivocal on the matter, he wrote: "Maybe yes and maybe no."[10(p478)]

Muscimol and Ibotenic Acid

The two psychoactive compounds in perhaps one of the world's most iconic mushrooms, *A. muscaria*, are muscimol and ibotenic acid. The red-capped *A. muscaria* is associated with video games like *Super Mario Bros.* and *Alice in Wonderland*, and it has long been used as an entheogen among Asiatic shamanistic cultures.[11] It can also be poisonous if taken in large quantities.[11]

Ibotenic acid is a prodrug to muscimol. While most ibotenic acid is converted to muscimol in the gastrointestinal tract, some remain unmetabolized. Ibotenic acid is neurotoxic in large amounts and is an agonist at *N*-methyl-D-aspartate (NMDA) receptors, which may cause hallucinations. Muscimol, which may be considered the essential principle of *A. muscaria*, is a nonselective γ-aminobutyric acid (GABA$_A$) agonist.[11] On account of its activity at GABA$_A$ receptors, some have theorized that it may help with neuropathic pain, though studies exploring this use are still preliminary.[12]

There is a notable increase in online interest for products containing *A. muscaria* extracts. Claims within gray literature suggest that *A. muscaria* can reduce anxiety and stress while improving sleep, but there is not a great deal of evidence to support these claims. Moreover, the online markets for products containing extracts from *A. muscaria* are not well regulated and may lack consistent concentrations of active ingredients. In other words, some products may contain virtually no *A. muscaria* extracts, while other ostensibly identical products may contain significantly higher concentrations of these extracts than advertised. The latter presents a far greater danger, as case reports suggest that overconsumption of *A. muscaria* can produce a host of unpleasant side effects, including ataxia, agitation, confusion, dizziness, time and space distortions, tachycardia, bradycardia, nausea, vomiting, and diarrhea.[13] These may last between 8 and 24 hours, though truly excessive consumption can lead to coma (the patient in the case report of Rampolli et al was in a coma for 72 hours), and potentially even death.[13]

Many of these risks can be significantly reduced with proper dosing and a better regulated market.

Miscellaneous Psychedelics of Potential Use

Psychedelics are frequently classified according to systems that take into account their chemical structure (phenethylamines, tryptamines, ergolines, and so on) or their subjective effects (classic psychedelics, entactogens, dissociatives, and so on), or some via some other criteria. The miscellaneous psychedelics in the later text have simply been organized alphabetically.

This is not a comprehensive list by any means, as there are too many psychedelic compounds contained within just the phenethylamine family to count. One hundred and seventy-nine of these compounds were famously (or perhaps infamously) described by Alexander Shulgin and Ann Shulgin in their book *PiHKAL: A Chemical Love Story* ("PiHKAL" serving as an acronym for phenethylamines I have known and loved), which is close to 1,000 pages in length. Their follow-up work, *TiHKAL: The Continuation* (tryptamines I have known and loved), covers 55 tryptamines and consists of another 800 pages.

The vast majority of the compounds described in both books were synthesized by Alexander Shulgin, who was an extremely accomplished chemist and one-time employee of Dow Chemical Company. He was also fond of experimenting with these compounds and taking thorough notes for posterity. Unfortunately, clinical research into these drugs has been limited and the full scope of their pharmacologic properties remains largely unknown, particularly for compounds that appear to have relatively mild psychedelic effects. Rather than simply list hundreds of drugs, I will focus on the following:

- 2,5-Dimethoxy-4-bromoamphetamine (DOB)
- 2,5-Dimethoxy-4-bromophenethylamine (2C-B)

- 2,5-Dimethoxy-4-ethylphenethylamine (2C-E)
- 2,5-Dimethoxy-4-ethylthiophenethylamine (2C-T-2)
- 2,5-Dimethoxy-4-methylamphetamine (DOM)
- 2,5-Dimethoxy-4-propylthiophenethylamine (2C-T-7)
- 2,5-Methoxy-4-iodoampheamine (DOI)
- 3-Methoxy-4,5-methylenedioxy-amphetamine (MMDA)
- 3,4-Methylenedioxy-amphetamine (MDA)
- 3,4,5-Trimethoxyamphetamine (TMA)
- 2,4,5-Trimethoxyamphetamine (TMA-2)

This listing includes five of Shulgin's "magical half dozen," which he claimed were mescaline (covered in Chapter 12), DOM, 2C-B, 2C-E, 2C-T-2, and 2C-T-7.

2,5-Dimethoxy-4-Bromoamphetamine

DOB is a long-acting psychedelic (16-30 hours), first synthesized by Shulgin in 1967.[14(p621)] It has shown activity primarily at serotonin receptors 5-HT$_{2B}$, 5-HT$_{2A}$, and 5-HT$_{2C}$.[15] Though DOB has been used as a research chemical, research into its activity in humans is very limited.

2,5-Dimethoxy-4-Bromophenethylamine

Since being synthesized by Shulgin, 2C-B has become one of the more popular "designer drugs" of the phenylethylamine family, with subjective effects similar to both MDMA and classic psychedelics like lysergic acid diethylamide (LSD). On account of its pleasurable effects, it has frequently been used in club settings.[16] Experiences are not always pleasant, and Shulgin describes individuals who have experienced dissociative states more akin to ketamine intoxication.[14(pp504-506)]

2C-B is active across a wide range of serotonin receptors (5-HT$_{2B}$, 5-HT$_{1D}$, 5-HT$_{2A}$, 5-HT$_{2C}$, 5-HT$_{1B}$, 5-HT$_{1E}$, 5-HT$_7$, 5-HT$_{1A}$, 5-HT$_6$) and adrenergic receptors (α_{2C}, α_{2A}, α_{2B}).[15] Given this profile and its subjective effects, 2C-B may have some clinical utility in psychedelic-assisted psychotherapy, particularly in conditions also treated by MDMA, but clinical trials are currently lacking.

2,5-Dimethoxy-4-Ethylphenethylamine

Also synthesized by Shulgin, 2C-E is a psychedelic phenylethylamine that produces significant somatic effects.[14(p517)] 2C-E is active across a wide range of serotonin receptors (5-HT$_{2B}$, 5-HT$_{2A}$, 5-HT$_{1D}$, 5-HT$_{2C}$, 5-HT$_{1B}$, 5-HT$_{1A}$, 5-HT$_7$, 5-HT$_{1E}$) and adrenergic receptors (α_{2C}, α_{2B}, α_{2A}), as well as at dopamine (D_3) receptors and muscarinic acetylcholine receptor M_5.[15] No clinical trials have been conducted with 2C-E.

2,5-Dimethoxy-4-Ethylthiophenethylamine

2C-T-2 was also synthesized by Shulgin. The compound is active at several serotonin receptors, particularly $5-HT_{2B}$, $5-HT_{2A}$, $5-HT_{2C}$, $5-HT_{1D}$, $5-HT_{1A}$, and $5-HT_{1E}$. It is also active at adrenergic receptors (especially α_{2C}).[15]

The subjective effects of 2C-T-2, as well as its relative 2C-T-7, make it a useful tool for introspection, according to Shulgin. He states that both have been used illicitly in a therapeutic context as follow-ups to psychedelic-assisted therapy with MDMA.[14(p560)] Unfortunately, no clinical trials have been conducted with 2C-T-2 at this time.

2,5-Dimethoxy-4-Methylamphetamine

DOM became notorious in the late spring of 1967 when it was distributed illicitly under the name STP (Serenity, Tranquility, and Peace) and led to the hospitalization of dozens of individuals in California. At the time, the *New York Times* reported that its effects lasted several days, was "much more powerful than LSD," and produced effects similar to BZ (3-quinuclidinyl benzilate),[17] a powerful anticholinergic that the Army studied as part of Operation Delirium and Project DORK.[18] By summer, the drug had been identified as DOM, which had been developed by Shulgin while he worked for the Dow Chemical Company, though he denied involvement in its sudden appearance on the streets in 1967.[14(pp53,56),19] According to Shulgin, the onset of DOM is relatively slow.[14(pp53,56)] Consequently, the reports of individuals feeling the effects of the drug for several days are likely not an exaggeration, as they likely doubled their dose upon not feeling the drug's effects in the time expected.

Like most other psychedelics, DOM is a selective partial agonist at $5-HT_{2A}$ receptors and is also a partial agonist at $5-HT_{2B}$ and $5-HT_{2C}$.[20] As it has enjoyed little clinical use in its history, any unique therapeutic benefits that DOM may have over more conventional classic psychedelics (eg, psilocybin, LSD) is unknown.

2,5-Dimethoxy-4-Propylthiophenethylamine

As noted above, 2C-T-7 may be a useful tool for introspection, according to Shulgin, and he claims that the drug has been used by undisclosed therapists following psychedelic-assisted therapy with MDMA.[14(p560)]

Unfortunately, no clinical trials have been conducted with 2C-T-7 at this time and a full pharmacologic profile of the drug is lacking, though evidence indicates that it is a partial agonist at 5-HT$_{2A}$ receptors.[21]

It should be noted that at least three deaths were linked to the use of 2C-T-7 in Japan in the early 2000s, when it was marketed under the name "Blue Mystic."

2,5-Methoxy-4-Iodoampheamine

DOI is an extremely potent 5-HT$_{2A}$ agonist and has been used in several studies involving animal models to map out the presence of serotonin receptors in the brain. In addition to being potent, it is long lasting, with an estimated duration of 16 to 30 hours.[14(p634)] While one may surmise that DOI could have clinical uses similar to other psychedelics, there is no clinical evidence to support that claim at this time.

Of note, DOI has also demonstrated potent inhibition of tumor necrosis factor in preclinical testing, suggesting that it may have some clinical utility outside of psychiatry as an anti-inflammatory.[22]

3-Methoxy-4,5-Methylendioxy-Amphetamine

Shulgin describes the duration of MMDA as "moderate" and notes that both he and Godon A. Alles of the University of California, Los Angeles independently synthesized the drug in 1962.[14(pp790,791)] Subjectively, MMDA has been described as having "primarily amphetamine-like activity with some LSD-like actions."[23] Shulgin described it as being relatively gentle for drugs of its class at moderate doses, with significant closed-eye visualizations ("brain movies") at higher doses that feel dreamlike.[14(p791)]

No clinical trials have been conducted with MMDA and a full pharmacologic profile of the drug is lacking.

3,4-Methylenedioxy-Amphetamine

Often referred to as the "love drug," MDA is an entactogen that acts on serotonin receptors (5-HT$_{2B}$, 5-HT$_7$, 5-HT$_{1A}$, 5-HT$_{2C}$), as well as adrenergic receptors (α_{2C}, α_{2B}, α_{2A}).[15] There is also evidence that it is active at 5-HT$_{2A}$ receptors.[24] MDA is also similar to MDMA in that it inhibits monoamine transporters for dopamine, serotonin, and norepinephrine (in descending order of potency).[25] Similarities to MDMA go beyond the pharmacology; the effects of the two are subjectively similar and MDA is often substituted for MDMA in illicit markets. Two distinctions between MDA and MDMA are that MDA appears to be slightly longer lasting and that its effects are more visual and less mentally stimulating.[25] It should be noted that MDA was used as an adjunct to psychotherapy from the 1960s through the 1980s, when it was banned at the same time as MDMA.[26-28]

Interest in MDA has returned within the last 15 years, with a study published in 2010 reporting that MDA increased self-reported measures of mystical-type experiences,[24] and a study from 2019 reporting that doses of 1.4 mg/kg of MDA were well tolerated in healthy volunteers.[29] Given its similar profile to MDMA, there is reason to believe that it could be a good candidate for psychedelic-assisted psychotherapy, but more clinical work needs to be performed to better understand its safety profile and pharmacokinetics.

3,4,5-Trimethoxyamphetamine

According to Shulgin, TMA was the first synthetic psychedelic phenethylamine found to be psychoactive in humans (in 1947).[30] An analog of mescaline, TMA is believed to be approximately twice the potency of its natural relative.[14(p23)]

Shulgin also notes that the effects are not particularly pleasant. While the term "psychotomimetic" was already outdated in the 1960, he believed it seemed apt for TMA given the drug's capacity to drain individuals of empathy.[14(pp22-25)]

TMA has a notably different pharmacologic profile than the other drugs discussed in this chapter, as it has shown activity not only at serotonin receptors ($5\text{-}HT_{2B}$, $5\text{-}HT_7$, $5\text{-}HT_{1A}$, $5\text{-}HT_{1B}$, $5\text{-}HT_{1D}$, $5\text{-}HT_{1E}$, $5\text{-}HT_{2C}$), but also σ receptors (σ-1 and σ-2), as well as adrenergic receptors (α_{2A} and α_{2C}).[15]

2,4,5-Trimethoxyamphetamine

The subjective effects of TMA-2 are far more pleasant than the subjective effects of TMA.[14(p886)] TMA-2 is also far more potent and long lasting than TMA, with the effects of a 20 to 40 mg dose lasting 8 to 12 hours.[14(p885)] Its primary pharmacologic targets are believed to be serotonin receptors ($5\text{-}HT_{2B}$, $5\text{-}HT_{2A}$, $5\text{-}HT_{2C}$).[15]

The drug is rarely encountered even in illicit settings, and its potential clinical utility has not been studied. Like many of the other drugs explored in this chapter, its subjective effects bear resemblance to both classic psychedelics and amphetamines, so it is possible that it could be used within a clinical setting in a manner akin to MDMA. However, until we have a better pharmacologic profile of this drug and all the other drugs mentioned in this chapter, their potential therapeutic uses, whether in psychedelic-assisted therapy or within another clinical context, remain unknown.

REFERENCES

1. Orton E, Liu R. Salvinorin A: a mini review of physical and chemical properties affecting its translation from research to clinical applications in humans. *Transl Perioper Pain Med*. 2014;1(1):9-11. PMID: 25346937; PMCID: PMC4208627.
2. MacLean KA, Johnson MW, Reissig CJ, Prisinzano TE, Griffiths RR. Dose-related effects of salvinorin A in humans: dissociative, hallucinogenic, and memory effects. *Psychopharmacology (Berl)*. 2013;226(2):381-392. doi:10.1007/s00213-012-2912-9. PMID: 23135605; PMCID: PMC3581702.
3. Ermakova AO, Dunbar F, Rucker J, Johnson MW. A narrative synthesis of research with 5-MeO-DMT. *J Psychopharmacol*. 2022;36(3):273-294. doi:10.1177/02698811211050543. PMID: 34666554; PMCID: PMC8902691.
4. Holmstedt B, Lindgren JE. Chemical constituents of pharmacology of South American snuffs. In: Efron DH, ed. *Ethnopharmacologic Search for Psychoactive Drugs: Proceedings of a Symposium held in San Francisco, California January 28-30, 1967*. Vol I. Synergetic Press; 2018:339-373.
5. Reckweg JT, van Leeuwen CJ, Henquet C, et al. A phase 1/2 trial to assess safety and efficacy of a vaporized 5-methoxy-N,N-dimethyltryptamine formulation (GH001) in patients with treatment-resistant depression. *Front Psychiatry*. 2023;14:1133414. doi:10.3389/fpsyt.2023.1133414. PMID: 37409159; PMCID: PMC10319409.
6. Davis AK, Barsuglia JP, Lancelotta R, Grant RM, Renn E. The epidemiology of 5-methoxy-N, N-dimethyltryptamine (5-MeO-DMT) use: benefits, consequences, patterns of use, subjective effects, and reasons for consumption. *J Psychopharmacol*. 2018;32(7):779-792. doi:10.1177/0269881118769063. PMID: 29708042; PMCID: PMC6248886.
7. Reckweg J, Mason NL, van Leeuwen C, Toennes SW, Terwey TH, Ramaekers JG. A phase 1, dose-ranging study to assess safety and psychoactive effects of a vaporized 5-methoxy-N, N-dimethyltryptamine formulation (GH001) in healthy volunteers. *Front Pharmacol*. 2021;12:760671. doi:10.3389/fphar.2021.760671. PMID: 34912222; PMCID: PMC8667866.
8. Davis AK, Xin Y, Sepeda N, Averill LA. Open-label study of consecutive ibogaine and 5-MeO-DMT assisted-therapy for trauma-exposed male Special Operations Forces Veterans: prospective data from a clinical program in Mexico. *Am J Drug Alcohol Abuse*. 2023;49(5):587-596. doi:10.1080/00952990.2023.2220874. PMID: 37734158.
9. Neumann J, Schulz N, Fehse C, et al. Cardiovascular effects of bufotenin on human 5-HT4 serotonin receptors in cardiac preparations of transgenic mice and in human atrial preparations. *Naunyn Schmiedebergs Arch Pharmacol*. 2023;396(7):1471-1485. doi:10.1007/s00210-023-02414-8. PMID: 36754881; PMCID: PMC10244282.
10. Shulgin A, Shulgin A. *TiHKAL: The Continuation*. Transform Press;2022.
11. Voynova M, Shkondrov A, Kondeva-Burdina M, Krasteva I. Toxicological and pharmacological profile of Amanita muscaria (L.) Lam.—a new rising opportunity for biomedicine. *Pharmacia*. 2020;67(4):317-323. doi:10.3897/pharmacia.67.e56112
12. Ramawad HA, Paridari P, Jabermoradi S, et al. Muscimol as a treatment for nerve injury-related neuropathic pain: a systematic review and meta-analysis of preclinical studies. *Korean J Pain*. 2023;36(4):425-440. doi:10.3344/kjp.23161. PMID: 37732408; PMCID: PMC10551397.
13. Rampolli FI, Kamler P, Carnevale Carlino C, Bedussi F. The deceptive mushroom: accidental *Amanita muscaria* poisoning. *Eur J Case Rep Intern Med*. 2021;8(3):002212. doi:10.12890/2021_002212. PMID: 33768066; PMCID: PMC7977045.
14. Shulgin A, Shulgin A. *PiHKAL: A Chemical Love Story*. Transform Press;2022.

15. Ray TS. Psychedelics and the human receptorome. *PLoS One*. 2010;5(2):e9019. doi:10.1371/journal.pone.0009019. Erratum in: *PLoS One*. 2010;5(3). doi:10.1371/annotation/e580a864-cf13-40c2-9bd9-b9687a6f0fe4. PMID: 20126400; PMCID: PMC2814854.
16. Caudevilla-Gálligo F, Riba J, Ventura M, et al. 4-Bromo-2,5-dimethoxyphenethylamine (2C-B): presence in the recreational drug market in Spain, pattern of use and subjective effects. *J Psychopharmacol*. 2012;26(7):1026-1035. doi:10.1177/0269881111431752. PMID: 22234927.
17. Lyons RD. A drug more potent than LSD widely distributed in California. *New York Times*. Published June 28, 1967. Accessed February 1, 2024. https://timesmachine.nytimes.com/timesmachine/1967/06/28/129284352.html?pageNumber=1
18. Khatchadourian R. Operation delirium. *The New Yorker*. Published December 9, 2012. Accessed February 1, 2024. https://www.newyorker.com/magazine/2012/12/17/operation-delirium
19. Schmeck HM Jr. U.S. identifies STP as chemical developed by Dow. *New York Times*. Published August 3, 1967. Accessed February 1, 2024. https://timesmachine.nytimes.com/timesmachine/1967/08/03/90386306.html?pageNumber=24
20. Sanders-Bush E, Burris KD, Knoth K. Lysergic acid diethylamide and 2,5-dimethoxy-4-methylamphetamine are partial agonists at serotonin receptors linked to phosphoinositide hydrolysis. *J Pharmacol Exp Ther*. 1988;246(3):924-928. PMID: 2843634.
21. Halberstadt AL, Luethi D, Hoener MC, Trachsel D, Brandt SD, Liechti ME. Use of the head-twitch response to investigate the structure-activity relationships of 4-thio-substituted 2,5-dimethoxyphenylalkylamines. *Psychopharmacology (Berl)*. 2023;240(1):115-126. doi:10.1007/s00213-022-06279-2. PMID: 36477925; PMCID: PMC9816194.
22. Flanagan TW, Sebastian MN, Battaglia DM, Foster TP, Maillet EL, Nichols CD. Activation of 5-HT2 receptors reduces inflammation in vascular tissue and cholesterol levels in high-fat diet-fed apolipoprotein E knockout mice. *Sci Rep*. 2019;9(1):13444. doi:10.1038/s41598-019-49987-0. PMID: 31530895; PMCID: PMC6748996.
23. Nozaki M, Vaupel DB, Bright LD, Martin WR. A pharmacological comparison of 3-methoxy-4,5-methylenedioxyamphetamine and LSD in the dog. *Drug Alcohol Depend*. 1978;3(3):153-163. doi:10.1016/0376-8716(78)90037-6. PMID: 668489.
24. Baggott MJ, Siegrist JD, Galloway GP, Robertson LC, Coyle JR, Mendelson JE. Investigating the mechanisms of hallucinogen-induced visions using 3,4-methylenedioxyamphetamine (MDA): a randomized controlled trial in humans. *PLoS One*. 2010;5(12):e14074. doi:10.1371/journal.pone.0014074. PMID: 21152030; PMCID: PMC2996283.
25. Oeri HE. Beyond ecstasy: alternative entactogens to 3,4-methylenedioxymethamphetamine with potential applications in psychotherapy. *J Psychopharmacol*. 2021;35(5):512-536. doi:10.1177/0269881120920420. PMID: 32909493; PMCID: PMC8155739.
26. Yensen R, Di Leo FB, Rhead JC, et al. MDA-assisted psychotherapy with neurotic outpatients: a pilot study. *J Nerv Ment Dis*. 1976;163(4):233-245. doi:10.1097/00005053-197610000-00002. PMID: 972325.
27. Climko RP, Roehrich H, Sweeney DR, Al-Razi J. Ecstacy: a review of MDMA and MDA. *Int J Psychiatry Med*. 1986-1987;16(4):359-372. doi:10.2190/dcrp-u22m-aumd-d84h. PMID: 2881902.
28. U.S. will ban 'ecstasy,' a hallucinogenic drug. *New York Times*. Published June 1, 1985. Accessed May 25, 2024. https://timesmachine.nytimes.com/timesmachine/1985/06/01/issue.html
29. Baggott MJ, Garrison KJ, Coyle JR, et al. Effects of the psychedelic amphetamine MDA (3,4-methylenedioxyamphetamine) in healthy volunteers. *J Psychoactive Drugs*. 2019;51(2):108-117. doi:10.1080/02791072.2019.1593560. PMID: 30967099.
30. Shulgin AT, Bunnell S, Sargent T III. The psychotomimetic properties of 3,4,5-trimethyoxyamphetamine. *Nature*. 1961;189:1011-1012. doi:10.1038/1891011a0

17
Patient Stories

As previous chapters have shown, there is a tremendous amount of variability with respect to the pharmacology of psychedelics. There is also no *typical* psychedelic experience. Even if there are great efforts made to maintain a consistent setting where the drugs are administered, each patient will enter treatment with a different mindset that will uniquely color the experience, and it is worth reiterating that these experiences run the gamut from blissful to deeply troubling. However, the more important point to keep in mind is that the therapeutic benefits of psychedelics are not always clearly tied to how enjoyable the experience was for the patient. Some patients will respond positively to the treatment even if it is deeply challenging while others may show limited symptom improvement following the treatment even if they describe feeling a sublime sense of love and serenity while under the acute effects of the drug.

To help make this point, I asked several patients who have used psychedelics to treat their psychiatric or neurologic conditions to describe their experiences in their own words. These stories will follow. However, it is important to note two things first.

One, this is not an endorsement. I do not tell my patients to take psychedelics. Most psychedelics cannot be prescribed because they are still Schedule I drugs. Depending on the jurisdiction, they may also be illegal unless administered as part of a clinical trial or at a retreat outside of the United States. Rather, I encourage my patients to inform me if they are using psychedelics because it is clinically relevant. Psychedelics can profoundly alter one's mood, spirituality, and outlook on life, and knowing that these alterations are not entirely organic helps me to better assess patients' status. For example, if a patient with a history of bipolar disorder comes into the office claiming to have had a spiritual awakening, knowing that they recently went to a psychedelic retreat and that the awakening was not entirely organic puts the claim in a dramatically different light. It is also clinically relevant because psychedelics can interfere with the efficacy and safety of medications the patient may currently be taking. Knowing that a patient plans to use psilocybin or ayahuasca allows the clinician to have an informed discussion, explaining any risks and adjusting their medication to avoid problematic drug-drug interactions.

Second, there is a deeply human side to the psychedelic experience that can be lost when one focuses exclusively on clinical studies and pharmacology. Hidden in the statistics are the stories of individual patients, which I will now share.

Patient 1, Psilocybin

Patient 1 is a 61-year-old male physician with no history of psychiatric illness. Patient does have a history of cluster headaches, which have occurred on and off for 20 years. As the patient notes in the succeeding text, the headaches tend to become more severe with increased psychosocial stress but can be mitigated with the use of psilocybin.

In the Patient's Own Words

I am a practicing physician and have been suffering from episodic cluster headaches for the past 20 years. In my case, they are seasonal, typically emerging at the onset of spring and fall. Over the years, I have utilized triptans and prophylactic high-dose calcium channel blockers with varying degrees of success. These medications, while occasionally effective, have come at the cost of considerable adverse effects. Inhalation of 100% oxygen usually aborted the cluster attack, but the availability of an oxygen tank and a nonrebreathing mask was not always guaranteed. I also turned to intranasal 4% topical lidocaine, which became my go-to medication due to its lack of systemic side effects. This method dulled the pain somewhat but never fully aborted the cluster attack. Despite these therapeutic strategies, my cluster cycles persisted, each lasting about 3 months.

In the fall of 2021, I experienced twice-daily cluster attacks despite being on a high dose of verapamil. Even oxygen had ceased to be effective. My neurologist recommended Emgality (galcanezumab-gnlm), but I decided to explore alternative remedies after reviewing its side effects. This led me to the literature on the use of psilocybin in treating and successfully aborting cluster cycles. I decided to give it a try. The protocol involved taking at least three doses of 1 g each of dried magic mushrooms, spaced 5 days apart, or continuing every 5 days until the cycle broke. One gram is considered a low dose for psychedelic effects. Since I was also advised to avoid traditional medications, particularly calcium channel blockers, I began tapering off verapamil.

I meticulously followed the instructions, preparing the tea, and took my first dose on an empty stomach in September of 2021. Within half an hour, I felt elated, as if I had consumed a beer. Remarkably, the heaviness in my head, a constant feature of my cluster cycle, dissipated within the next hour. For the next 2 days, I experienced no headaches. However, the headaches returned on the third day, signaling it was time for my second dose.

After my second dose, I enjoyed two headache-free days before they returned once again. I took my third dose at the prescribed 5-day interval. While at work the following day, I experienced a profound realization about how my job might be contributing to my headaches by creating a significant work-life imbalance.

The next day, I had a headache while seeing patients—an unusual timing for my attacks. I had to cancel the rest of my appointments, leaving me with little doubt that I was suffering from burnout.

For my fourth dose, I increased the amount to 1.5 g. The next day, my headache was of much lower intensity and more tolerable. Subsequently, I continued to increase the dose by 0.5 g with each session until I reached 2.5 g. The psychedelic effects became more pronounced with each dose. I felt enveloped in Nature's loving embrace. A realization struck me: We are utterly lonely in the universe, yet the vast darkness of space cradles us like a womb, shielding us from harm. Paradoxically, this darkness is the source of light, needing an object to reflect or manifest. I embraced this darkness, allowing it to fill me inside and out. My headaches had become a secondary concern as I embarked on a journey of self-discovery.

Please note that my higher psychedelic doses—2 g and above—were taken outdoors in Nature. My experience with a 3-g dose was extraordinarily beautiful, even magical. The fall foliage was at its peak, and I was by a lakeside near my home. I experienced a phenomenal time distortion—a few seconds felt like a few hours. Time seemed to dilate into an ever-deepening present moment, which felt like an eternity.

Eventually, my cluster headache cycle broke, and I was truly free from the excruciating pain. But more importantly, these experiences filled me with a profound sense of awe. I realized that the best antidote to my burnout was this sense of awe.

The following year, I started taking prophylactic doses—500 mg weekly for 6 to 8 weeks—in spring and fall, and for the most part, I remained headache-free. In the fall of 2023, I did not take the mushrooms prophylactically and experienced a cluster attack, but I managed to terminate it with three weekly doses of 2 g each.

Patient 2, Psilocybin

Patient 2 is a 37-year-old female of South Asian descent who is married with a stable career. Patient had experienced psychiatric symptoms since high school that included anxiety, panic episodes, depression, and a mix of both obsessions and compulsions, despite a trial of numerous psychotropics that include antidepressant and antianxiety medications without success. The patient has also reported an extended history of chronic pain and migraines, as well as sleep problems that date back many years. Of note, the patient was also diagnosed with attention-deficit/hyperactivity disorder (ADHD) during high school and since that time has intermittently taken stimulants.

At the time of the first consultation, patient reported poor sleep, low mood, lack of self-esteem, excessive worrying/rumination, and some suicidal ideation, with symptoms of an eating disorder. The patient described fixating on obsessions and compulsions, as well as engaging in repetitive behaviors. Medications included stimulants for ADHD, alprazolam (Xanax) for anxiety, and a selective serotonin reuptake inhibitor (SSRI).

In the Patient's Own Words

Before

When I was young, I saw depictions of mushrooms as one of those scandalous drugs—reserved for hippies from the 1960s and the like. As I got older, I learned more and more about the complex reality of mushrooms: their integral role in our ecosystem, their rich diversity, and a little secret some of them contained known as psilocybin; a secret many refer to as magic.

As an exhaustive researcher, not by choice, I delved into the history of what made this compound so magical. What I found was far from the stereotypes we had perhaps too easily accepted as truth: artists across the spectrum and across time vouching for the creativity they unlocked; depictions of mushrooms in ancient paintings, spanning cultures; rave reviews from many in Silicon Valley touting the benefits of microdosing; and many psychologists, such as Timothy Leary, who worked hard to highlight the potential therapeutic benefits of this emerging drug.

When I was in graduate school studying clinical psychology, a peer of mine told me excitedly about her thesis on psilocybin and mental illness. After I divulged to her my struggles with depression and mental illness, she said it might help me on my journey to accept my brain. I knew then it was something I would do; but I also knew that I was not ready yet, emotionally or mentally, to delve into it. I had some more work to do. So, I did just that, and at the age of 28, decided to take the leap.

During

It's difficult to explain an experience that feels like a shift in reality, a fever dream, or an unlocking of something in your brain that you didn't know existed. My disclaimer, and one I believe in firmly, is this: Every person's experience with psilocybin will be uniquely their own, yet once done, will make them part of an inexplicable collective that is now aware of another plane of existence.

My relationship with psilocybin has been, as cliché as it may be, one of clarity, inspiration, and acceptance. By the time I tried it, I had made peace with many of my demons, or faced my shadow self, as some may say. This might be why the only negative part of my trips has been slight stomach discomfort and annoying spells of yawning in the beginning. Once it settled in, it's like I saw life in the colors I knew existed (but had a tendency of evading me). There was no internal turmoil, but rather internal peace, a strange understanding that I am exactly who I am, who I was, who I come from, and who I will be. It lessened the constant noise in my head, leaving space for that being in me to just—exist. This may sound simple, but for those who struggle with mental illness, this is indeed magic.

A large part of my experience was, and is, dynamic, vivid visuals. I would not call them hallucinations because there is no loss of reality or control. Instead, I'd say it turns the world around me into a painting. When I sit in the grass, it grows around me. When I gaze at the clouds, they tell me stories of the world. When I gaze at the stars, the barrier between earth and the universe is broken for us to become one. When I face a tree, it embodies my ancestors and sends me messages from beyond. When I stare at paintings or focus on songs or read books—even ones I've known countless times before—they give me context, relaying messages and feelings the artists perhaps intended to leave behind.

The other part of it is emotional. As someone who sits on one extreme end of the highly sensitive spectrum, psilocybin felt like a homecoming. It did not force me into introspection or internal work; it allowed me relief from my usual level of it. It did not make me cry because I was scared; it let me do my usual daily cry without inhibition or fear of judgment.

After

I've found that even when I am not actively taking psilocybin, the visual stimulation has remained. If I stare at a painting long enough, I can see the brush strokes moving. My meditation practice has become easier. The traits I value within myself are ones I have become sure of. It has, lastingly, deepened my love for people, art, and history, cracking open my creativity in a new way. Above all, every time I do it, I feel my brain healing just a little bit more.

While it can be a daunting, sometimes even a draining endeavor for some, I believe the results are comparable to other drugs we commonly use for treatments of mental illnesses. More research, availability, and access, as well as careful prescribing and titration, may lead to a transformation in the way we approach treatments. I'm hopeful and eager to witness our understanding and usage of psilocybin evolve; even more so to continue reaping its magical benefits.

Patient 3, Psilocybin (Microdose)

Patient 3 is a single, White male aged 33 years with bipolar disorder ("BP" throughout the patient's narrative). Patient is currently working in the real estate space, but at the time of first consultation, he was unemployed and was receiving help from his family as he struggled to regain his bearings.

In hindsight, the patient has experienced symptoms of mania and hypomania since his teens, but only became cognizant of his condition upon experiencing a major depressive episode in his early 20s. During his late 20s, patient experienced mood cycling with a more significant manic episode followed by a severe depressive episode. During the former, the patient was gregarious, hypersexual, and willing to take major risks (such as letting go of a stable job). During depressive episodes, the patient reported being asocial, apathetic, unmotivated, indecisive with cognitive slowing, and also experienced anxiety as well as disturbed sleep.

Patient's drug use history includes casual marijuana and occasional cocaine use. Additionally, the patient reported using a combination of Benadryl and melatonin for sleep. He had never seen a psychiatrist before and at the time was under the care of a nurse practitioner (NP) and being prescribed a subtherapeutic dose of lamotrigine (Lamictal).

The patient's current treatment regimen includes a mood stabilizer and an atypical antipsychotic that have been combined with lifestyle changes. Currently, the patient is asymptomatic and is in full remission.

In the Patient's Own Words

I'm very much of the mindset that to tackle BP and live your best life (as the kids would say) is to address it with a robust, holistic, self-aware lifestyle, along with any psychiatric medicine that may be needed. Always looking for ways to improve my self-care plan, I came across microdosing in 2019 and decided to give it a try. I used psychedelics throughout my 20s and have always been drawn to them for a multitude of reasons. I view psychedelics as "medicine," so I thought I would give it a try.

In the summer of 2019, I had a few bad months of depression, anxiety, and little sleep. I thought I was doing a good job managing it, but it was obvious that something needed to change. My psychiatrist upped my lamotrigine (Lamictal) dosage, and it helped to raise my floor, but I wasn't fully back and felt like there was more improvement possible. In November 2019, I started following Paul Stamets' protocol of lion's mane mushrooms, psilocybin and niacin. Shortly after starting, I noticed an overall improvement in my mood, disposition, sociability, and physical performance.

I still have my normal fluctuations, but they are far less severe and far more manageable with a regular microdosing protocol. It's been 5 years since I started, and I would recommend it to anyone that's seeking more balance and addressing our tendencies with a holistic solution. My advice for everyone dealing with BP and other mood disorders is that you need to be locked in to actively monitoring and managing your behavior. *Your plan for success can't be to just take a pill.* This, unfortunately, requires a lot more self-care, but if you do, you can live up to your full potential.

Patient 4, Ayahuasca

Patient 4 describes their 2015 experience with ayahuasca while at a retreat in Iquitos, Peru. At the time, the patient was 30 years old. He is a single, White male who is unemployed but domiciled as a result of family support. The patient has a history of unspecified mood disorder and substance use.

Prior to consultation, the patient had recently been discharged from inpatient care following a period of psychosis and mania. The patient reported grandiosity, restlessness, insomnia, paranoia, being easily distracted, and vague visual hallucinations. According to the patient, they were also receiving some subliminal messages. Patient denied experiencing suicidality, obsessions, or compulsions during either manic or major depressive episodes.

The patient had long expressed ambivalence about treatment with psychotropic medications but has been more open to holistic forms of healing. Since his experience with ayahuasca, he has become less resistant to the idea of using more conventional psychotropics for mood stabilization and ketamine during depressive episodes. As a result, he has shown significant improvement and is currently stable and in remission.

One important point is that the patient refers to ayahuasca as a plant and Ayahuasca as an entity. This is a common practice within many cultures within the Amazon basin and has been adopted by many individuals outside of the region who use plant-based psychedelics.

In the Patient's Own Words

I arrived at the lodge in the worst mental shape of my life. Debilitating depression had plagued me for over 2 years, making every moment an absolute slog. I went to Iquitos hoping for a solution, as life was becoming impossible to bear. My experience was divided into four ceremonies over the course of a week at the lodge. In each ceremony, our group of 20 would be seated around the perimeter of a large tent and come up one by one to ritualistically drink the cup of ayahuasca served by the shaman. After drinking my cup, I sat back down on my cushion, vomited the bowl within reach, closed my eyes, and waited for the effects to kick in. The first session was an absolute disappointment. I waited and waited but nothing happened. I worried that my body was somehow immune to ayahuasca's effects, and this nonexperience in the midst of my depression was absolutely devastating.

My second ceremony a couple of days later, however, was absolutely astounding. About 45 minutes after drinking my cup, my view became filled with geometric shapes, and I found myself floating gently down a psychedelic river, guided by a voice that seemed to be my higher consciousness. I was taken through various moments of my life as the voice analyzed and reframed them, giving me a sense of acceptance and understanding that had previously eluded me. As some negative thoughts began to accumulate, I projectile vomited into the nearby bowl and synchronously felt the negativity expel from my body.

By the end of this journey, I had a distinct feeling that everything was okay, and I was simply glad to be alive. I woke up the next morning feeling upbeat and completely free of depression. This feeling, however, proved to be short lived, and, despite my newfound understanding, I sank back down into depression by the afternoon. The previous night's experience became nothing but a memory, information without my heart attached. It was a frustrating experience but a big improvement over the first session.

My third session was horrible. It felt like a sensory tour of a nasty swamp, with disgusting, closeup imagery of animal anatomy accompanied by putrid smells. There was no insight attached to this, just 5 hours of visceral misery. The next morning, I felt like this was Ayahuasca's message to not take the positive experiences for granted, as it could inspire as much as it could disgust. My final ceremony was a return to the brilliance of the second, except instead of a psychedelic river, I was gliding through space, filled with memories and elements of my life. It felt like a celebration of hope, reframing weaknesses as strengths and bringing out the value of my life's experiences. Once again, the experience became but a memory by the following day, and, overall, I left Iquitos largely unchanged. The ceremonies had been a respite from my misery but far from life changing or life fixing.

Patient 5, Ketamine

Patient 5 is a White male in his 30s with a long history of dysthymia and major depression (ie, double depression). The most salient of the patient's symptoms could be described as neurovegetative, as he was apathetic, asocial, reluctant to speak (alogia), or even eat. The latter symptom became so pronounced that he was diagnosed with an eating disorder and sent to several specialized clinics to address the said disorder. Following inpatient treatment, the patient was referred for ongoing care. It became clear that his most pronounced symptom of poor appetite was secondary to severe depression, requiring a combination of antidepressants in addition to ketamine therapy which led to complete remission, and as a result, he was able to finish college and graduate.

Since our first meeting, the patient has undergone multiple ketamine sessions and continues to receive maintenance ketamine treatment once per month or once every 2 months in conjunction with an SSRI and bupropion (Wellbutrin).

In the Patient's Own Words

My experience with ketamine starts after years of treatment-resistant depression, inpatient hospitalizations, therapy, and a myriad of medications. A traumatic instance of electroconvulsive therapy (ECT), where the paralytic agent worked but the anesthesia did not, brought me to ketamine infusions. Originally, when presented with a choice between ECT and ketamine in the hospital, I deferred to my doctors who had more familiarity with ECT. I wish I hadn't. My first round of ECT kept me out of the hospital for 6 months. I didn't complete my second round due to the aforementioned complications. Ketamine's benefits have persisted far beyond that.

Treatment-resistant depression makes it clear that our existence has physical limitations. While therapy was beneficial, negative thought patterns were solidified in my brain. I needed a reprieve from this to effectively apply the skills learned in therapy. Ketamine gave me that. It bought me time to rewire my brain.

Seeing what the brain is capable of experiencing during my ketamine sessions completely washed away the deep-seated conviction that the way I saw life and the world while depressed was objective. Since then, my baseline mood is in a satisfactory place. Like anyone, I go through highs and lows, but the depth of the lows is miniscule compared to when I was sick. My baseline is neutral rather than anhedonia.

Ketamine doesn't magically solve problems. It does give an opportunity to implement changes in your life from a clean state. This is only temporary in my experience. I still benefit from follow-up infusions but not to the extent I did. When tolerance is built up to ketamine, it doesn't have the same impact. It's crucial to utilize the clean slate as best you can while you have it. If you do, it can have profound impacts on your psyche. It is much easier to maintain a healthy mind than fixing deep, catatonic depression. It's important to seek support if depression starts to take hold again, before it crystalizes again.

Conclusion

As these stories reveal, each person will respond to the psychedelic experience in their own way. Many individuals will feel as though the experience has given them insight into their personal mindset, which can be beneficial for patients with psychiatric conditions. Similarly, many patients with psychiatric ailments like mood or anxiety disorders may experience symptom improvements, but, as has been stressed throughout this book, this is not universally true and, more importantly, the use of psychedelics is optimized when paired with psychotherapy, as the modality of psychotherapy provides a safe and therapeutic environment for patients.

18

Conclusion

After a review of the clinical evidence involving psychedelic-assisted psychotherapy, it is difficult to not feel a sense of optimism. The use of these drugs has provided patients struggling with some of the most difficult-to-treat conditions in psychiatry the opportunity to heal rather than just manage their symptoms with daily medication regimens. Moreover, there is a strong theoretical framework to help explain these benefits, as well as a growing body of evidence to indicate that such benefits persist for extended periods of time, particularly among individuals who have "peak" or mystical-type experiences while under the influence of psychedelics.

What often gets lost in the media narrative, but not in the serious clinical work being conducted with these substances, is that psychotherapy is integral to the treatment modality. Clinicians are not simply handing out bags of psychedelic mushrooms to patients and saying, "Take two and call me in the morning." Rather, psychotherapy is complementary to psychedelic drugs, which may be best conceptualized as extremely potent potentiators capable of promoting metaplasticity, neuritogenesis, spinogenesis, and synaptogenesis.[1,2] Without the proper set, setting, and support from therapists or other knowledgeable guides, the full efficacy of psychedelics cannot be realized. This is not to diminish these drugs, but rather to emphasize that the two components play interrelated and necessary roles.

This message needs to be repeated again and again because there is a growing narrative that simply taking psychedelic drugs will make individuals happier, healthier, less stressed, more creative, and more in touch with their emotions. These kinds of statements are not supported by clinical evidence, as there is no evidence to support unguided and uncontrolled psychedelic use for the treatment of any condition. As discussed in Chapter 7, the evidence in favor of microdosing is weak.[3] There may even be some association between microdosing and valvular heart disease.

Discouraging this narrative is imperative for several reasons. First and foremost, the unmonitored use of psychedelics is dangerous. Individuals who are under the influence of psychedelics may behave in a reckless or irresponsible manner without supervision. While it is true that treatment with ketamine and esketamine (Spravato) may occur without concomitant psychotherapy, these drugs are meant to be administered within a clinical setting because individuals under the influence of ketamine and esketamine may not have full awareness of their surroundings.

Secondly, it can be very difficult to tell if certain psychedelics are adulterated when purchased on the illicit market. This may not be a major concern when one is consuming peyote or psilocybin mushrooms, but powders claiming to be MDMA (3,4-methylenedioxymethamphetamine), 2C-B (2,5-dimethoxy-4-bromophenethylamine), or even ibogaine may also contain any number of inert or toxic substances, including heroin, fentanyl, or xylazine. According to one study that collected 718 samples of powdered drugs between May 2021 and June 2023 (64% methamphetamine and 36% cocaine) from 77 harm reduction programs across 25 states, fentanyl was found in 12.5% of methamphetamine samples and 14.8% of cocaine samples.[4]

Third, the use of psychedelics in uncontrolled environments can be psychologically traumatic. Not every psychedelic experience is filled with kaleidoscopic colors, celestial visions, and a sense of unity with the cosmos. Some psychedelic experiences can be deeply disturbing, and individuals benefit from having experienced guides on hand to help them through acute challenges. Moreover, support through preparatory and integrative sessions can help make even difficult experiences therapeutically beneficial. When psychedelics are administered in a medical facility, therapists can take additional precautions before and during the psychedelic session, such as administering anxiolytics or using medications such as a 5-HT_{2A} antagonist to abort the session.

Finally, psychedelics may not help everyone, especially individuals with severe and persistent mental illnesses such as schizophrenia and bipolar disorder with psychotic features. Undergoing proper screening ensures that people with contraindications who will be adversely affected by these drugs do not receive them. Similarly, screening by a medical professional can help identify concomitant medications that should be discontinued before the use of psychedelics. For example, selective serotonergic reuptake inhibitors (SSRIs), serotonin and norepinephrine reuptake inhibitors (SNRIs), tricyclic antidepressants (TCAs), and haloperidol (to name just a few) may attenuate or otherwise modify the effects of classic psychedelics, while concomitant administration with lithium may increase risk of seizures.[5-7]

These are potent drugs, and they deserve proper respect. It is something that indigenous peoples and shamanistic cultures have known for generations, and it is something that medical science should keep in mind as we begin to utilize these drugs in treating psychiatric conditions. A great deal of hope and optimism currently surrounds psychedelics, but more research is still needed to determine how to best use them.

There were many commentators from the 1950s or possibly even the early 1960s who proclaimed that the future of psychedelics medicine was bright, and, from their perspectives, they were correct. The future did seem bright, and the same can be said as of summer 2024. Psychedelic-assisted psychotherapy is proving to be effective in the treatment of several conditions for which even first-line treatments often prove woefully ineffective. We owe it to our patients to develop safe and cost-effective protocols for administering these drugs in a way that optimizes patients' experiences and provides a path to healing.

REFERENCES

1. Ly C, Greb AC, Cameron LP, et al. Psychedelics promote structural and functional neural plasticity. *Cell Rep*. 2018;23(11):3170-3182. doi:10.1016/j.celrep.2018.05.022. PMID: 29898390; PMCID: PMC6082376.
2. Nardou R, Sawyer E, Song YJ, et al. Psychedelics reopen the social reward learning critical period. *Nature*. 2023;618(7966):790-798. doi:10.1038/s41586-023-06204-3. PMID: 37316665; PMCID: PMC10284704.
3. Cavanna F, Muller S, de la Fuente LA, et al. Microdosing with psilocybin mushrooms: a double-blind placebo-controlled study. *Transl Psychiatry*. 2022;12(1):307. doi:10.1038/s41398-022-02039-0. PMID: 35918311; PMCID: PMC9346139.
4. Wagner KD, Fiuty P, Page K, et al. Prevalence of fentanyl in methamphetamine and cocaine samples collected by community-based drug checking services. *Drug Alcohol Depend*. 2023;252:110985. doi:10.1016/j.drugalcdep.2023.110985. PMID: 37826988; PMCID: PMC10688611.

5. Barbut Siva J, Barba T, Kettner H, et al. Interactions between classic psychedelics and serotonergic antidepressants: effects on the acute psychedelic subjective experience, well-being and depressive symptoms from a prospective survey study. *J Psychopharmacol*. 2024;38(2):145-155. doi:10.1177/02698811231224217. PMID: 38281075; PMCID: PMC10863370.
6. Rucker JJH, Iliff J, Nutt DJ. Psychiatry & the psychedelic drugs. Past, present & future. *Neuropharmacology*. 2018;142:200-218. doi:10.1016/j.neuropharm.2017.12.040. PMID: 29284138.
7. Nayak SM, Gukasyan N, Barrett FS, Erowid E, Erowid F, Griffiths RR. Classic psychedelic coadministration with lithium, but not lamotrigine, is associated with seizures: an analysis of online psychedelic experience reports. *Pharmacopsychiatry*. 2021;54(5):240-245. doi:10.1055/a-1524-2794. PMID: 34348413.

About the Author

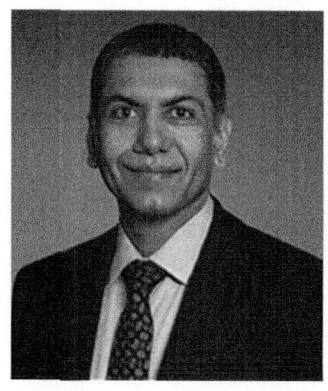

Samoon Ahmad, MD is a clinical professor of psychiatry at NYU Grossman School of Medicine and recently completed 30 years of service at Bellevue Hospital Center serving as the unit chief of inpatient psychiatry. A graduate of Allama Iqbal Medical College in Lahore, Pakistan, where he trained in Internal Medicine, General Surgery, and Cardiology, Dr Ahmad completed his psychiatric training at Bellevue Hospital/NYU Medical Center, serving as chief resident in his final year. Upon completion, he became an attending at Bellevue and joined the faculty of the NYU School of Medicine. Dr Ahmad supervises and mentors trainees, and lectures globally on various topics, including antipsychotics, obesity, metabolic disorders, and medical marijuana. He is a Diplomate of the American Board of Psychiatry and Neurology, a Distinguished Life Fellow of the American Psychiatric Association, and an International Associate member of the Royal College of Psychiatrists.

During his tenure, Dr Ahmad has served as director of the Division of Continuing Medical Education (CME), on the board of Governors of Bellevue Psychiatric Society, and on various committees including Grand Rounds, CME Advisory, CME Task Force, Educational Steering, Bellevue Collaboration Council, and Bellevue Psychiatry's Oversight Committee. He developed the Bellevue Hospital Psychiatry Department's Integrated Systems Conference, based on the morbidity and mortality conference in medicine, to better coordinate services and treatment in the department. He was recognized for 25 years of distinguished service at Bellevue and was named Bellevue's Physician of the Year in Psychiatry (2014) for his continued pursuit of clinical excellence, leadership, and dedication at the institution.

Dr Ahmad's research has focused primarily on the prevalence of metabolic abnormalities in the chronically mentally ill, specifically the association of psychiatric medications, diet, physical activity, and obesity. He has conducted other research on the role of faith, religion, and resilience in disasters. His documentary "The Wrath of God: A

Faith Based Survival Paradigm" about the aftermath of the earthquake in Pakistan was awarded "The Frank Ochberg Award for Media and Trauma" by the International Society for Traumatic Stress Studies.

Dr Ahmad specializes in the psychopharmacologic treatment of psychotic, mood, anxiety, and substance use disorders. He is the founder of Integrative Center for Wellness in New York City. He is an author, contributor, and consulting editor for several medical textbooks. His most recent books are the seventh edition of *Kaplan & Sadock's Pocket Handbook of Clinical Psychiatry* (2024), the eighth edition of *Kaplan & Sadock's Pocket Handbook of Psychiatric Drug Treatment* (2023), and *Coping with COVID-19: The Medical, Mental and Social Consequences of the Pandemic* (2022). He also coauthored *Medical Marijuana: A Clinical Handbook* (2021) and previous editions of the *Pocket Handbook of Clinical Psychiatry*. He lives in New York City with his wife and son, and enjoys photography, travel, classic cars, and vinyl in his spare time.

Index

Note: Page numbers followed by *f* indicate figures; page numbers followed by *t* indicate tables.

A

Addiction Research Foundation, 35
Adjustment disorder, with anxiety, 108
Aeruginascin, 128
Affective disorders, 96–100
  bipolar disorder, 96–98
  major depressive disorder, 98–100
  persistent depressive disorder, 100
Alcohol use disorder, 113, 142–144
  and lysergic acid diethylamide, 34–35
Alcoholics Anonymous, 35
Alpert, Richard, 38–39
α-amino-3-hydroxy-5-methyl-4-isoxazolepropionic acid (AMPA), 86, 125
Alzheimer disease, 165–166
Amazon, 173–174
American Indian Religious Freedom Act of 1978, 57
American Psychiatric Association (APA), 235
Amphetamine, 271, 276
Anorexia nervosa, 109–110, 145
  and menopause, 110
  types of, 110
Anxiety disorders, 100–103, 253–254
  adjustment disorder with, 108
  causes of, 101
  generalized, 102
  panic, 102, 103*t*
  psilocybin, 141–142
  signs and symptoms, 100, 101*t*
  social, 102
  terminal diagnosis, 102
APA. *See* American Psychiatric Association
Aristotle, 19
Aromatic-L-amino acid decarboxylase (AADC), 175
Arylcyclohexylamine, 231
Atypical psychedelics, 7–8, 84
Aurelius, Marcus, 19
Ayahuasca, 69
  patient stories, 306–308

B

Baeocystin, 128
Barger, George, 30
BDD. *See* Body dysmorphic disorder

BDI. *See* Beck Depression Inventory
BDNF. *See* Brain-derived neurotrophic factor
Beck Depression Inventory (BDI), 132, 165
Benzodiazepines, 260
Beringer, Kurt, 29
Binge eating disorder, 112
Bipolar disorder, 96–98, 252–253
Bipolar I disorder, 97
Bipolar II disorder, 97
Body dysmorphic disorder (BDD), 105
Borderline personality disorder, 257
Brain
  alterations in functional connectivity, 89–90
  consciousness, 86–88, 87*f*
  hierarchical, 86–88
    default mode network and compression, 88
  5-HT$_{2A}$ receptors, 85–86
  microdosing, 91–92
  REBUS (RElaxed Beliefs Under pSychedelics) model, 87
  reopening of critical windows, 90–91
Brain-derived neurotrophic factor (BDNF), 86, 125, 175, 181–182, 220, 239, 277
Breakthrough status, 52–53
Buddy drug, 232–233
Bufotenin, 289, 292
Bulimia nervosa, 110–111
  lifetime prevalence of, 111
  treatment, 111
  types of, 110

C

cAMP. *See* Cyclic adenosine 3,5-monophosphate
Cannabis use disorder, 113
Cardiovascular disease, psilocybin, 149
CBT. *See* Cognitive behavioral therapy
CDC. *See* Centers for Disease Control and Prevention
Celexa. See Citalopram
Centers for Disease Control and Prevention (CDC), 112
Central nervous system (CNS), 216, 238–239
Certainty, 65
Chlorpromazine, 33

317

Citalopram (Celexa), 136
Classic psychedelics, 7–8, 84, 86, 89, 90, 91, 92
Clinical Global Impression-Severity (CGI-S) scores, 136, 250
Clinical studies, 50–52, 51f
  requirements for, 52
Cluster headaches, 165
CNS. *See* Central nervous system
Cocaine, 271
Cocaine use disorder, 113
Cognitive behavioral therapy (CBT), 144
Columbus, Christopher, 172
Comfort, defined, 78
COMP360, 120, 131
Concord Prison Experiment, 40
Consciousness, 86–88, 87f
Consciousness Explained (Dennett), 87, 87f
Controlled Substances Act of 1970 (CSA), 4, 46–53, 121, 156, 157, 213
Corssen, Guenter Dr., 231–232
Cortico-striatal-thalamo-cortical (CSTC) pathway, 89–90
Cortisol, 277
Coulter, John Merle, 194
COVID-19 pandemic
  anxiety disorder, 101
  major depressive disorder, 98
Craig, L. C., 27
CSA. *See* Controlled Substances Act of 1970
CSTC pathway. *See* Cortico-striatal-thalamo-cortical pathway
CYB003, 131
Cybin, 137
Cyclic adenosine 3,5-monophosphate (cAMP), 276
Cyclothymia. *See* Cyclothymic disorder
Cyclothymic disorder, 96, 97
CYP3A4, 216, 259, 272
CYP2B6, 259
Cytochrome P450 enzyme 2D6 (CYP2D6), 210, 271, 272

D
Dale, Henry Hallett, 30–31
de Lima, Oswaldo Gonçalves, 174
de Sahagún, Bernardino, 20
DEA. *See* U.S. Drug Enforcement Agency (DEA)
Decriminalization, 53–55
Default mode network (DMN), 64
  disruption, brain, 88–89
Dehydroepiandrosterone (DHEA), 277
Dehydronorketamine, 238
Dennett, Daniel, 87

Depression
  major depressive disorder, 98–100
  persistent depressive disorder, 100
  psilocybin, 141–142
  following terminal diagnosis, 100
  treatment-resistant, 99–100
Depressive episode, 97
Descheduled, drug, 49
  criticism of, 49–50
DHE. *See* Dihydroergotamine (DHE)
DHEA. *See* Dehydroepiandrosterone (DHEA)
Diagnostic and Statistical Manual of Mental Disorders (DSM-5-TR), 96, 255
  diagnostic criteria, 72
Dihydroergotamine (DHE), 165
3,4-dihydroxyamphetamine (HHA), 272
3,4-dihydroxymethamphetamine (HHMA), 272
2,5-dimethoxy-4-bromoamphetamine, 294
2,5-dimethoxy-4-bromophenethylamine (2C-B), 270–271, 294
2,5-dimethoxy-4-ethylphenethylamine, 294–295
2,5-dimethoxy-4-ethylthiophenethylamine, 295
2,5-dimethoxy-4-iodoamphetamine (DOI), 270–271
2,5-dimethoxy-4-methylamphetamine, 295
2,5-dimethoxy-4-propylthiophenethylamine, 295–296
Dissociative anesthetic, 231–232
DMN. *See* Default mode network (DMN)
DMT. *See* N,N-dimethyltryptamine (DMT)
Doblin, Rick, 121
DOI. *See* 2,5-dimethoxy-4-iodoamphetamine (DOI)
Domino, Edward Dr., 231–232
The Doors of Perception (Huxley), 5, 37
Dopamine, 267
DPD. *See* Drinks per drinking day (DPD)
Drinks per drinking day (DPD), 143
Drug Abuse Control Amendments of 1965, 42
Drug scheduling, 48t
Dysthymia. *See* Persistent depressive disorder

E
Eating disorders, 109–112, 256–257
  anorexia nervosa, 109–110
  binge, 112
  bulimia nervosa, 110–111
  defining features of, 109
  exercise, 109
Ego dissolution, 22
Ego-dissolving transcendental, 243
Eleusinian Mysteries, 19
Ellis, Havelock, 28–29, 194

INDEX   319

Empathogen, 268
Entactogens, 70–71, 268
Entheogen, 209
Entropy, defined, 89
Ergot, 29–30
  medicinal uses, 30–31
  poisoning, 29–30
Escitalopram (Lexapro), 136
  vs. psilocybin, 139–140
Esketamine (Spravato), 61, 229–230
Ethanol, 260
Eticyclidine, 231
Ewell, Erwin, 194
Exercise, 109
Extrovertive mystical experience, 66

F
FDA. See U.S. Food and Drug Administration (FDA)
Fluoxetine (Prozac), 136
Food, Drug, and Cosmetic Act, 33, 42
Frederking, Walter, 29

G
GDNF. See Glial-derived neurotrophic factor
Generalized anxiety disorder, 102
George Washington University, 194
Glial-derived neurotrophic factor (GDNF), 175, 181
Global Assessment of Functioning, 132
Glutamate, 86
Good Friday Experiment, 40–41, 67, 129
GRID-Hamilton Depression Rating Scale (GRID-HAMD) score, 138
Grob, Charles, 270
Grof, Stanislav, 229

H
HADS. See Hospital Anxiety and Depression Scale
Hallucinogen Persisting Perception Disorder (HPPD), 72
Haloperidol, 313
Hamilton Anxiety Rating Scale (HAM-A), 142, 164
Hamilton Depression Scale (HAM-D), 132
Handovsky, Hans, 292
Harbor University of California Los Angeles (UCLA) Medical Center, 270
Heffter, Arthur, 27
Helmuth, Richard, 27
HHA. See 3,4-dihydroxyamphetamine
HHMA. See 3,4-dihydroxymethamphetamine

HMA. See 4-hydroxy-3-methoxyamphetamine
HMMA. See 4-hydroxy-3-methoxymethamphetamine
Hoffer, Abram, 77
Hofmann, Albert, 3–4, 31, 121, 156
  bicycle day, 31–33
Hospital Anxiety and Depression Scale (HADS), 142
HPPD. See Hallucinogen Persisting Perception Disorder
5-HT$_{2A}$ receptors, 85, 90
  distribution and activation, 85–86
Huxley, Aldous, 5, 195
4-hydroxy-3-methoxyamphetamine (HMA), 272
4-hydroxy-3-methoxymethamphetamine (HMMA), 272
4-hydroxy-N,N,N-trimethyltryptamine (4-HO-TMT), 128
5-hydroxy-N,N-dimethyltryptamine (bufotenin), 292
6-hydroxy-norketamine, 238
Hypomanic episode, 97

I
Ibogaine, 14, 70, 269
  dosage and administration, 225–226
  history of, 210–214
    in Europe, 212
    iboga and the Bwiti tradition, 210–212
    iboga trade, 214
    Lotsof, Howard, legacy of, 212–214
  pharmacology, 214–221
    description, 214–215, 215f
    pharmacodynamics, 216–220, 218–219t
    pharmacokinetics, 215–216
    route of administration, 215
    subjective effects, 221
  potential uses, 221–224
    opioid withdrawal, 222
    posttraumatic stress disorder, 223–224
    substance use disorders, 223
  precautions and adverse events, 224–225
  special populations, 225
  therapeutic indications, 221
Ibogamine, 214
Illicit substance abuse, 113
Indolethylamine-N-methyltransferase (INMT), 175–176
Informed consent, 81
Ingersoll, Robert G., 194
INMT. See Indolethylamine-N-methyltransferase (INMT)

Introvertive mystical experience, 66
16-item Quick Inventory of Depressive Symptomatology-Self Report (QIDS-SR-16), 139–140

J
Jacobs, W. A., 27
James, William, 65
Jay, Mike, 56, 197
John Barry, 4
Johns Hopkins Medicine, 137–138
Journeys into the Bright World (1978), 233

K
Kefauver-Harris Amendments (1962), 33, 42
Ketalar. See Ketamine
Ketamine (Ketalar), 69–70, 235
  dosage and clinical guidelines, 260–261
  drug interactions, 259
  esketamine risk evaluation and mitigation strategy, 261
  history of, 230–235
    from "buddy drug" to club drug, 232–233
    early days, 231–232
    precursors, 230–231
    psychiatry, acceptance in, 234–235
  off-label uses, 251–257
    anxiety disorders, 253–254
    bipolar disorders, 252–253
    borderline personality disorder, 257
    eating disorders, 256–257
    major depressive disorder, 252
    obsessive-compulsive disorders, 254
    postpartum depression, 252
    posttraumatic stress disorder, 254–255
    substance use disorders, 255–256
  patient stories, 308–309
  pharmacology, 235–243
    description, 236
    pharmacodynamics, 238–243, 240–242t
    pharmacokinetics, 236–238
    route of administration, 236, 237t
  precautions and adverse effects, 258–259
  pregnant and nursing women, 259
  psychedelic-assisted psychotherapy, 257
  therapeutic indications, 244–251
    suicidal ideation, 244–251, 245–250t
    treatment-resistant depression, 244–251, 245–250t
Ketamine-assisted psychotherapy, 78
Ketamine psychedelic psychotherapy (KPP), 234
Kolp, Eli, 234
κ-opioid receptors (KORs), 290

KPP. See Ketamine psychedelic psychotherapy
Krupitsky's model, 234

L
The Lancet, 194
LD_{50}, 162, 166, 182, 200, 201t
Leary, Timothy, 4, 38–40
Legalization, 53–55
Lexapro. See Escitalopram
Liebowitz Social Anxiety Scale (LSAS), 281
Lilly, John, 233
Lithium, 33
Lodge, David, 234
Lotsof, Howard, 212–214
LSAS. See Liebowitz Social Anxiety Scale
LSD. See Lysergic acid diethylamide
Lysergic acid diethylamide (LSD), 27, 29–33, 97, 174, 179, 183, 190–191, 195, 199, 201, 206, 269, 280
  and alcohol use disorder, 34–35
  dosage and administration, 168–169
  history of, 155–158
  Hofmann, Albert and, 31–33
  pharmacology, 158–163
    description, 158, 158f
    pharmacodynamics, 160–162, 161t
    pharmacokinetics, 159–160
    route of administration, 159
    somatic effects, 163
    subjective effects, 162–163
    tolerance, dependence, and withdrawal, 162
  potential uses, 163–166
    adult attention-deficit/hyperactivity disorder, 165
    Alzheimer disease, 165–166
    cluster headaches, 165
    depression, 164–165
    generalized anxiety disorder, 163–164
    palliative care, 164
    substance use disorders, 164
  precautions and adverse effects, 166–168
    drug interactions, 166–168, 167t, 168t
    risk of overdose, 166
  precursors to, 29–31
  synthesis of, 13
  therapeutic indications, 163
  use in pregnancy and lactation, 168

M
MADRS score. See Montgomery-Åsberg Depression Rating Scale (MADRS) score
"Magic" mushrooms, 38. See also Psilocybin
Major depressive disorder (MDD), 96, 98–100, 252

INDEX **321**

COVID-19 pandemic, 98
depression following terminal diagnosis, 100
etiology, 98–99
heterogeneity, 99
prevalence of, 98
symptoms, 98
treatment, 99
treatment-resistant depression, 99–100
Manic episode, 96–97
Manske, Frederick, 27
MAO. *See* Monoamine oxidase
MAOI. *See* Monoamine oxidase inhibitor (MAOI)
MAPS. *See* Multidisciplinary Association for Psychedelic Studies (MAPS)
Mash, Deborah C., 213
MDA. *See* 3,4-methylenedioxyamphetamine
MDD. *See* Major depressive disorder
MDMA. *See* 3,4-methylenedioxymethamphetamine
MEQ. *See* Mystical Experience Questionnaire
Mescaline, 14
  dosage and administration, 206
  early studies, 27–29
  history of, 192–195
  pharmacology, 195–202
    description, 196–197, 196f
    pharmacodynamics, 199–201, 200t, 201t
    pharmacokinetics, 198–199
    route of administration, 197
    somatic effects, 202
    subjective effects, 201–202
  potential uses, 202–203
  precautions and adverse effects, 203–206, 204t
  drug interactions, 205–, 205t
  risk of overdose, 203–205
  pregnant and nursing women, 206
  therapeutic indications, 202
Mescaline: A Global History of the First Psychedelic, 56, 197
Methamphetamine, 276
18-methoxycoronaridine (18-MC), 214
2,5-methoxy-4-iodoampheamine, 296
3-methoxy-4,5-methylendioxy-amphetamine, 296
5-methoxy-*N*,*N*-dimethyltryptamine (5-MeO-DMT), 222, 290–291
3,4-methylenedioxyamphetamine (MDA), 269, 272, 296–297
3,4-methylenedioxymethamphetamine (MDMA), 104
  dosage and clinical guidelines, 284–285
  drug interactions, 28t, 283–284, 283t
  history of, 268–270
  pharmacology of, 270–278, 271f
    description, 271
    pharmacodynamics, 273–278, 274–276t
    pharmacokinetics, 271–273
    route of administration, 271
  potential uses, 278–281
    autism spectrum disorders, social anxiety disorders in adults, 281
    eating disorders, 281
    palliative care, 280–281
    posttraumatic stress disorder, 279–280
  precautions and adverse effects, 282
  pregnant and nursing women, 282
  synthesis of, 13
  therapeutic indications, 278
Methylsafrylamin, 268
Methysergide, 165
Metzinger, Thomas, 88
Metzner, Ralph, 268
Microdosing, 91–92
Miscellaneous psychedelics
  5-hydroxy-*N*,*N*-dimethyltryptamine (bufotenin), 292
  5-methoxy-*N*,*N*-dimethyltryptamine, 290–291
  miscellaneous psychedelics of potential use, 293
  2,4,5-trimethoxyamphetamine, 297–298
  2,5-dimethoxy-4-bromoamphetamine, 294
  2,5-dimethoxy-4-bromophenethylamine, 294
  2,5-dimethoxy-4-ethylphenethylamine, 294–295
  2,5-dimethoxy-4-ethylthiophenethylamine, 295
  2,5-dimethoxy-4-methylamphetamine, 295
  2,5-dimethoxy-4-propylthiophenethylamine, 295–296
  2,5-methoxy-4-iodoampheamine, 296
  3-methoxy-4,5-methylendioxy-amphetamine, 296
  3,4-methylenedioxy-amphetamine, 296–297
  3,4,5-trimethoxyamphetamine, 297
  muscimol/ibotenic acid, 292–293
  salvinorin A, 290
Monoamine oxidase (MAO), 171, 177, 179
Monoamine oxidase inhibitor (MAOI), 14, 171–172, 177–179, 186
Montgomery-Åsberg Depression Rating Scale (MADRS) score, 8–9, 132–134, 136, 250
Mood disorders. *See* Affective disorders
Moore, Marcia, 233
Morgan, Francis, 28, 194

322 INDEX

Morphium, 27
Multidisciplinary Association for
    Psychedelic Studies (MAPS), 79, 270
Muscimol/ibotenic acid, 292–293
Mystical experience, 64–67
  characteristics of, 66
  elements, 65
  extrovertive, 65
  introvertive, 65–66
  organic, 67–68
    psychedelic-induced, 67–68
  shortcut to, 42–43
Mystical Experience Questionnaire (MEQ), 61
Mysticism Scale (M-scale), 61
Mysticism Scale-Lifetime, 130

N

N-methyl-D-aspartate (NMDA) receptors, 125, 217, 230, 232, 238–239
N,N-Dimethyltryptamine (DMT)/ayahuasca, 69
  dosage and administration, 187
  endogenous, 175–176
    biosynthesis, 175–176, 176t
    prevalence, 176
  history of, 173–174
  pharmacology, 177–184
    description, 177–178, 177f
    pharmacodynamics, 179–182, 180–181t
    pharmacokinetics, 178–179
    route of administration, 178
    somatic effects, 184
    subjective effects, 182–184
  potential dangers, 185–187
    adverse effects, 186
    drug interactions, 186, 187t
    pregnant and nursing women, 186
    risk of overdose, 186
  potential uses, 185
    major depressive disorder, 185
    substance use disorders, 185
    therapeutic indications, 185
NAC. *See* Native American Church
National Center for Health Statistics (NCHS), 101
National Institute on Drug Abuse (NIDA), 52, 213
Native American Church (NAC), 190, 195, 203
NCHS. *See* National Center for Health Statistics
NDE. *See* Near-death experience
Near-death experience (NDE), 68, 172, 175, 183–184, 243
  psychedelic-induced, 68
NEO Personality Inventory, 130
Nichols, David E., 268
NIDA. *See* National Institute on Drug Abuse
NMDA. *See* N-methyl-D-aspartate (NMDA)
N,N-dimethyltryptamine (DMT), 14
Noetic quality, 65
Nonordinary states of consciousness (NOSCs), 6, 21, 64–68, 89, 229, 233, 240, 241–242t, 257
  benefits of, 22–23
  mystical experience, 64–67
  near-death experiences, 68
  organic mystical experiences, 67–68
  psychedelic-induced mystical experiences, 67–68
  psychedelic-induced near-death experiences, 68
Norbaeocystin, 128
Norepinephrine, 267
Noribogaine, 214, 220
Norketamine, 237
NOSCs. *See* Nonordinary states of consciousness (NOSCs)

O

Obsessive-compulsive disorder (OCD), 103–104, 144–145, 254
  etiology of, 104
  prevalence of, 104
  symptoms of, 103–104
OCD. *See* Obsessive-compulsive disorder
Oneirophrenic, 210
Opioid use disorder, 113
Opioids, 260, 271
Osmond, Humphrey, 34, 5, 77

P

Pahnke-Richards MEQ, 66
Pahnke, Walter, 40
Palliative care, 114
PANAS. *See* Positive and Negative Affect Schedule
Panic disorder, 102
  signs and symptoms, 103t
Parker, Quanah, 56
Paroxetine (Paxil), 136
Patient Health Questionnaire 9-item (PHQ-9), 250
Paxil. See Paroxetine
PDD. *See* Percentage of drinking days
Percentage of drinking days (PDD), 143
Percentage of heavy drinking days (PHDD), 143

INDEX 323

Perry, Matthew, 230
Persistent depressive disorder, 100
Persisting Effects Questionnaire, 130
Peyote use, history of, 56–57
PHDD. *See* Percentage of heavy drinking days
4-phosphoryloxy-*N*,*N*-dimethyltryptamine.
  See Psilocybin
PiHKAL: A Chemical Love Story (PiHKAL), 293
Plato, 19
Polytherapy, 224
Positive and Negative Affect Schedule (PANAS), 130
Postpartum depression, 252
Premenstrual dysphoric disorders, 96
Prentiss, Daniel Webster, 28, 194
Prolactin, 277
Prozac. See Fluoxetine
Psilocin
  binding affinity, 126*t*
  in brain dynamics and functional connectivity, 127
  chemical structure, 125*f*
  mechanism of action, 125
Psilocybe, 120
Psilocybin, 13, 97, 119–150, 190
  acute effects, 119
  administration of, 127
  adverse effects, 147–148
  anorexia nervosa, 145
  anxiety and depression, 141–142
  bipolar II disorder, 140–141
  body dysmorphic disorder, 146
  chemical structure, 125*f*
  cluster headaches, 146
  defined, 119
  depression, 131–140
    Compass Pathways studies, 133–136, 135*t*
    Cybin, 137
    early research, 132
    Heffter Research Institute (Zurich), 139
    Johns Hopkins Medicine, 137–138
    response and remission rates to CYB003, 137T
    Usona Institute studies, 132–133
  description, 122–123
  dosage and administration, 149
  drug interactions, 147–148, 147*t*, 148*t*
  history, 120–122
  for hyperactivity, 127
  16-item Quick Inventory of Depressive Symptomatology-Self Report (QIDS-SR-16), 139–140
  major depressive disorder, 140–141

  migraines, 146
  mystical-type experiences, 129–130
  obsessive-compulsive disorder, 144–145
  patient stories, 301–306
  pharmacodynamics, 125–128
    mechanism of action, 125, 127
    therapeutic index, 127
    tolerance, dependence, and withdrawal, 127–128
  pharmacokinetics, 123–124
    absorption, 123–124
    bioavailability, 124
    distribution, 124
    elimination and excretion, 124
    metabolism, 124
  pharmacology, 122–130
  potential uses, 131–146
  precautions, 147–148
  psychotropic compounds
    aeruginascin, 128
    baeocystin, 128
    norbaeocystin, 128
  route of administration, 123
  somatic effects, 128–129
  special populations, 148–149
  subjective effects, 129–130
  substance use disorders, 142–144
    alcohol, 142–144
    tobacco, 144
  vs. escitalopram, 139–140
Psychedelics
  1800s to 1950, 26–33
    early studies with mescaline, 27–29
    ergot, 29–30
    lysergic acid diethylamide (LSD), 29–33
  1950 to 1970, 33–43
    alcohol use disorder, LSD and, 34–35
    Good Friday Experiment, 40–41
    model psychosis and M-substance, 34
    one bright may morning, 37–38
    psilocybin, arrival of, 38
    psychedelic-assisted psychotherapy, 36–37
    psycholytic treatment, 36–37
    set and setting, 35–36
    shortcut to mystical experiences, 42–43
    Timothy Leary and extra-scientific uses of psychedelics, 38–40
    turning off, 41–42
  after 1970, 43–44
  adulterated, 312
  archaeological record, 14–16
    ancient artworks, 16, 16–18*f*
  -assisted psychotherapy, 75–83

Psychedelics (*continued*)
  atypical, 84
  brain, 84–93
  classic, 84, 86, 89, 91, 92
  clinical history, 26–44
  experience, 60–73
  global history of, 13–24
  historical record, 18–21
  introduction, 1–11
  ketamine, 229–262
  ibogaine, 209–226
  lysergic acid diethylamide, 155–169
  3,4-Methylenedioxymethamphetamine, 267–285
  mescaline, 190–206
  miscellaneous psychedelics, 289–298
  N, N-dimethyltryptamine (DMT)/ayahuasca, 171–188
  patient stories, 300–310
  potential clinical indications, 95–115
  psilocybin, 119–150
  regulations, 46–58
  shamanism, 21–22
  in uncontrolled environments, 312
Psychedelic-assisted psychotherapy, 8–9, 75–83, 313
  1950 to 1970, 36–37
  consent agreements, 81–82
  posttreatment and integration, 80
  psychedelics in clinic, 76–77
  scalability, 82
  setting, 77–79
  support, 79–80
  vs. psycholytic paradigm, 77
Psychedelic experience
  emotional effects, 63
  Hallucinogen Persisting Perception Disorder (HPPD), 72
  increased suggestibility, 71
  nonordinary state of consciousness (NOSC), 64–68
    mystical experience, 64–67
    near-death experiences, 68
    organic mystical experiences, 67–68
    psychedelic-induced mystical experiences, 67–68
    psychedelic-induced near-death experiences, 68
  onset, peak, and comedown experiences, 61, 62t
  sensory effects, 62–63
    closed-eye visualizations, 63
    open-eye visualizations, 62–63
  subjective differences, 68–71

ayahuasca, 69
entactogens, 70–71
ibogaine, 70
ketamine, 69–70
N, N-dimethyltryptamine, 69
Psychedelic renaissance, 190
Psychoanalysis, 33
PTSD. *See* Posttraumatic stress disorder (PTSD)
PubMed, 190

Q

QIDS. *See* Quick Inventory of Depressive Symptoms (QIDS)
Quick Inventory of Depressive Symptoms (QIDS), 132

R

Reardon, Sara, 2
REBUS (RElaxed Beliefs Under pSychedelics) model, 87
Regulations, 46–58
  breakthrough status, 52–53
  clinical studies, 50–52, 51f
  requirements for, 52
  Controlled Substances Act of 1970 (CSA), 46–53
  decriminalization, 53–55
  drug scheduling, 48t
  enforcement, 49
  legalization, 53–55
  religious freedom, 55–57
    peyote use, history of, 56–57
    Religious Freedom Restoration Act, 57
  rescheduling/descheduling, 49
    criticism of, 49–50
  supported adult use, 54–55
Religious Freedom Restoration Act, 57
REMS. *See* Risk Evaluation and Mitigation Strategy (REMS)
Rescheduled, drug, 49
  criticism of, 49–50
Richard, William A., 76, 121
Rigveda, 18
Risk Evaluation and Mitigation Strategy (REMS), 230, 261
Roquet, Salvador, 234

S

Sacred Knowledge (Richards), 76
Salvinorin A, 290
Sartre, Jean-Paul, 202
Schizophrenomimetic/psychomimetic, 231–232

Schultes, Richard Evan, 194
The Scientist (1978), 233
SDS. *See* Sheehan Disability Scale (SDS) score
Selective serotonergic reuptake inhibitors (SSRIs), 313
Serotonergic psychedelics, 85
Serotonin, 85, 267
Serotonin and norepinephrine reuptake inhibitors (SNRIs), 313
Serotonin, chemical structure, 125*f*
Serotonin syndrome, 186, 187*t*
Serotonin transporters (SERTs), 217
Sertraline (Zoloft), 136
SERTs. *See* Serotonin transporters (SERTs)
Sertürner, Friedrich Wilhelm, 27
Set, defined, 6–7
Setting, defined, 7, 77–78
Shamanism, 21–22
Sheehan Disability Scale (SDS) score, 132–133, 250, 280
Shulgin, Alexander, 268–269, 293
Shulgin, Ann, 293
Smith, Huston, 18
Smythies, John, 34
Snaith-Hamilton Pleasure Scale, 132
SNRIs. *See* Serotonin and norepinephrine reuptake inhibitors (SNRIs)
Social anxiety disorder, 102
Späth, Ernst, 29
Spielberger's State-Trait Anxiety Inventory (STAI), 132
Spiritual Transcendence Scale, 130
Spravato. See Esketamine
SSRIs. *See* Selective serotonergic reuptake inhibitors (SSRIs)
STAI. *See* Spielberger's State-Trait Anxiety Inventory (STAI)
STAI. *See* State-Trait Anxiety Inventory (STAI) trait scores
State-Trait Anxiety Inventory (STAI) trait scores, 280–281
Stevens, Calvin, 231
Stimulant use disorder, 113
Stoll, Arthur, 156–157
Substance use disorders, 112–114, 142–144, 223, 255–256
  alcohol, 113, 142–144
  cannabis, 113
  cocaine, 113
  opioid, 113
  signs and symptoms of, 113
  stimulant, 113
  tobacco, 113, 144
Suicidal ideation, 244–251, 245–250*t*

Suicidality, 114–115
Support, defined, 7
SUSTAIN-3 study, 244, 250–251, 250*t*
Szára, Stephen, 174

T
Tabernanthalog, 214
Tabernanthe iboga, 209, 210
Tachyphylaxis, 86
TCAs. *See* Tricyclic antidepressants (TCAs)
Timothy Leary, 121
TMPA. *See* 3,4,5-trimethoxyphenylacetic acid (TMPA)
Tobacco use disorder, 113, 144
Trace amine-associated receptor 1 (TAAR1), 272, 277
Transiency, 65
Trauma- and stressor-related disorders, 105–108
  adjustment disorder with anxiety, 108
  clusters and specific events, 106*t*
  posttraumatic stress disorder, 105, 107–108
Treatment-resistant depression, 99–100, 244–251, 245–250*t*
Tricyclic antidepressants (TCAs), 313
2,4,5-trimethoxyamphetamine, 297–298
3,4,5-trimethoxyamphetamine, 297
3,4,5-trimethoxyphenylacetic acid (TMPA), 198, 199
Triptans, 165
TrkB. *See* Tropomyosin-related kinase B (TrkB) receptors
Tropomyosin-related kinase B (TrkB) receptors, 86
Tryptamine, 125, 175
Tryptophan, chemical structure, 125*f*

U
UCLA. *See* Harbor University of California Los Angeles (UCLA) Medical Center
Unipolar depression, 98
U.S. Drug Enforcement Agency (DEA), 49, 233, 267
U.S. Food and Drug Administration (FDA), 120, 156, 213, 229–230, 232, 233, 235, 236, 267, 270, 278

V
Valvular heart disease (VHD), symptoms of, 92
VHD. *See* Valvular heart disease (VHD), symptoms of
Viibryd. See Vilazodone
Vilazodone (Viibryd), 136
Voacangine, 214

W

Wasson, R. Gordon, 18, 38, 121
Whiskey root, 27
Wilson, Bill, 35
Winkelman, Michael, 21
World Mental Health Survey, 102

Y

Yale-Brown Obsessive Compulsive Disorder Scale (YBOCS), 144
Yale-Brown Obsessive Compulsive Disorder Scale Modified for Body Dysmorphic Disorder (BDD-YBOCS), 146
YBOCS. *See* Yale-Brown Obsessive Compulsive Disorder Scale (YBOCS)

Z

Zoloft. See Sertraline